Quick Find Guide

Sixth Edition

Fundamentals of Periodontal Instrumentation

& Advanced Root Instrumentation

Jill S. Nield-Gehrig, RDH, MA

Dean, Emeritus, Division of Allied Health & Public Service Education
Asheville-Buncombe Technical Community College
Asheville, North Carolina

Visiting Professor
Dental Education Programs
South Florida Community College
Avon Park, Florida

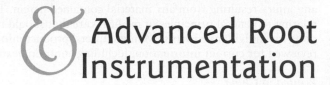

Philadelphia • Baltimore • New York • London
Buenos Aires • Hong Kong • Sydney • Tokyo

Aquisitions Editor: John Goucher
Managing Editor: Kevin C. Dietz
Marketing Manager: Hilary Henderson
Production Editor: Jennifer P. Ajello
Designer: Doug Smock
Compositor: Maryland Composition, Inc.
Printer: R.R. Donnelley & Sons—Shenzhen

351 West Camden Street
Baltimore, MD 21201

530 Walnut Street
Philadelphia, PA 19106

Printed in China

Library of Congress Cataloging-in-Publication Data

Nield-Gehrig, Jill S. (Jill Shiffer)
    Fundamentals of periodontal instrumentation & advanced root instrumentation / Jill S.
Nield-Gehrig.—6th ed.
        p. ; cm.
    Includes bibliographical references and index.
    ISBN 978-0-7817-6992-1
        1. Dental instruments and apparatus. 2. Dental hygiene. I. Title. II. Title: Fundamentals of
periodontal instrumentation and advanced root instrumentation.
    [DNLM: 1. Dental Prophylaxis—instrumentation. 2. Dental Prophylaxis—methods.
3. Root Planing—instrumentation. 4. Root Planing—methods. WU 113 N6673fa 2008]
    RK681.N53 2008
    617.6'01—dc22

                                                                           2006048833

To purchase additional copies of this book, call our customer service department at (800) 638-
3030 or fax orders to (301) 223-2320. International customers should call (301) 223-2300.

Visit Lippincott Williams & Wilkins on the Internet: http://www.LWW.com. Lippincott
Williams & Wilkins customer service representatives are available from 8:30 am to 6:00 pm,
EST.

09 10 11
6 7 8 9 10

Registered Trademarks

American Eagle Instruments, Inc.
Gracey +3 Access Curettes
Gracey +3 Deep Pocket Curettes

DentalView, Inc.
Perioscopy System (dental endoscope)

DENTSPLY Preventive Care:
Cavitron ultrasonic scalers
ProphyJet
JetShield

EMS (Electro Medical Systems)
Piezon Master 400

The Florida Probe

Hu-Friedy Mfg. Company, Inc.
After Five Curettes
After Five 11/12 Explorer
O'Hehir Debridement Curettes
Mini Five Curettes
Satin Steel instrument handle
Vision Curvette instrument series

KaVo America Corporation
KaVo Sonicflex scaler

Kilgore International, Inc.
Dental hygiene and periodontal typodonts
Acrylic tooth models
Dental manikin systems

Parkell USA
Burnett Power Tip

SportsHealth Power Putty

SurgiTel/General Scientific Corporation
SurgiTel Telescopic magnification system

Liability Statement

The author, editors, and publisher have made every effort to confirm the accuracy of the information presented and to describe generally accepted practices at the time of publication. However, as new information becomes available, changes in instrumentation techniques and patient treatment may become necessary. It is the responsibility of the reader to verify the information found here from independent sources. This publication contains information relating to general principles of dental healthcare and should not be construed as specific instructions for individual clinicians or patients. Not all recommendations for positioning and instrumentation are suitable for all clinicians and patients. The author, editors, and publisher are not responsible for errors or omissions or for any consequences from the application of the information in this book and make no warranty, express or implied, with respect to the contents of this publication.

Preface for Course Instructors

Fundamentals of Periodontal Instrumentation is a detailed instructional guide to periodontal instrumentation that takes students from the basic skills—patient positioning, intraoral finger rests, and basic instrumentation—all the way to advanced techniques—assessment of periodontal patients and instrumentation of the root branches of multi-rooted teeth, root concavities, and furcation areas.

The foremost instructional goal of *Fundamentals* is to make it easy for students to learn and faculty to teach instrumentation. The sixth edition retains the features that have made it the market-leading textbook on periodontal instrumentation and adds many new features designed to facilitate learning and teaching.

Faculty Resource CD

The Faculty Resource CD has a collection of instructional aids for use in teaching instrumentation.

1. **PowerPoint Slides.** The PowerPoint slides were designed so as to be user-friendly for a wide variety of software versions and equipment.
   - You may customize the slide design by saving the slides to the computer hard drive and using the formatting features of your slide presentation software, such as the slide design, slide color scheme, or slide background feature.
   - You may add effects, such as progressive disclosure, to the slides by using the custom animation feature of your slide presentation software.
2. **Test Bank.** The test bank questions can be used for quizzes, combined to make up unit tests, or combined to create midterm and final examinations.
3. **Instructor Guide.** The instructor guide includes:
   - Critical thinking activities found in the *Practical Focus* section of each chapter.
This instructor guide includes suggestions for leading classroom discussions.
   - A list of phrases that facilitate the teaching of instrumentation.
   - Guidelines for introduction of alternate and advanced techniques.

Textbook Features

1. **Module outlines.** Each chapter begins with a module outline that provides an overview of content and makes it easier to locate material within the module. The outline provides the reader with an organizational framework with which to approach new material.
2. **Learning objectives** assist students in recognizing and studying important concepts in each chapter.

3. **Step-by-step format.** The clear, step-by-step self-instructional format allows the learner to work independently—fostering student autonomy and decision-making skills. The learner is free to work at his or her own pace spending more time on a skill that he or she finds difficult and moving on when a skill comes easily. The self-instructional format relieves the instructor from the task of endlessly repeating basic information, and frees him or her to demonstrate instrumentation techniques, observe student practice, and facilitate the process of skill acquisition.

4. **Key terms** are listed at the start of each module. One of the most challenging tasks for any student is learning a whole new dental vocabulary and gaining the confidence to use new terms with accuracy and ease. The key terms list assists students in this task by identifying important terminology and facilitating the study and review of terminology in each instructional module.

5. **Study aids**—boxes, tables, and flow charts—visually highlight and reinforce important content and permit quick reference during technique practice and at-home review.

6. **Critical thinking activities**—in the *Practical Focus* sections of the book—encourage students to apply concepts to clinical situations, facilitate classroom discussion, and promote the development of student problem-solving skills.

7. **Case-based patient experiences** allow students to apply instrumentation concepts to patient cases.

8. **A Glossary of instrumentation terms** provides quick access to instrumentation terminology.

9. **Skill evaluation checklists** guide student practice, promote student self-assessment skills, and provide benchmarks for faculty evaluation of skill attainment. Use of the student self-evaluation portion of the evaluation forms should be encouraged. The self-evaluation process helps students to develop the ability to assess their own level of competence rather than relying on instructor confirmation of skill attainment.

Module Format and Sequencing

The book is divided into six major content areas:

Part 1: Basic Skills
Part 2: Elements of the Instrument Stroke
Part 3: Patient Assessment
Part 4: Debridement with Hand-Activated Instruments
Part 5: Advanced Instrumentation Techniques
Part 6: Supplementary Instrumentation

From an instructional viewpoint, it is important to note that *each major instrument classification is addressed in a stand-alone module*—sickle scalers, universal curets, and area-specific curets. Each stand-alone module provides complete step-by-step instruction in the use of an instrument classification. For example, the module on universal curets provides complete instruction on the use of universal curets. This chapter does not rely on the student having studied the previous module on sickle scalers before beginning the universal curet module. This stand-alone module structure means that it is not necessary to cover the instrument modules in any particular order or even to include all of the modules. If sickle scalers, for example, are not part of the school's instrument kit, this module does not need to be included in the course outline.

PART 1—BASIC SKILLS

Part 1—Basic Skills—covers the fundamental skills of position, grasp, mirror use, and finger rests. These basic skills are introduced first to allow the learner to perfect them before tackling the use of instruments. Incorrect performance of one or more of these basic skills is the most common cause of poor skill attainment in instrumentation. These distinct instructional modules underscore for the learner the importance and universal application of these basic skills. A student who masters and consistently applies these skills will learn instrumentation with greater efficiency and ease.

PART 2—ELEMENTS OF THE INSTRUMENTATION STROKE

Part 2—Elements of the Instrument Stroke—introduces the principles involved in stroke production—adaptation, angulation, activation, pivot, handle roll, and instrumentation strokes. The three modules in this section guide the student through the steps involved in using any instrument to engage and remove calculus and provide technique practice independent of concerns about a particular instrument's design.

PART 3—PATIENT ASSESSMENT

Part 3—Patient Assessment—provides detailed step-by-step instructions on the use of probes and explorers. Modules 11 and 12 cover basic probing and exploring techniques for use in healthy sulci and shallow pockets. The use of probes and explorers in deep periodontal pockets is covered in Part 5 of the book.

PART 4—DEBRIDEMENT WITH HAND-ACTIVATED INSTRUMENTS

Part 4—Debridement with Hand-Activated Instruments—contains detailed step-by-step instructions on the use of the major classifications of calculus removal instruments. Calculus removal instruments are discussed according to classification—universal curets—rather than by specific design name—Columbia 13/14. This instructional approach helps students to realize that they are learning to use *types of instruments* rather than how to use the *specific instruments in a school kit*. It is unfortunate that so many graduate clinicians are reluctant to use any instruments other than those that they used while in school. Emphasis on instrument design characteristics—rather than on specific instruments in the school's instrument kit—provides clinicians with concepts that apply while learning about instruments in school and to new instrument designs in the future.

PART 5—ADVANCED INSTRUMENTATION TECHNIQUES

Part 5—Advanced Instrumentation Techniques—is a new five-chapter section that guides students step-by-step through the challenging advanced techniques required for the assessment and instrumentation of root surfaces within deep periodontal pockets. Advanced probing techniques for periodontal assessment are covered in Module 21. Module 22 introduces instruments for use with periodontal patients and provides a step-by-step technique practice in exploring techniques for root surfaces with deep periodontal pockets. Module 23 has step-by-step instructions on advanced instrumentation within periodontal pockets, including instrumentation of the root branches of multi-rooted teeth, root concavities, and furcation areas. Module 24 covers ultrasonic and sonic instrumentation. Module 25 discusses the debridement of dental implants.

PART 6—SUPPLEMENTARY INSTRUMENTATION

Part 6—Supplementary Instrumentation—contains Module 26, an optional module, which covers cosmetic polishing procedures. This module discusses rubber cup polishing and air-powder techniques for stain removal.

Feedback From Students and Faculty

I appreciate the enthusiastic comments and suggestions from educators and students about previous editions of *Fundamentals*, and welcome continued input. Mastering the psychomotor skill of periodontal instrumentation is a very challenging process. It is my sincere hope that this textbook will help students to acquire the psychomotor skills that—combined with clinical experience—will lead to excellence in periodontal instrumentation.

Jill S. Nield-Gehrig, RDH, MA

Acknowledgments

It is gratifying to be a member of a profession that includes so many individuals who strive for excellence in teaching. I am most grateful to all of the outstanding educators who shared their comments and suggestions for improving this edition. I thank all who generously gave their time, ideas, and resources, and gratefully acknowledge the special contributions of the following individuals:

- **Rebecca Sroda, RDH, MA,** Director of Dental Education at South Florida Community College, who created the Faculty Resource CD for this edition.

- **Cynthia Biron, RDH, EMT, MA,** of *DH-Meth-Ed* dental hygiene education consulting services, for her recommendations for the 6th edition.

- **Charles D. Whitehead,** a highly skilled medical illustrator, who created all the wonderful full color illustrations for the book.

- **Dee Robert Gehrig,** P.E., Gehrig Photographic Studio—the talented individual who created the hundreds of photographs for this book.

- The following individuals who were extremely generous with their time and knowledge—**Susan Boyden, Karen Neiner,** and **Patricia Parker** of Hu-Friedy Manufacturing; **Dave Salender** of Parkell USA; **Leann Keefer** of Dentsplay Preventive Care. A very special "thank you" to **Craig Kilgore,** President, Kilgore International, Inc. for providing the periodontal typodonts used throughout the book.

- And finally, and with great thanks, my wonderful team at Lippincott Williams and Wilkins, without whose guidance and support this book would not have been possible: **John Goucher, Kevin Dietz, Jennifer Clements, Jennifer Ajello, and Hilary Henderson.**

Jill S. Nield-Gehrig, RDH, MA

Contents

PART 2: ELEMENTS OF THE INSTRUMENT STROKE

PART 3: PATIENT ASSESSMENT

PART 4: DEBRIDEMENT WITH HAND-ACTIVATED INSTRUMENTS

PART 5: ADVANCED INSTRUMENTATION TECHNIQUES

PART 6: SUPPLEMENTARY INSTRUMENTATION

Module 1

Mathematical Principles and Anatomic Descriptors

Module Overview

This module contains a review of the mathematical principles and anatomic descriptors used in periodontal instrumentation. None of these concepts or terms is difficult, and you have probably studied them in the past. You should, however, review them now to be sure that you have a clear understanding of each principle or descriptor.

Module Outline

Key Terms

Angle	Vertical	Apical
90-degree angle	Oblique	Coronal
Right angle	Horizontal	Midline
45-degree angle	Cross section	Line angle
Parallel	Millimeter	
Perpendicular	Long axis	

Learning Objectives

1. Identify a 90-degree angle found in an everyday object. Create a 45-degree angle using two textbooks.

2. Draw two parallel lines. Draw two perpendicular lines.

3. Define the terms vertical, oblique, and horizontal.

4. Define the term cross section. Select an object and describe its shape in cross section.

5. Select a word from a page in a textbook. Measure the length of the word in millimeters.

6. Define the term "long axis of a tooth."

7. Using a typodont tooth, demonstrate "apical to" and "coronal to."

8. Define the terms midline, aspect, and sextant.

9. Using a tooth model, name and identify (locate) the four line angles.

10. Using a tooth model, name and identify the three tooth surfaces included in the facial aspect of the tooth.

Section 1
Mathematical Principles

GEOMETRIC ANGLES

An angle is formed by two straight lines that meet at an endpoint. The size of an angle is measured in degrees using a protractor. The 90-degree angle and the 45-degree angle are common reference points in instrumentation. For example, the cutting edge of an instrument meets the tooth surface at an angle that is greater than 45 degrees but less than 90 degrees. Review the everyday examples of 90-degree and 45-degree angles shown below.

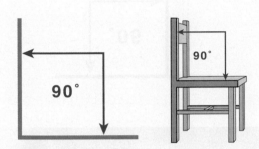

A 90-Degree Angle. The seat of this chair is at a 90-degree angle to the chair back. A right angle is another term for a 90-degree angle.

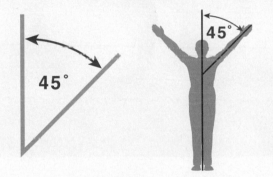

A 45-Degree Angle. This man is holding his arms at a 45-degree angle to the midline of his body.

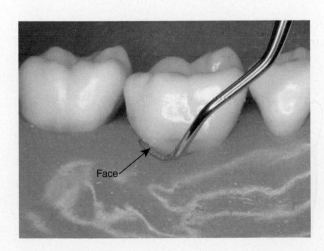

Face

Angulation for Calculus Removal. For effective calculus removal, it is important to establish the correct angulation between the instrument face and the tooth surface. The correct angulation for calculus removal is an angle that is greater than 45 degrees and less than 90 degrees.

PARALLEL AND PERPENDICULAR

To correctly position a periodontal instrument, you need to understand the terms parallel and perpendicular.

Parallel Lines. Parallel lines are lines that run in the same direction and never meet or intersect one another.

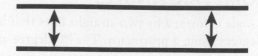

Perpendicular Lines. Perpendicular lines are two lines that intersect (meet) to form a 90-degree angle.

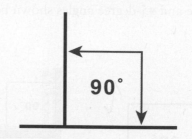

Shank Position. The shank of this periodontal instrument is positioned parallel to the long axis of the second premolar tooth.

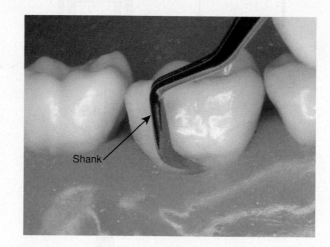

Shank

LINES

The three orientations that lines may have are vertical, oblique, and horizontal. To correctly move the instrument over the tooth, you need to understand these terms.

Stroke Direction. During instrumentation, instrument strokes may be made across the tooth surface in a vertical, oblique, or horizontal direction. Horizontal instrumentation strokes also are referred to as circumferential strokes because these strokes are made around the circumference of the tooth.

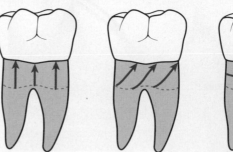
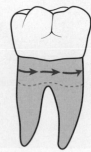

CROSS SECTION

A cross section is exposed by cutting through an object, usually at right angles to its longest dimension. If you can imagine a knife cutting through a pencil at a 90-degree angle to its length, you will have a good idea of what a cross section looks like.

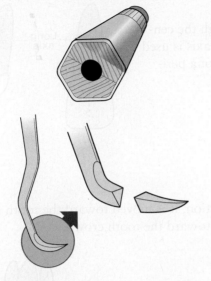

Hexagonal Cross Section. A typical lead pencil is hexagonal in cross section.

Triangular Cross Section. The working-end of certain periodontal instruments is triangular in cross section. Other periodontal instruments have working-ends that are semi-circular in cross section.

MILLIMETER MEASUREMENTS

A millimeter is a unit of length equal to one thousandth of a meter or 0.0394 inch. The abbreviation for millimeters is mm. The anatomic features of the teeth are often measured in millimeters.

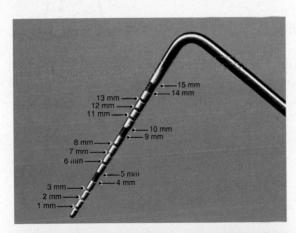

A Periodontal Probe. A probe is a periodontal instrument that is similar to a miniature ruler. The probe is marked in millimeter units and is used for making intraoral measurements.

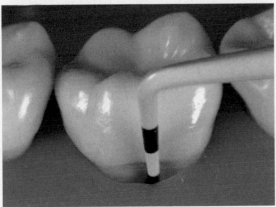

Pocket Depth. Using a periodontal probe, the depth of a periodontal pocket is measured in millimeters. Periodontal pockets are 4 mm or greater in depth.

Section 2
Anatomic Descriptors

LONG AXIS

The long axis is an imaginary straight line that passes through the center of a tooth and divides the tooth symmetrically. The long axis is used as a reference point when selecting the correct working-end of a periodontal instrument.

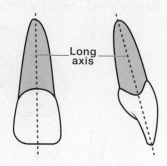

APICAL AND CORONAL

If the working-end of an instrument moves in an apical direction, it is moved toward the tooth apex. If the working-end moves in a coronal direction, it is moved toward the tooth crown.

Apical. Point 3 is located apical to the cemento-enamel junction (CEJ) on both illustrations.

Coronal. Point 4 is coronal to the CEJ on both illustrations.

For both teeth shown here, moving from point 3 to point 4 is moving in a coronal direction. When removing calculus with a hand instrument, the cutting edge is placed apical to the calculus deposit, and the instrumentation stroke is made in a coronal direction.

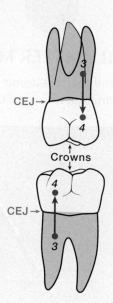

MIDLINE AND LINE ANGLE

The crown of an anterior tooth can be divided in half by an imaginary line called the midline. The crown of a posterior tooth can be divided into surfaces at imaginary lines called line angles.

Midline. The crown of an anterior tooth may be divided into two equal halves at the midline. Instrumentation of an anterior tooth is initiated (started) at the midline of the tooth.

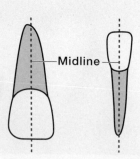

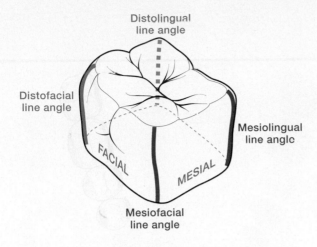

Distolingual
line angle

Distofacial
line angle

Mesiolingual
line angle

FACIAL   MESIAL

Mesiofacial
line angle

Line Angle. A line angle is an imaginary line formed where two tooth surfaces meet.

Each tooth has four line angles:

1. Mesiofacial line angle
2. Distofacial line angle
3. Mesiolingual line angle
4. Distolingual line angle

Instrumentation of a posterior tooth often is initiated at the distofacial or distolingual line angle of the tooth.

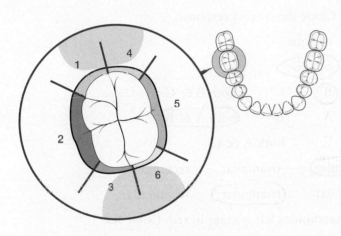

ASPECT

Facial and Lingual Aspects. A tooth, sextant, quadrant, or dental arch may be divided into two aspects: (1) a facial aspect and (2) a lingual aspect.

The facial aspect of a tooth is subdivided into three areas: (1) distofacial area, (2) facial surface, and (3) mesiofacial area.

The lingual aspect of a tooth is subdivided into three areas: (4) distolingual area, (5) lingual area, and (6) mesiolingual area.

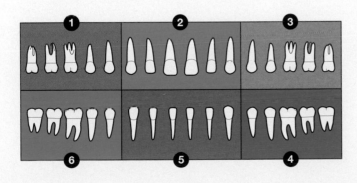

SEXTANT

For purposes of identification, the dentition may be divided into six areas. Each area is referred to as a sextant. There are two anterior sextants and four posterior sextants in the dental arch:

1. Maxillary right posterior sextant
2. Maxillary anterior sextant
3. Maxillary left posterior sextant
4. Mandibular left posterior sextant
5. Mandibular anterior sextant
6. Mandibular right posterior sextant

Section 3
Skill Application

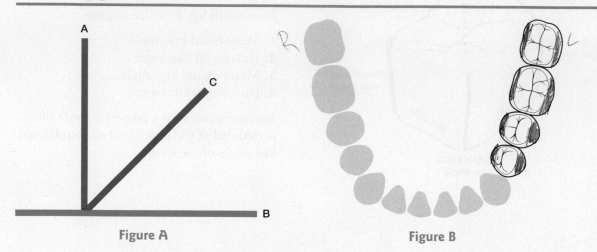

Figure A

Figure B

Questions 1 to 5 refer to **Figure A.** Directions: Circle the correct response.

1. Line A is: ~~vertical~~   horizontal   oblique

2. Line C is: vertical   horizontal   ~~oblique~~

3. Line(s) at 90-degree angle to Line A: ~~B~~   C   both B & C

4. Line(s) at 45-degree angles to Line C: A   B   ~~both A & B~~

5. Line(s) perpendicular to Line B: ~~A~~   C   both A & C

6. Shape of a baseball in cross section: ~~circular~~   triangular   rectangular

7. Shape of a pyramid in cross section: circular   ~~triangular~~   rectangular

8. On Figure B, color the *facial aspect* of the mandibular left sextant in red. Color the *lingual aspect* in blue.

Principles of Positioning

Module Overview

This module introduces the principles of positioning for periodontal instrumentation. Correct positioning techniques help to (1) prevent clinician discomfort and injury, (2) permit a clear view of the tooth being worked on, (3) allow easy access to the teeth during instrumentation, and (4) facilitate efficient treatment of the patient.

Module Outline

| Section 6 | **Skill Application** | 42 |

Practical Focus
Skill Evaluation Module 2: Position, Mandibular Sextants
Skill Evaluation Module 2: Position, Maxillary Sextants

Key Terms

Work-related musculoskeletal
   disorder
Repetitive task
Ergonomics

Supine position
Neutral position
Nondominant hand
Dominant hand

Anterior surfaces toward
Anterior surfaces away
Posterior aspects facing toward
Posterior aspects facing away

Learning Objectives

1. Develop an appreciation of evidence-based knowledge of positioning in the dental environment.

2. Understand the relationship between neutral position and the prevention of musculoskeletal problems.

3. Demonstrate operation of the clinician chair and the patient chair.

4. Demonstrate correct patient position relative to the clinician.

5. State the reason why it is important that the top of the patient's head is even with top edge of the chair headrest. Demonstrate how to correctly position a patient who is short in the dental chair so that (a) the patient is comfortable and (b) you have good vision and access to the oral cavity.

6. Position equipment so that it enhances neutral positioning.

7. Demonstrate correct clinician and patient position in each of the mandibular and maxillary treatment areas while maintaining neutral positioning.

8. Recognize incorrect position and describe how to correct the problem.

Section 1
Evidence-Based Knowledge of Positioning

INTRODUCTION TO WORK-RELATED MUSCULOSKELETAL DISORDERS

In simple terms, a work-related musculoskeletal disorder (WMD) is an injury—affecting the musculoskeletal, peripheral nervous, and neurovascular systems—that is caused or aggravated by prolonged repetitive forceful or awkward movements, poor posture, ill-fitting chairs and equipment, or a fast-paced workload. According to the U.S. Bureau of Labor Statistics, musculoskeletal disorders result in more than 60 percent of all newly reported occupational injuries.[1] The result is injury to the muscles, nerves, and tendon sheaths of the back, shoulders, neck, arms, elbows, wrists, and hands that can cause loss of strength, impairment of motor control, tingling, numbness, or pain. Work-related musculoskeletal disorders are a common complaint of practicing dentists and dental hygienists.[2–8]

The human body was not designed to maintain the same body position or engage in fine hand movements hour after hour, day after day. B.A. Silverstein, in an article in the *British Journal of Industrial Medicine,* defined a repetitive task as a task that involves the same fundamental movement for more than 50 percent of the work cycle.[9] Periodontal instrumentation would certainly be categorized as a repetitive task under this definition. More than 50 percent of the time is spent performing very controlled, fast motions. Periodontal instrumentation requires excessive upper body immobility while the tendons and muscles of the forearms, hands, and fingers overwork. The dental healthcare professional has a high risk of musculoskeletal injury when repetitive motions are combined with forceful movements, awkward postures, and insufficient recovery time.[9–12] Fortunately, injury to the muscles, tendons, and nerves can be prevented in most cases. This module presents strategies for the prevention of musculoskeletal injuries.

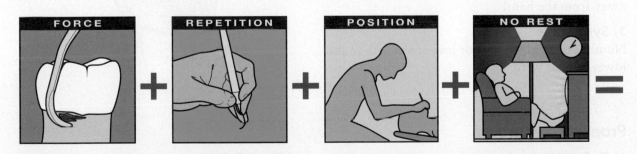

MUSCULOSKELETAL INJURY

MUSCULOSKELETAL DISORDERS SEEN IN DENTAL HEALTHCARE PROVIDERS

Carpal Tunnel Syndrome (CTS)

1. Definition
A painful disorder of the wrist and hand caused by compression of the median nerve within the carpal tunnel of the wrist

2. Causes
The nerve fibers of the median nerve originate in the spinal cord in the neck; therefore, poor posture can cause symptoms of CTS. Other causes include repeatedly bending the hand up, down, or from side to side at the wrist and continuously pinch-gripping an instrument without resting the muscles.

3. Symptoms
Numbness, pain, tingling in the thumb, index, and middle fingers

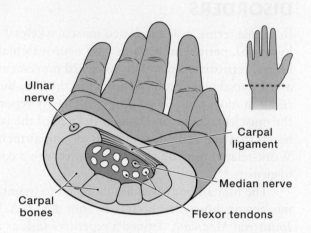

Ulnar Nerve Entrapment

1. Definition
A painful disorder of the lower arm and wrist caused by compression of the ulnar nerve of the arm as it passes through the wrist

2. Causes
Bending the hand up, down, or from side to side at the wrist and holding the little finger a full span away from the hand

3. Symptoms
Numbness, tingling, and/or loss of strength in the lower arm or wrist

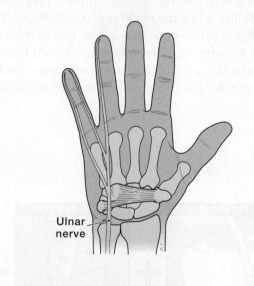

Pronator Syndrome

1. Definition
A painful disorder of the wrist and hand caused by compression of the median nerve between the two heads of the pronator teres muscle

2. Causes
Holding the lower arm away from the body

3. Symptoms
Similar to those of carpal tunnel syndrome

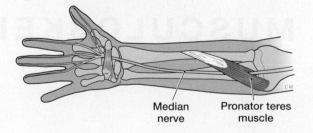

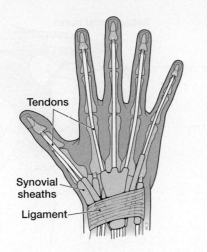

Tendinitis

1. Definition
A painful inflammation of the tendons of the wrist resulting from strain

2. Causes
Repeatedly extending the hand up or down at the wrist

3. Symptoms
Pain in the wrist, especially on the outer edges of the hand, rather than through the center of the wrist

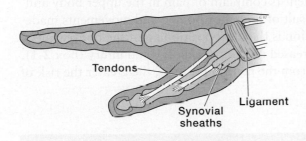

Tenosynovitis

1. Definition
A painful inflammation of the tendons on the side of the wrist and at the base of the thumb

2. Causes
Hand twisting, forceful gripping, bending the hand back or to the side

3. Symptoms
Pain on the side of the wrist and the base of the thumb; sometimes movement of the wrist yields a crackling noise

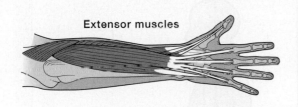

Extensor Wad Strain

1. Definition
A painful disorder of the fingers as a result of injury of the extensor muscles of the thumb and fingers

2. Causes
Extending the fingers independently of each other

3. Symptoms
Numbness, pain, and loss of strength in the fingers

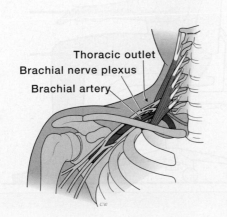

Thoracic Outlet Syndrome

1. Definition
A painful disorder of the fingers, hand, and/or wrist as a result of the compression of the brachial nerve plexus and vessels between the neck and shoulder

2. Causes
Tilting the head forward, hunching the shoulders forward, and continuously reaching overhead

3. Symptoms
Numbness, tingling, and/or pain in the fingers, hand, or wrist

Rotator Cuff Tendinitis

1. Definition
A painful inflammation of the muscle tendons in the shoulder region

2. Causes
Holding the elbow above waist level and holding the upper arm away from the body

3. Symptoms
Severe pain and impaired function of the shoulder joint

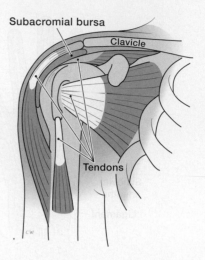

NEUTRAL POSITION FOR THE CLINICIAN

Research indicates that over 80 percent of dental hygienists complain of pain in the upper body and back.[2] This musculoskeletal pain often is the direct result of body positioning and movements made by dental hygienists in their daily work. Neutral position is the ideal positioning of the body while performing work activities and is associated with decreased risk of musculoskeletal injury (Box 2-1). It is generally believed that the more a joint deviates from the neutral position, the greater the risk of injury.

Box 2-1. Neutral Seated Position

1. Forearms parallel to the floor
2. Weight evenly balanced
3. Thighs parallel to the floor
4. Hip angle of 90°
5. Seat height positioned low enough so that you are able to rest the heels of your feet on the floor

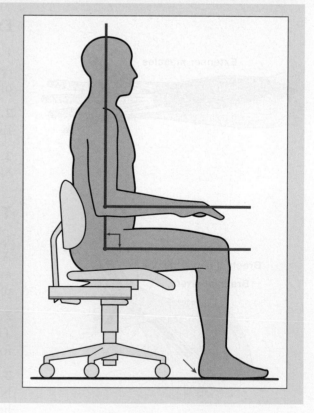

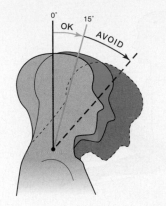

Neutral Neck Position

GOAL:

- Head tilt of 0° to 15°
- The line from eyes to the treatment area should be as near to vertical as possible

AVOID:

- Head tipped too far forward
- Head tilted to one side

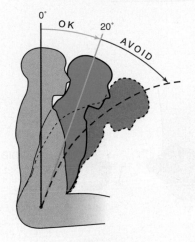

Neutral Back Position

GOAL:

- Leaning forward slightly from the waist or hips
- Trunk flexion of 0° to 20°

AVOID:

- Overflexion of the spine (curved back)

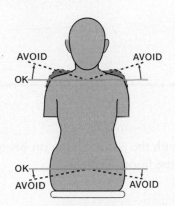

Neutral Shoulder Position

GOAL:

- Shoulders in horizontal line
- Weight evenly balanced when seated

AVOID:

- Shoulders lifted up toward ears
- Shoulders hunched forward
- Sitting with weight on one hip

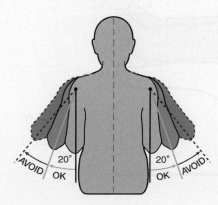

Neutral Upper Arm Position

GOAL:

- Upper arms hang parallel to the long axis of torso
- Elbows at waist level held slightly away from body

AVOID:

- Greater than 20° of elbow abduction away from the body
- Elbows held above waist level

Neutral Forearm Position

GOAL:

- Parallel to the floor
- Raised or lowered, if necessary, by pivoting at the elbow joint

AVOID:

- Angle between forearm and upper arm of less than 60°

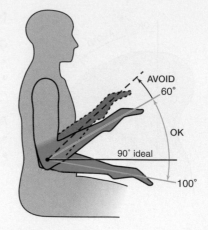

Neutral Hand Position

GOAL:

- Little finger-side of palm slightly lower than thumb-side of palm
- Wrist aligned with forearm

AVOID:

- Thumb-side of palm rotated down so that palm is parallel to the floor
- Hand and wrist bent up or down

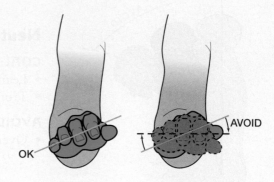

Section 2
Patient Position

SUPINE PATIENT POSITION

Supine position—the position of the patient during dental treatment, with the patient lying on his or her back in a horizontal position and the chair back nearly parallel to the floor (Table 2-1).

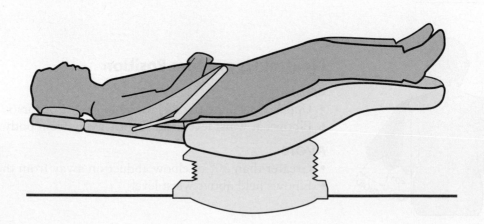

TABLE 2-1.	The Supine Patient Position

Recommended Position

Body	The patient's heels should be slightly higher than the tip of the nose. This position maintains good blood flow to the head. An apprehensive patient is more likely to faint if positioned with the head higher than the heels.
	The chair back should be nearly parallel to the floor for maxillary treatment areas.
	The chair back may be raised slightly for mandibular treatment areas.
Head	The top of the patient's head should be even with the upper edge of the headrest. If necessary, ask the patient to slide up in the chair to assume this position.
Headrest	If the headrest is adjustable, raise or lower it so that the patient's neck and head are aligned with the torso.

PATIENT HEAD POSITION

The patient's head position is an important factor in determining whether the clinician can see and access the teeth in a treatment area. Unfortunately, a clinician may ignore this important aspect of patient positioning, contorting his or her body into an uncomfortable position instead of asking the patient to change head positions. Working in this manner not only causes stress on the clinician's musculoskeletal system but also makes it difficult to see the treatment area. Remember that the patient is only in the chair for a limited period of time while the clinician spends hours at chairside day after day. The patient should be asked to adjust his or her head position to provide the clinician with the best view of the treatment area (Table 2-2).

TABLE 2-2.	Basic Positioning of the Patient's Head

Recommended Position

Position on Headrest	To be able to see and reach the patient's mouth comfortably, the top of the patient's head must be even with the end of the headrest.
Mandibular Areas	Ask your patient to open the mouth and tilt the head downward. The term for this patient head position is the **chin-down position**.
Maxillary Areas	Ask your patient to open the mouth and position the head in a neutral position. The term for this patient head position is the **chin-up position**.

Section 3
Clinician and Equipment Position

THE ADJUSTABLE CLINICIAN CHAIR

Ergonomics is the science of adjusting the design of tools, equipment, tasks, and environments for safe, comfortable, and effective human use. Blood circulation to your legs, thighs, and feet is maintained by adjusting the clinician chair to a proper height. Minimize stress on your spine by moving the chair back closer to or farther away from the seat so that your upper arms and torso are aligned with the long axis of your body.

Each clinician who uses the chair should readjust it to fit his or her own body. A chair that is adjusted correctly for another person may be uncomfortable for you. Just as each driver of the family car must change the position of the driver's seat and mirrors, you should adjust the clinician chair height and seat back to conform to your own body proportions and height.

The chair should have the following design characteristics[13]:

1. **Legs**—five legs for stability; casters for easy movement
2. **Height**
   * Should allow clinician to sit with thighs parallel to the floor. A seat height range of 14 to 20 inches accommodates both tall and short clinicians.
   * Should be easily adjustable from a seated position.
3. **Seat**
   * Front edge of seat should have a waterfall shape (rounded front edge).
   * Should not be too heavily padded; thick padding requires constant minor readjustments to maintain balance.
   * When seated with the back against the backrest, the seat length should not impinge on the back of the clinician's knees. A seat length of 15 to 16 inches fits most clinicians.
4. **Backrest**
   * Should be adjustable in both vertical and horizontal directions so that it can be positioned to touch the lumbar region of the back when comfortably seated.
   * Angle between the seat and the chair back should be between 85 and 100 degrees.

PATIENT POSITION RELATIVE TO THE CLINICIAN

The first component in avoiding fatigue and injury is proper positioning of the patient in relation to the seated clinician (Boxes 2-2 and 2-3). While working, the clinician must be able to gain access to the patient's mouth and the dental unit without bending, stretching, or holding his or her elbows above waist level.

Box 2-2. Establishing Neutral Position in Relation to the Patient

1. First, adjust the height of the clinician chair to establish a hip angle of 90°.

2. Next, lower the patient chair until the tip of the patient's nose is below the clinician's waist level. Your elbow angle should be at 90° when your fingers are touching the teeth in the treatment area.

3. **AVOID** placing your legs under the *back* of the patient chair—in this position the patient will be too high and you will need to raise your arms to reach the patient's mouth. It is acceptable to place your legs under the *headrest* of the chair.

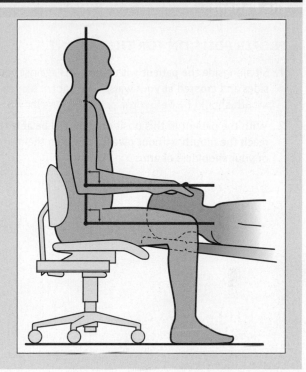

Common Positioning Error

The most common positioning error made by clinicians during periodontal instrumentation is positioning the patient too high in relation to the clinician.

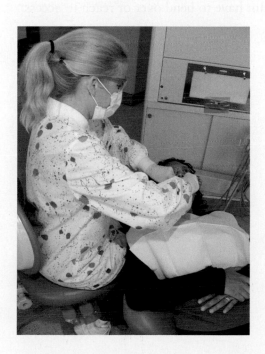

Incorrect Positioning—Patient Too High. Note how this clinician must hold her elbows up in a stressful position to reach the patient's mouth.

This error is often the result of a misconception that the clinician can see better if the patient is closer. Actually, the reverse is true; the clinician has improved vision of the mouth when the patient is in a lower position.

Box 2-3. Easy Technique for Establishing Neutral Position in Relation to the Patient

PROPER POSITION FOR THE PATIENT

1. Sit alongside the patient with your arms against your sides and crossed at your waist. The patient's open mouth should be *below* the point of your elbow.

2. With the patient in this position, you will be able to reach the mouth without placing stress on the muscles of your shoulders or arms.

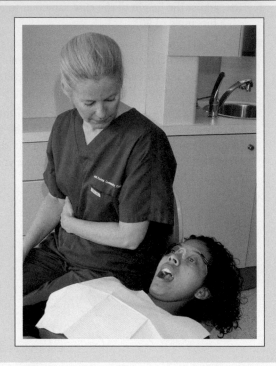

EQUIPMENT POSITION RELATIVE TO THE CLINICIAN

The second component in avoiding fatigue and injury is proper positioning of the dental equipment in relation to the clinician. It is important that the clinician not have to bend over or reach to access dental instruments or equipment.

Position for Mandibular Teeth

1. **Dental Light.** Position the dental light directly above the patient's head. The light should be as far above the patient as possible while still remaining within easy reach. In this position, the light beams will shine directly down into the patient's mouth.

2. **Bracket Table.** If the dental unit has a bracket table, it should be positioned as low as possible so that the clinician can easily view the instruments resting on it. Instruments should be within easy reach.

3. **Patient Chair.** Position the patient chair so that your elbow angle is at a 90-degree angle when your fingers rest on the mandibular teeth.

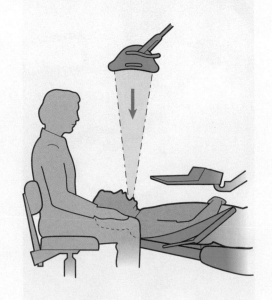

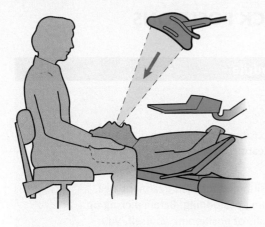

Light Position for Maxillary Teeth

1. **Dental Light.** Position the dental light above the patient's chest. Tilt the light so that the light beams shine into the patient's mouth at an angle. Position the light as far away from the patient's face as possible while still keeping it within easy reach.

2. **Patient Chair.** When instrumentation moves from the mandibular to the maxillary teeth, lower the *entire* patient chair (not just the chair back) until your elbow angle is at a 90-degree angle when your fingers rest on the maxillary teeth.

TABLE 2-3.	Summary Sheet: Relationship to Patient and Equipment
Clinician Chair	Your thighs should be parallel to the floor and you should be able to rest your heels on the floor.
	Your legs and the stool base should form a tripod, somewhat like the legs of a three-legged stool. This tripod formation creates a very stable position from which to work.
Height of Patient Chair	TEST FOR PROPER NEUTRAL POSITION: Fold your arms across your waist. The tip of the patient's nose should be lower than your elbows.
Clinician	You should not have to raise your elbows above waist level when working in the patient's mouth.
	Your *lower arms* should be in a horizontal position or raised slightly so that the angle formed between your lower and upper arms is slightly less than 90 degrees. In this position, your muscles are well positioned to control fine wrist and finger movements.
	Your shoulders should be level and should not be hunched up toward your ears.
Bracket Table	Position it slightly above the patient's body. The lower the tray level, the easier it will be for you to see the periodontal instruments resting on it.
Dental Light	Position the light as far away from the patient's face as possible while still keeping it within easy reach.

DIRECTIONS FOR PRACTICING THE CLOCK POSITIONS

Box 2-4. Directions for Sections 4 and 5 of this Module

POSITION FOR TREATMENT AREAS OF THE MOUTH

1. The next two sections of this module contain instructions for positioning yourself to obtain the best possible access to each of the treatment areas. For some treatment areas, there is a range of clock positions in which you can sit.

2. For this module, you should concentrate on mastering your positioning for each treatment area. Work without dental instruments and just concentrate on learning positioning. Before picking up a periodontal instrument, you should master the large motor skills of positioning yourself, your patient, and the dental equipment to facilitate neutral position.

3. As you practice each clock position, position your arms and hands as described in this module. You will use both of your hands for periodontal instrumentation, the periodontal instrument is held in your dominant hand, and the mirror is held in your **non**dominant hand. For this module, practice placing the fingertips of your hands as shown in the illustration for each clock position.

4. You will not be able to obtain a clear view of all the teeth as you practice positioning in this module. In Modules 4, 5, and 6, you will learn to use a dental mouth mirror to view these "hidden" tooth surfaces.

5. When practicing on a classmate, use universal precautions for infection control.

RIGHT- AND LEFT-HANDED SECTIONS

The remainder of this module is divided into right- and left-handed sections.

Right-handed Clinicians: Refer to Section 4 on the following page.

Left-handed Clinicians: Turn to Section 5 on page 32.

Section 4
Position for RIGHT-Handed Clinician

Instrumentation of the various treatment areas may be accomplished from one of four basic clinician positions. The four basic clinician positions are usually identified in relation to a 12-hour clock face:

1. 8 o'clock position—to the front of the patient's head
2. 9 o'clock position—to the side of the patient's head
3. 10 to 11 o'clock position—near the corner of the patient headrest
4. 12 o'clock position—behind the patient's head

The four clock positions are described in detail on the following pages.

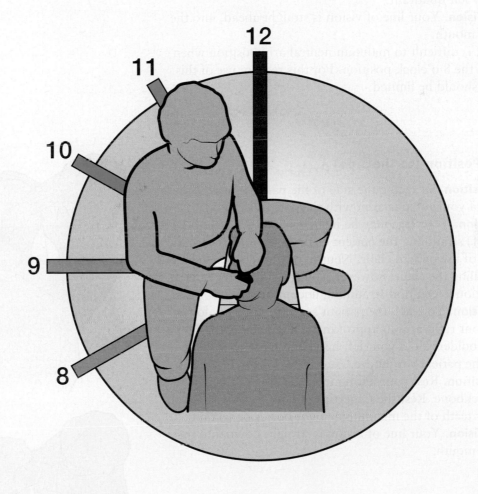

CLOCK POSITIONS

8 o'clock Position (to the Front)

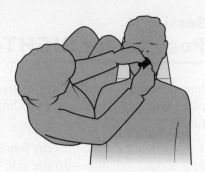

1. **Torso Position.** Sit facing the patient with your hip in line with the patient's upper arm.
2. **Leg Position.** Your thighs should rest against the side of the patient chair.
3. **Arm Position.** To reach the patient's mouth, hold your arms slightly away from your sides. Hold your lower right arm over the patient's chest. NOTE: Do not rest your arm on the patient's head or chest.
4. **Hand Position.** Rest the side of your left hand in the area of the patient's right cheekbone and upper lip. Rest the finger-tips of your right hand on the *anterior teeth* in the patient's maxillary left quadrant.
5. **Line of Vision.** Your line of vision is straight ahead, into the patient's mouth.
6. **NOTE:** It is difficult to maintain neutral arm position when seated in the 8 o'clock position. For this reason, use of this position should be limited.

9 o'clock Position (to the Side)

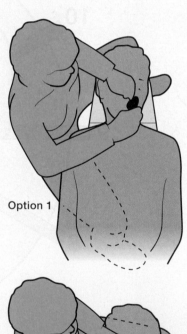

1. **Torso Position.** Sit facing the side of the patient's head. The midline of your torso is even with the patient's mouth.
2. **Leg Position.** Your legs may be in either of two acceptable po-sitions: (1) straddling the patient chair or (2) underneath the *headrest* of the patient chair. Neutral position is best achieved by straddling the chair; however, you should use the alterna-tive position if you find straddling uncomfortable.
3. **Arm Position.** To reach the patient's mouth, hold the lower half of your right arm in approximate alignment with the pa-tient's shoulder. Hold your left hand and wrist over the re-gion of the patient's right eye.
4. **Hand Position.** Rest your left hand in the area of the patient's right cheekbone. Rest the fingertips of your right hand on the premolar teeth of the mandibular right posterior sextant.
5. **Line of Vision.** Your line of vision is straight down into the patient's mouth.

Option 1

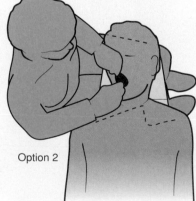

Option 2

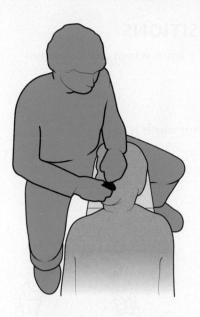

10 to 11 o'clock Position (Near Corner of Headrest)

1. **Torso Position.** Sit at the top right corner of the headrest; the midline of your torso is even with the temple region of the patient's head.
2. **Leg Position.** Your legs should straddle the corner of the headrest.
3. **Arm Position.** To reach the patient's mouth, hold your right hand directly across the corner of the patient's mouth. Hold your left hand and wrist above the patient's nose and forehead.
4. **Hand Position.** Rest your left hand in the area of the patient's left cheekbone. Rest the fingertips of your right hand on the premolar teeth of the mandibular left posterior sextant.
5. **Line of Vision.** Your line of vision is straight down into the mouth.

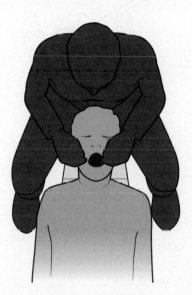

12 o'clock Position (Behind Patient)

1. **Torso Position.** Sit behind the patient's head; you may sit anywhere from the right corner of the headrest to directly behind the headrest.
2. **Leg Position.** Your legs should straddle the headrest.
3. **Arm Position.** To reach the patient's mouth, hold your wrists and hands above the region of the patient's ears and cheeks.
4. **Hand Position.** Place the fingertips of your left hand on the anterior teeth in the maxillary left quadrant. Rest the fingertips of your right hand on the anterior teeth in the mandibular right quadrant.
5. **Line of Vision.** Your line of vision is straight down into the patient's mouth.

RIGHT-Handed Clinician

QUICK START GUIDE TO LEARNING CLOCK POSITIONS

Directions: Follow the simple steps outlined below and you will quickly learn which clock position to use for each treatment area of the mouth.

Quick Start Guide to Anterior Tooth Surfaces

1. **Divide Each Anterior Tooth in "Half".** For instrumentation, an anterior tooth is divided into two halves at the midline of the tooth.
2. **Sit at 8:00.**
3. **Determine Surfaces Closest to You.**

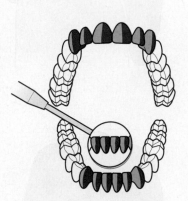

Anterior Surfaces Toward You when you sit at 8:00 are instrumented from the 8:00 to 9:00 position.

Anterior Surfaces Away From You when you sit at 8:00 are instrumented from the 12:00 position.

Quick Start Guide to Posterior Sextants

1. **Divide Each Sextant into Aspects.** For instrumentation, each sextant is divided into aspects. One clock position is used for the facial aspect of a sextant. Another clock position is used for the lingual aspect of a sextant.
2. **Sit at 9:00.**
3. **For EACH SEXTANT, determine the Aspect Facing Toward You.** For example, look at the mandibular right posterior sextant.
   - The facial aspect of the mandibular right posterior sextant is facing toward 9:00.
   - The lingual aspect of the mandibular right posteriors is facing away from 9:00.

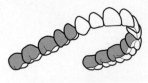

Posterior Aspects Facing Toward You when seated at 9:00 are instrumented from the 9:00 position.

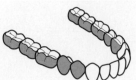

Posterior Aspects Facing Away From You when seated at 9:00 are instrumented from the 10:00-11:00 position.

RIGHT-Handed Clinician

FLOW CHART: SEQUENCE FOR PRACTICING POSITIONING

For successful periodontal instrumentation, it is important to proceed in a step-by-step manner. A useful saying to help you remember the step-by-step approach is "Me, My Patient, My Light, My Nondominant Hand, My Dominant Hand."

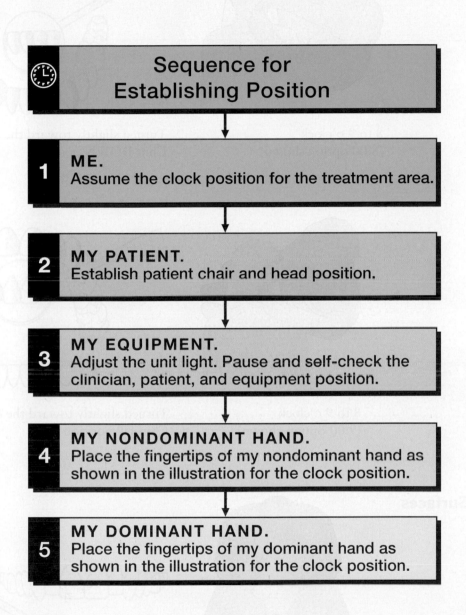

Sequence for Establishing Position

1 ME.
Assume the clock position for the treatment area.

2 MY PATIENT.
Establish patient chair and head position.

3 MY EQUIPMENT.
Adjust the unit light. Pause and self-check the clinician, patient, and equipment position.

4 MY NONDOMINANT HAND.
Place the fingertips of my nondominant hand as shown in the illustration for the clock position.

5 MY DOMINANT HAND.
Place the fingertips of my dominant hand as shown in the illustration for the clock position.

RIGHT-Handed Clinician

POSITIONING FOR THE ANTERIOR SEXTANTS

Anterior Surfaces
TOWARD

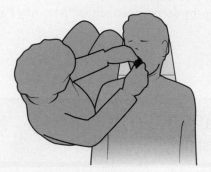

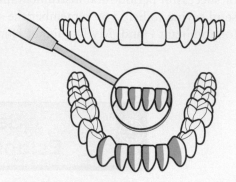

8 to 9 o'clock
(8:00 option shown)

Turned slightly toward the clinician
Chin-DOWN position

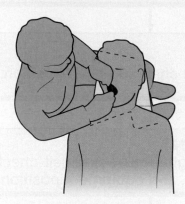

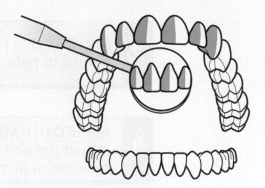

8 to 9 o'clock
(9:00 option shown)

Turned slightly toward the clinician
Chin-UP position

Anterior Surfaces
AWAY

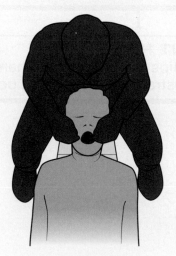

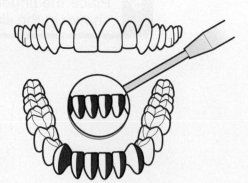

12 o'clock position

Turned slightly toward the clinician
Chin-DOWN position

Anterior Surfaces AWAY

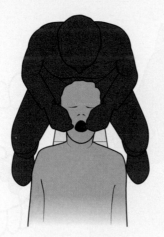

12 o'clock position

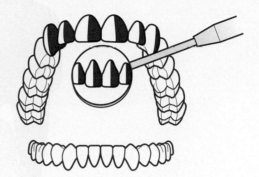

Turned slightly toward the clinician
Chin-UP position

POSITIONING FOR THE POSTERIOR SEXTANTS

Posterior Aspects Facing TOWARD

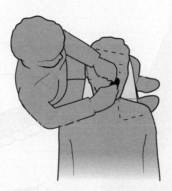

9 o'clock
(Option 1 for 9:00)

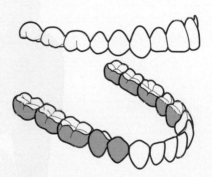

Turned slightly away from the clinician
Chin-DOWN position

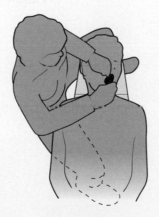

9 o'clock
(Option 2 for 9:00)

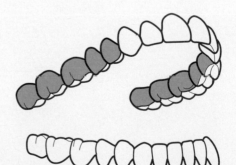

Turned slightly away from the clinician
Chin-UP position

Posterior Aspects
Facing AWAY

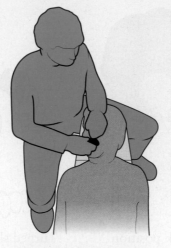

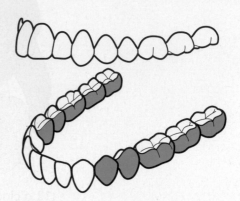

10 to 11 o'clock

Turned toward the clinician
Chin-DOWN position

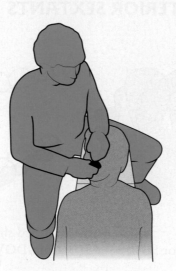

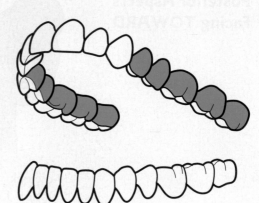

10 to 11 o'clock

Turned toward the clinician
Chin-UP position

REFERENCE SHEET: POSITION FOR THE RIGHT-HANDED CLINICIAN

Photocopy this page and use it for quick reference as you practice your positioning skills. Place the photocopied reference sheet in a plastic page protector for longer use.

TABLE 2-4.	Positioning Summary	
Treatment Area	**Clock Position**	**Patient Head Position**
Mandibular Arch—Anterior surfaces toward	8–9:00	Slightly toward, Chin DOWN
Maxillary Arch—Anterior surfaces toward	8–9:00	Slightly toward, Chin UP
Mandibular Arch—Anterior surfaces away	12:00	Slightly toward, Chin DOWN
Maxillary Arch—Anterior surfaces away	12:00	Slightly toward, Chin UP
Mandibular Arch—Posterior aspects facing toward	9:00	Slightly away, Chin DOWN
Maxillary Arch—Posterior aspects facing toward	9:00	Slightly away, Chin UP
Mandibular Arch—Posterior aspects facing away	10–11:00	Toward, Chin DOWN
Maxillary Arch—Posterior aspects facing away	10–11:00	Toward, Chin UP

NOTE: This ends the section for the RIGHT-Handed Clinician.
Turn to page 42 for Section 6: Skill Application.

RIGHT-Handed Clinician

Section 5
Position for LEFT-Handed Clinician

Instrumentation of the various treatment areas may be accomplished from one of four basic clinician positions. The four basic clinician positions are usually identified in relation to a 12-hour clock face:

1. 4 o'clock position—to the front of the patient's head
2. 3 o'clock position—to the side of the patient's head
3. 2 to 1 o'clock position—near the corner of the patient headrest
4. 12 o'clock position—behind the patient's head

The four clock positions are described in detail on the following pages.

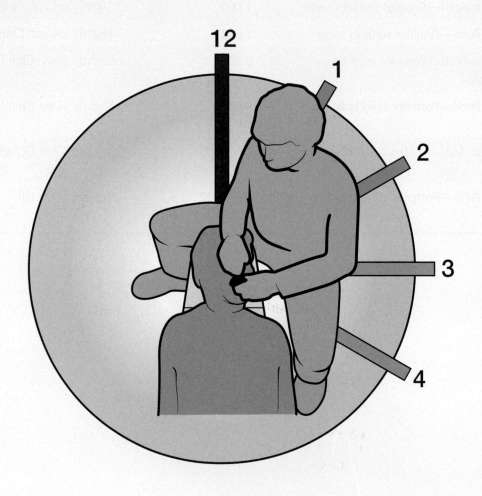

CLOCK POSITIONS

4 o'clock Position (to the Front)

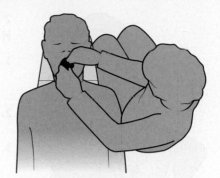

1. **Torso Position.** Sit facing the patient with your hip in line with the patient's upper arm.
2. **Leg Position.** Your thighs should rest against the side of the patient chair.
3. **Arm Position.** To reach the patient's mouth, hold your arms slightly away from your sides. Hold your lower left arm over the patient's chest. The side of your right hand rests in the area of the patient's left cheekbone and upper lip. NOTE: Do not rest your arm on the patient's head or chest.
4. **Line of Vision.** Your line of vision is straight ahead, into the patient's mouth.
5. **Hand Position.** Rest the side of your right hand in the area of the patient's left cheekbone and upper lip. Rest the fingertips of your left hand on the anterior teeth in the patient's maxillary right quadrant.
6. **NOTE:** It is difficult to maintain neutral arm position when seated in the 4 o'clock position. Use of this position should be limited.

3 o'clock Position (to the Side)

1. **Torso Position.** Sit facing the side of the patient's head. The midline of your torso is even with the patient's mouth.
2. **Leg Position.** Your legs may be in either of two acceptable positions: (1) straddling the patient chair or (2) underneath the *headrest* of the patient chair. Neutral position is best achieved by straddling the chair; however, you should use the alternative position if you find straddling uncomfortable.
3. **Arm Position.** To reach the patient's mouth, hold the lower half of your left arm in approximate alignment with the patient's shoulder. Hold your right hand and wrist over the region of patient's left eye.
4. **Hand Position.** Rest your right hand in the area of the patient's left cheekbone. Rest the fingertips of your left hand on the premolar teeth of the mandibular left posterior sextant.
5. **Line of Vision.** Your line of vision is straight down into the mouth.

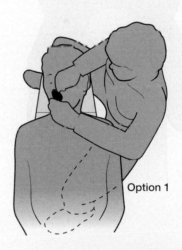

Option 1

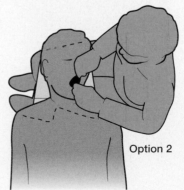

Option 2

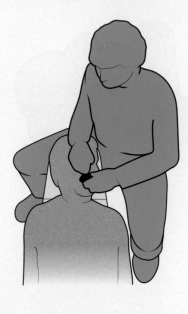

2 to 1 o'clock Position (Near Corner of Headrest)

1. **Torso Position.** Sit at the top left corner of the headrest; the midline of your torso is even with the temple region of the patient's head.
2. **Leg Position.** Your legs should straddle the corner of the headrest.
3. **Arm Position.** To reach the patient's mouth, hold your left hand directly across the corner of the patient's mouth. Hold your right hand and wrist above the patient's nose and forehead.
4. **Hand Position.** Rest your right hand in the area of the patient's right cheekbone. Rest the fingertips of your left hand on the premolar teeth of the mandibular right posterior sextant.
5. **Line of Vision.** Your line of vision is straight down into the mouth.

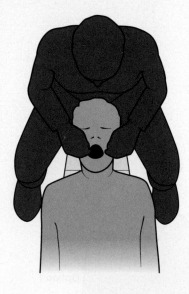

12 o'clock Position (Directly Behind Patient)

1. **Torso Position.** Sit directly behind the patient's head; you may sit anywhere from the left corner of the headrest to directly behind the headrest.
2. **Leg Position.** Your legs should straddle the headrest.
3. **Arm Position.** To reach the patient's mouth, hold your wrists and hands above the region of the patient's ears and cheeks.
4. **Hand Position.** Place the fingertips of your right hand on the anterior teeth in the maxillary right quadrant. Rest the fingertips of your left hand on the anterior teeth in the mandibular left quadrant.
5. **Line of Vision.** Your line of vision is straight down into the patient's mouth.

QUICK START GUIDE TO LEARNING CLOCK POSITIONS

Directions: Follow the simple steps outlined below and you will quickly learn which clock position to use for each treatment area of the mouth.

Quick Start Guide to Anterior Tooth Surfaces

1. **Divide Each Anterior Tooth in "Half".** For instrumentation, an anterior tooth is divided into two halves at the midline of the tooth.
2. **Sit at 4:00.**
3. **Determine Surfaces Closest to You.**

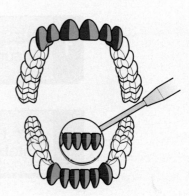

Anterior Surfaces Toward You when you sit at 4:00 are instrumented from the 4:00 to 3:00 position.

Anterior Surfaces Away From You when seated at 4:00 are instrumented from the 12:00 position.

Quick Start Guide to Posterior Sextants

1. **Divide Each Sextant into Aspects.** For instrumentation, each sextant is divided into aspects. One clock position is used for the facial aspect of a sextant. Another clock position is used for the lingual aspect of a sextant.
2. **Sit at 3:00.**
3. **For EACH SEXTANT, determine the Aspect Facing Toward You.** For example, look at the mandibular left posterior sextant.
   - The facial aspect of the mandibular left posterior sextant is facing toward 3:00.
   - The lingual aspect of the mandibular left posteriors is facing away from 3:00.

Posterior Aspects Facing Toward You when you sit at 3:00 are instrumented from the 3:00 position.

Posterior Aspects Facing Away From You when you sit at 3:00 are instrumented from the 2 to 1 o'clock position.

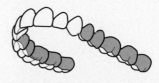

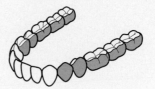

LEFT-Handed Clinician

FLOW CHART: SEQUENCE FOR PRACTICING POSITIONING

For successful periodontal instrumentation, it is important to proceed in a step-by-step manner. A useful saying to help you remember the step-by-step approach is "Me, My Patient, My Light, My Nondominant Hand, My Dominant Hand."

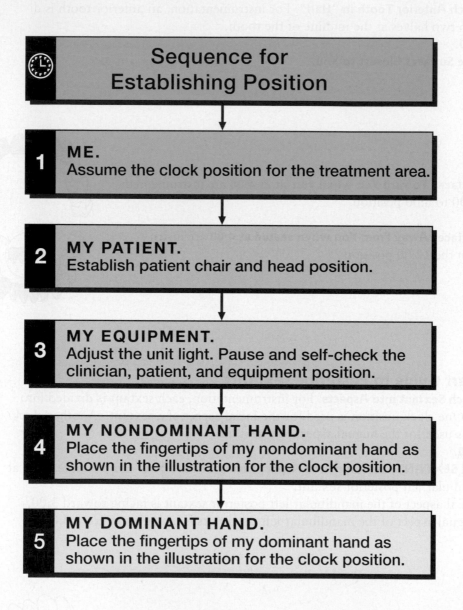

Sequence for Establishing Position

1 ME.
Assume the clock position for the treatment area.

2 MY PATIENT.
Establish patient chair and head position.

3 MY EQUIPMENT.
Adjust the unit light. Pause and self-check the clinician, patient, and equipment position.

4 MY NONDOMINANT HAND.
Place the fingertips of my nondominant hand as shown in the illustration for the clock position.

5 MY DOMINANT HAND.
Place the fingertips of my dominant hand as shown in the illustration for the clock position.

LEFT-Handed Clinician

POSITIONING FOR THE ANTERIOR SEXTANTS

Anterior Surfaces TOWARD

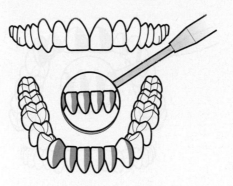

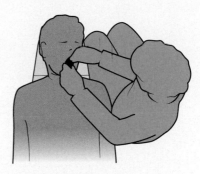

Turned slightly toward the clinician
Chin-DOWN position

4 to 3 o'clock
(4:00 option shown)

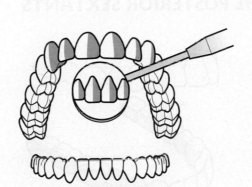

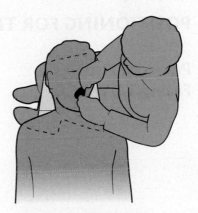

Turned slightly toward the clinician
Chin-UP position

4 to 3 o'clock
(3:00 option shown)

Anterior Surfaces AWAY

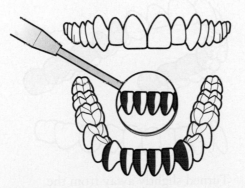

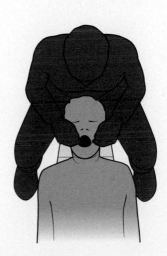

Turned slightly toward the clinician
Chin-DOWN position

12 o'clock position

Anterior Surfaces
AWAY

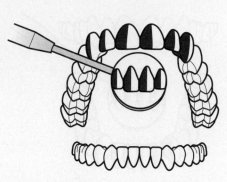

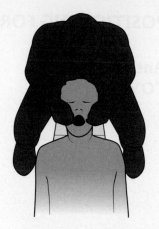

Turned slightly toward the clincian
Chin-UP position

12 o'clock position

POSITIONING FOR THE POSTERIOR SEXTANTS

Posterior Aspects
Facing TOWARD

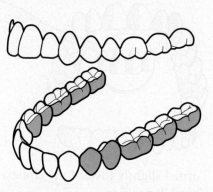

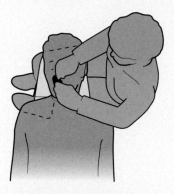

Turned slightly away from the
clinician
Chin-DOWN position

3 o'clock
(Option 1 shown)

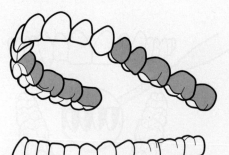

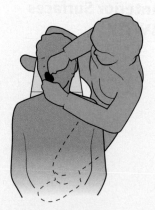

Turned slightly away from the
clinician
Chin-UP position

3 o'clock
(Option 2 shown)

Posterior Aspects
Facing AWAY

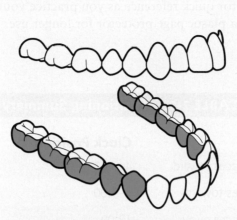

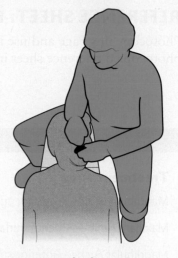

Turned toward the clinician
Chin-DOWN position

2 to 1 o'clock

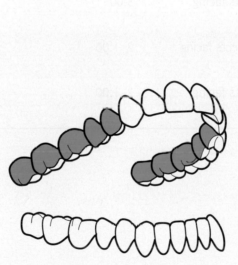

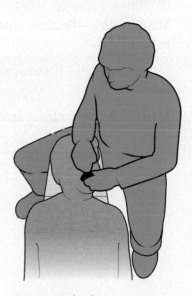

Turned toward the clinician
Chin-UP position

2 to 1 o'clock

REFERENCE SHEET: POSITION FOR THE LEFT-HANDED CLINICIAN

Photocopy this page and use it for quick reference as you practice your positioning skills. Place the photocopied reference sheet in a plastic page protector for longer use.

TABLE 2-5. Positioning Summary		
Treatment Area	**Clock Position**	**Patient Head Position**
Mandibular Arch—Anterior surfaces toward	4–3:00	Slightly toward, Chin DOWN
Maxillary Arch—Anterior surfaces toward	4–3:00	Slightly toward, Chin UP
Mandibular Arch—Anterior surfaces away	12:00	Slightly toward, Chin DOWN
Maxillary Arch—Anterior surfaces away	12:00	Slightly toward, Chin UP
Mandibular Arch—Posterior aspects facing toward	3:00	Slightly away, Chin DOWN
Maxillary Arch—Posterior aspects facing toward	3:00	Slightly away, Chin UP
Mandibular Arch—Posterior aspects facing away	2–1:00	Toward, Chin DOWN
Maxillary Arch—Posterior aspects facing away	2–1:00	Toward, Chin UP

LEFT-Handed Clinician

NOTE: This ends the section for the LEFT-Handed Clinician. Turn to page 42 for Section 6: Skill Application.

REFERENCES

1. Silverstein, B.A., *et al.*, *Work-related musculoskeletal disorders: comparison of data sources for surveillance*. Am J Ind Med, 1997. 31(5): p. 600-8.

2. Jacobsen, N., and A. Hensten-Pettersen, *Occupational health problems among dental hygienists*. Community Dent Oral Epidemiol, 1995. 23(3): p. 177-81.

3. Jacobsen, N., T. Derand, and A. Hensten-Pettersen, *Profile of work-related health complaints among Swedish dental laboratory technicians*. Community Dent Oral Epidemiol, 1996. 24(2): p. 138-44.

4. Moen, B.E. and K. Bjorvatn, *Musculoskeletal symptoms among dentists in a dental school*. Occup Med (Lond), 1996. 46(1): p. 65-8.

5. Reitemeier, B., *Psychophysiological and epidemiological investigations on the dentist*. Rev Environ Health, 1996. 11(1-2): p. 57-63.

6. Rundcrantz, B.L., B. Johnsson, and U. Moritz, *Cervical pain and discomfort among dentists. Epidemiological, clinical and therapeutic aspects. Part 1. A survey of pain and discomfort*. Swed Dent J, 1990. 14(2): p. 71-80.

7. Rundcrantz, B.L., B. Johnsson, and U. Moritz, *Pain and discomfort in the musculoskeletal system among dentists. A prospective study*. Swed Dent J, 1991. 15(5): p. 219-28.

8. Rundcrantz, B.L., *Pain and discomfort in the musculoskeletal system among dentists*. Swed Dent J Suppl, 1991. 76: p. 1-102.

9. Silverstein, B.A., L.J. Fine, and T.J. Armstrong, *Hand wrist cumulative trauma disorders in industry*. Br J Ind Med, 1986. 43(11): p. 779-84.

10. Latko, W.A., *et al.*, *Development and evaluation of an observational method for assessing repetition in hand tasks*. Am Ind Hyg Assoc J, 1997. 58(4): p. 278-85.

11. Kilbom, S., *et al.*, *Musculoskeletal disorders: work-related risk factors and prevention*. Int J Occup Environ Health, 1996. 2(3): p. 239-246.

12. Silverstein, B.A., L.J. Fine, and T.J. Armstrong, *Occupational factors and carpal tunnel syndrome*. Am J Ind Med, 1987. 11(3): p. 343-58.

13. Occhipinti, E., *et al.*, *Criteria for the ergonomic evaluation of work chairs*. Med Lav, 1993. 84(4): p. 274-85.

The Skill Application Section begins on the following page.

Section 6
Skill Application

PRACTICAL FOCUS

Your course assignment is to visit a local dental office and photograph a clinician at work to assess position. Your photographs are shown below. (1) Evaluate each photograph for clinician, patient, and equipment position. (2) For each incorrect positioning element, describe: (a) how the problem could be corrected and (b) the musculoskeletal problems that could result from each positioning problem.

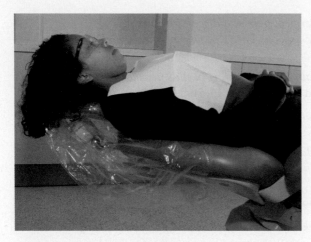

Photo 1

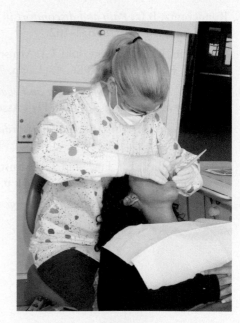

Photo 3

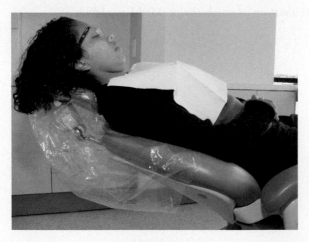

Photo 2

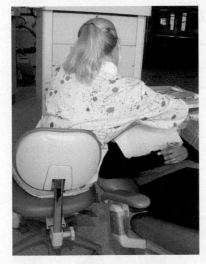

Photo 4

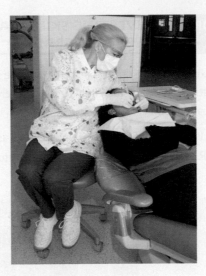

Photo 5

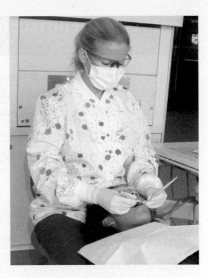

Photo 6

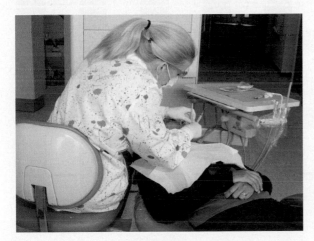

Photo 7

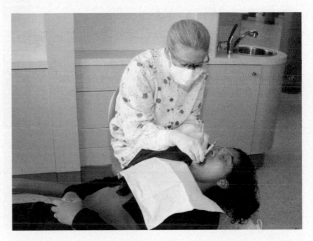

Photo 8

NOTE TO COURSE INSTRUCTOR

CONVERTING SKILL EVALUATION TO A PERCENTAGE GRADE

If you like, the Skill Evaluations in this textbook can comprise a percentage of the student's overall course grade. To determine a percentage grade for a Skill Evaluation, divide the total number of **S**'s received by the Total Points Possible for the evaluation. An example of a graded evaluation form is shown below.

DIRECTIONS FOR STUDENT: Use **Column S.** Evaluate your skill level as: **S** (satisfactory) or **U** (unsatisfactory).

DIRECTIONS FOR EVALUATOR: Use **Column E.** Indicate: **S** (satisfactory) or **U** (unsatisfactory). Each **S** equals I point, each **U** equals 0 points.

	Area 1		Area 2		Area 3		Area 4		Area 5		Area 6	
CRITERIA:	S	E	S	E	S	E	S	E	S	E	S	E
Adjusts clinician chair correctly		S		S		S		S		S		S
Positions patient chair correctly		S		S		S		S		S		S
Ensures that patient's head is even with top of headrest		S		S		S		S		S		S
Positions bracket table within easy reach		S		U		S		S		U		S
Positions unit light at arm's length		S		S		U		S		S		S
Assumes recommended clock position		S		S		S		U		S		U
Asks patient to adjust head position		U		U		S		S		S		S
Adjusts patient chair so that clinician's elbows are at waist level when fingers touch teeth in treatment area		S		S		S		S		S		S
Maintains neutral position		U		U		S		U		S		U
Directs unit light to illuminate treatment area		S		S		S		S		S		S
OPTIONAL GRADE PERCENTAGE CALCULATION Total **S**'s in each **E** column.		8		7		9		8		9		8

Sum of **S**'s ____49____ divided by Total Points Possible (**60**) equals the Percentage Grade ____82____ %

SKILL EVALUATION MODULE 2	POSITION, MANDIBULAR SEXTANTS

Student: _____

Evaluator: _____

Date: _____

Area 1 = anterior sextant, facial aspect
Area 2 = anterior sextant, lingual aspect

Area 3 = right posterior sextant, facial aspect
Area 4 = right posterior sextant, lingual aspect

Area 5 = left posterior sextant, facial aspect
Area 6 = left posterior sextant, lingual aspect

DIRECTIONS FOR STUDENT: Use **Column S**. Evaluate your skill level as: **S** (satisfactory) or **U** (unsatisfactory).

DIRECTIONS FOR EVALUATOR: Use **Column E**. Indicate: **S** (satisfactory) or **U** (unsatisfactory). Each **S** equals 1 point, each **U** equals 0 points.

CRITERIA:	Area 1 S	E	Area 2 S	E	Area 3 S	E	Area 4 S	E	Area 5 S	E	Area 6 S	E
Adjusts clinician chair correctly												
Positions patient chair correctly												
Ensures that patient's head is even with top of headrest												
Positions bracket table within easy reach												
Positions unit light at arm's length												
Assumes recommended clock position												
Asks patient to adjust head position												
Adjusts patient chair so that clinician's elbows are at waist level when fingers touch teeth in treatment area												
Maintains neutral position												
Directs unit light to illuminate treatment area												
OPTIONAL GRADE PERCENTAGE CALCULATION Total **S**'s in each **E** column.												

Sum of **S**'s _____ divided by Total Points Possible (**60**) equals the Percentage Grade _____%

SKILL EVALUATIONS—NOTE TO COURSE INSTRUCTOR

The Skill Evaluation pages for all modules are designed so that these forms may be torn from the book without loss of text content. If you like, the forms may be used for evaluation and then removed for your records at completion of each module or completion of the course.

SKILL EVALUATION MODULE 2   POSITION, MANDIBULAR SEXTANTS

Student: _____

EVALUATOR COMMENTS

_____

_____

_____

_____

_____

_____

_____

_____

_____

_____

_____

_____

_____

_____

_____

_____

Box for sketches pertaining to written comments.

SKILL EVALUATION MODULE 2 | **POSITION, MAXILLARY SEXTANTS**

Student: _____

Area 1 = anterior sextant, facial aspect
Area 2 = anterior sextant, lingual aspect

Evaluator: _____

Area 3 = right posterior sextant, facial aspect
Area 4 = right posterior sextant, lingual aspect

Date: _____

Area 5 = left posterior sextant, facial aspect
Area 6 = left posterior sextant, lingual aspect

DIRECTIONS FOR STUDENT: Use **Column S**. Evaluate your skill level as: **S** (satisfactory) or **U** (unsatisfactory).
DIRECTIONS FOR EVALUATOR: Use **Column E**. Indicate: **S** (satisfactory) or **U** (unsatisfactory). Each **S** equals 1 point, each **U** equals 0 points.

CRITERIA:	Area 1		Area 2		Area 3		Area 4		Area 5		Area 6	
	S	E	S	E	S	E	S	E	S	E	S	E
Adjusts clinician chair correctly												
Positions patient chair correctly												
Ensures that patient's head is even with top of headrest												
Positions bracket table within easy reach												
Positions unit light at arm's length												
Assumes recommended clock position												
Asks patient to adjust head position												
Adjusts patient chair so that clinician's elbows are at waist level when fingers touch teeth in treatment area												
Maintains neutral position												
Directs unit light to illuminate treatment area												
OPTIONAL GRADE PERCENTAGE CALCULATION Total **S**'s in each E column.												

Sum of **S**'s _____ divided by Total Points Possible (**60**) equals the Percentage Grade _____%

SKILL EVALUATIONS—NOTE TO COURSE INSTRUCTOR

The Skill Evaluation pages for all modules are designed so that these forms may be torn from the book without loss of text content. If you like, the forms may be used for evaluation and then removed for your records at completion of each module or completion of the course.

SKILL EVALUATION MODULE 2   POSITION, MAXILLARY SEXTANTS

Student: _____

EVALUATOR COMMENTS

_____
_____
_____
_____
_____
_____
_____
_____
_____
_____
_____
_____
_____
_____
_____
_____

Box for sketches pertaining to written comments.

Module 3

Instrument Grasp

Module Overview

This module introduces the correct grasp for holding a periodontal instrument. It begins by explaining the parts of a periodontal instrument and proper glove selection for instrumentation. Covered next is the correct finger placement for the modified pen grasp. This module also contains exercises designed to help develop and maintain the strength of the hand muscles.

Module Outline

Key Terms

Handle
Shank
Working-end
Modified pen grasp

Learning Objectives

1. Given a variety of periodontal instruments, identify the parts of each instrument.

2. Understand the relationship among correct finger position in the modified pen grasp, the prevention of musculoskeletal problems, and the control of a periodontal instrument during instrumentation.

3. Demonstrate correct finger position for the modified pen grasp.

4. Describe the function each finger serves in the modified pen grasp.

5. Recognize incorrect finger position in the modified pen grasp and describe how to correct the problem(s).

6. Select the correct glove size for your hands and explain how the glove size selected meets the criteria for proper glove fit.

7. Understand the relationship between proper glove fit and the prevention of musculoskeletal problems in the hands.

8. Perform exercises for improved hand strength.

Section 1
Instrument and Finger Identification

A correct instrument grasp requires precise finger placement on the instrument (Table 3-1). To follow the instructions for the grasp, you must be able to identify (1) the parts of a periodontal instrument and (2) the fingers for use in the modified pen grasp.

PARTS OF THE PERIODONTAL INSTRUMENT

Handle—the part of a periodontal instrument used for holding the instrument.

Shank—a rod-shaped length of metal located between the handle and the working-end of a dental instrument. The shank is an extension device that increases the length of the instrument so that the working-end can be positioned on the tooth root. Look closely at the instrument handle; usually you will be able to see a line or edge where the handle joins the shank. The shank is generally much smaller in diameter than the handle. The shank may be straight, or it may be bent in one or more places.

Working-End—the part of a dental instrument that does the work of the instrument. The working-end begins where the instrument shank ends. The shank is circular and smooth, but the working-end is shaped or flattened on some of its surfaces. The working-end may terminate in a sharp point or a rounded surface. It may be thin and wirelike or look somewhat like a tiny measuring stick. In some cases, the working-end is a small mirror. An instrument may have one or two working-ends.

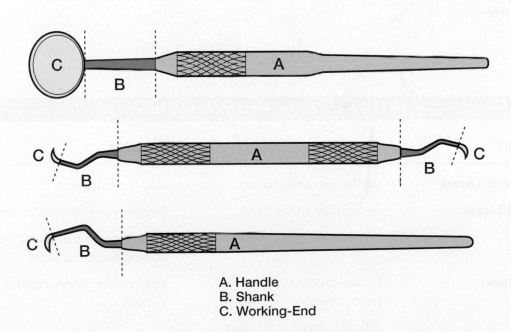

A. Handle
B. Shank
C. Working-End

FINGER IDENTIFICATION FOR THE GRASP

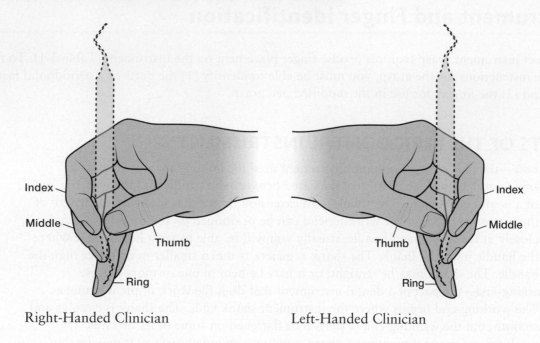

Index

Middle

Thumb

Ring

Right-Handed Clinician

Index

Middle

Thumb

Ring

Left-Handed Clinician

Finger Identification and Placement in Modified Pen Grasp. The index finger and thumb hold the instrument handle. The middle finger rests on the instrument shank. The ring finger advances ahead of the other fingers to act as a support for the hand and instrument.

TABLE 3-1. Finger Placement and Function		
Digit(s)	**Placement**	**Function**
Index and Thumb	On the instrument handle	Hold the instrument
Middle Finger	Rests lightly on the shank	Helps to guide the working-end
		Feels vibrations transmitted from the working-end to the shank
Ring Finger	On oral structure; often a tooth surface	Stabilizes the hand for control and strength
	Advances ahead of the other fingers in the grasp	
Little Finger	Near ring finger, held in a natural, relaxed manner	Has no function in the grasp

Section 2
Grasp for Periodontal Instrumentation

THE MODIFIED PEN GRASP

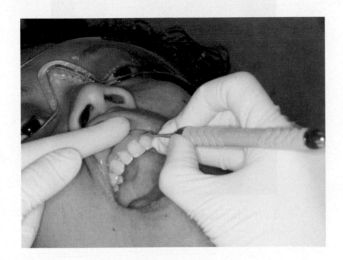

The Modified Pen Grasp. The modified pen grasp is the recommended grasp for holding a periodontal instrument. This grasp allows precise control of the working-end, permits a wide range of movement, and facilitates good tactile conduction.

RIGHT-Handed Clinician: Modified Pen Grasp

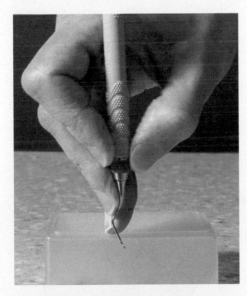

Right-Handed Clinician: Side View

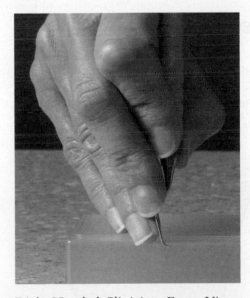

Right-Handed Clinician: Front View

LEFT-Handed Clinician: Modified Pen Grasp

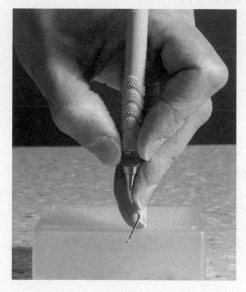

Left-Handed Clinician: Side View

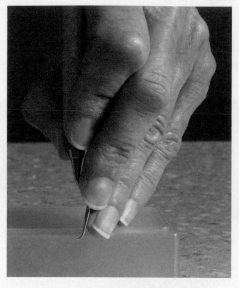

Left-Handed Clinician: Front View

FINE-TUNING YOUR GRASP

Successful instrumentation technique depends to a great degree on the precise placement of each finger of your dominant hand in the modified pen grasp. Use the illustrations below and the Summary Sheet on the next page to fine-tune your grasp.

Finger Placement in the Grasp

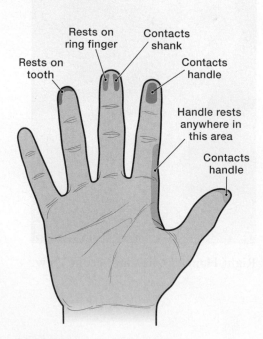

RIGHT-Handed Clinician

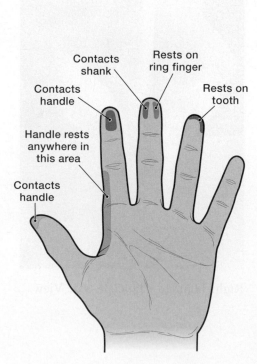

LEFT-Handed Clinician

TABLE 3-2.	Summary Sheet: Correct Finger Placement

Digit	Recommended Position
Index and Thumb	The finger pads rest opposite each other at or near the junction of the handle and the shank.
	The fingers do not overlap; there is a tiny space between them.
	These fingers should hold the handle in a relaxed manner. If your fingers are blanched, you are holding too tightly.
	The index finger and thumb curve outward from the handle in a C-shape; this position places the finger pads on the handle in the best position for instrumentation.
	These fingers should not bend inward toward the handle in a U-shape. This U-shape causes the pads to lift off of the handle, making it difficult to roll the instrument during instrumentation.
Middle	One side of the finger pad rests lightly on the instrument shank. The other side of the finger pad rests against (or slightly overlaps) the ring finger.
	Not used to hold the instrument. You should be able to lift your middle finger off the shank without dropping the instrument. If you drop the instrument, then you are incorrectly using the middle finger to help hold the instrument.
Ring	Fingertip, not the pad, of the dominant hand balances firmly on the tooth to support the weight of the hand and instrument. When grasping the dental mirror, the rest may be on a tooth or against the patient's lip or cheek area.
	The ring finger of the dominant hand advances ahead of the other fingers in the grasp. It is held straight and upright to act as a strong support beam for the hand. The finger should not feel tense, but it should not be held limply on the tooth.
Little	This finger should be held in a relaxed manner.

CORRECT GRASP FOR PRECISE CONTROL

The correct grasp allows the clinician to achieve precise control of the working-end during instrumentation. The examples shown below illustrate how the grasp can facilitate or hinder instrumentation.

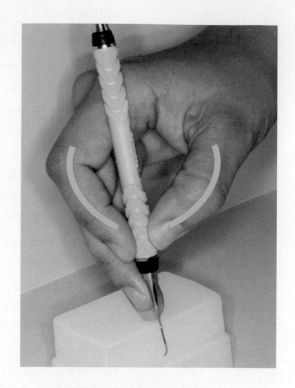

Correct Grasp. The finger placement of this grasp assists the clinician during instrumentation. This grasp allows the clinician to roll the instrument handle between the fingers in a precise manner. The handle roll is used to position the working-end against the tooth surface in an exact manner.

- **Soft C-Shape.** The index finger and thumb form a soft C-shape.
- **Finger Pads.** The finger pads contact the handle allowing precise control of the instrument.

Incorrect Grasp. The finger placement of this grasp hinders the clinician during instrumentation. This grasp makes it extremely difficult to roll the instrument handle between the fingers. It will be difficult to control the position of the working-end with this grasp.

- **U-Shape.** The index finger and thumb should not curve inward toward the handle, as shown here.
- **Pads Not in Contact.** A U-shaped grasp causes the finger pads to lift off of the handle, making it difficult to roll the instrument handle between the fingers.

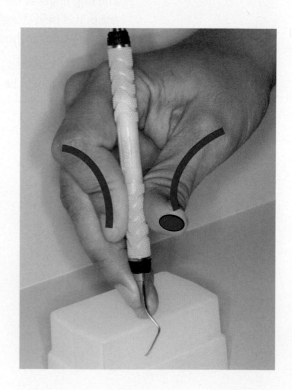

PROPER GLOVE FIT FOR INSTRUMENTATION

Proper glove fit is important in avoiding muscle strain during instrumentation. In fact, surgical glove-induced injury is a type of musculoskeletal disorder that is caused by improperly fitting gloves. Symptoms include numbness, tingling or pain in the wrist, hand, and/or fingers. This disorder is caused by wearing gloves that are too tight or by wearing ambidextrous gloves. It is best to wear right- and left-fitted gloves that are loose fitting across the palm of the hand and wrist.

Correct Glove Fit. Gloves should be loose fitting across the palm and wrist areas of the hand. The index finger of your opposite hand should slip easily under the wrist area of the gloved hand.

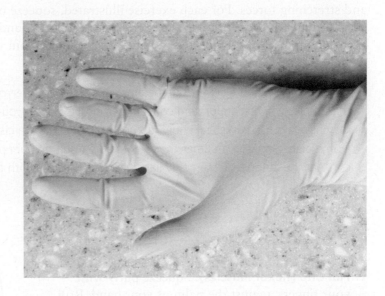

Incorrect Glove Fit. Gloves that are tight fitting across the palm and/or wrist area of your hand can cause muscle strain during instrumentation.

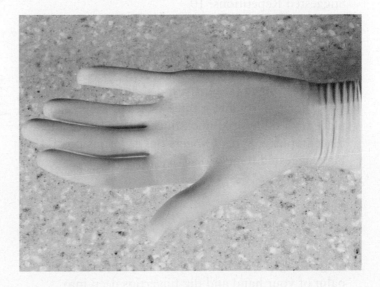

Section 3
Exercises for Improved Hand Strength

Well-conditioned muscles have improved control and endurance, allow for freer wrist movement, and reduce the likelihood of injury. The hand exercises shown here will help you to develop and maintain muscle strength for instrumentation.

Directions: These exercises use Power Putty, a silicone rubber material that resists both squeezing and stretching forces. For each exercise illustrated, squeeze or stretch the Power Putty for the suggested number of repetitions. The exercise set, for both hands doing all nine exercises, should take no more than 10 to 20 minutes. When exercising, maintain your hands at waist level.

> **CAUTION:**   Not all exercise programs are suitable for everyone; discontinue any exercise that causes you discomfort and consult a medical expert. If you have or suspect that you may have a musculoskeletal injury, do not attempt these exercises without the permission of a physician. Any user assumes the risk of injury resulting from performing the exercises. The creators and authors disclaim any liabilities in connection with the exercises and advice herein.

1. **Full Grip (flexor muscles).** Squeeze putty with your fingers against the palm of your hand. Roll it over and around in your hand, and repeat as rapidly and with as much strength as possible. Suggested Repetitions: 10

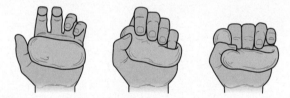

2. **All Finger Spread (extensor and abductor muscles).** Form putty into a thick pancake shape and place on a tabletop. Bunch fingertips together and place in putty. Spread fingers out as fast as possible. Suggested Repetitions: 3

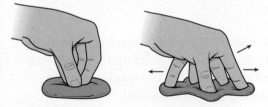

3. **Fingers Dig (flexor muscles).** Place putty in the palm of your hand and dig fingertips deep into the putty. Release the fingers, roll putty over and repeat. Suggested Repetitions: 10

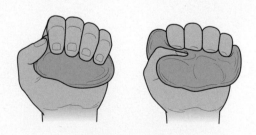

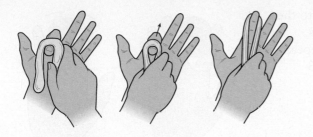

4. **Finger Extension (extensor muscles).** Close one finger into palm of hand. Wrap putty over tip of finger and hold loose ends with the other hand. As quickly as possible, extend finger to a fully opened position. Regulate difficulty by increasing or decreasing thickness of putty wrapped over the fingertip. Repeat with each finger. Suggested Repetitions: 3

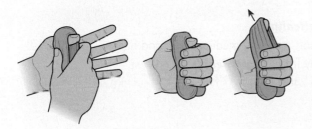

5. **Thumb Press (flexor muscles).** Form putty into a barrel shape and place in the palm of your hand. Press your thumb into the putty with as much force as you can. Reform putty and repeat. Suggested Repetitions: 5

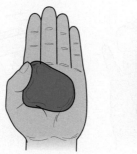
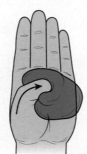

6. **Thumb Extension (extensor muscles).** Bend your thumb toward the palm of the hand; wrap putty over the thumb tip. Hold the loose ends down and extend the thumb open as quickly as possible. Regulate difficulty by increasing or decreasing the thickness of putty wrapped over tip of thumb. Suggested Repetitions: 3

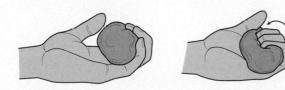

7. **Fingers Only (flexor muscles).** Lay putty across fingers and squeeze with fingertips only. Keep the palm of your hand flat and open. Rotate putty with thumb and repeat. Suggested Repetitions: 10

8. **Finger Scissors (adductor muscles).** Form putty into the shape of a ball and place between any two fingers. Squeeze fingers together in scissorlike motion. Repeat with each pair of fingers. Suggested Repetitions: 3

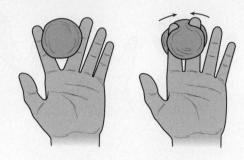

9. **Finger Splits (abductor muscles).** Mold putty around any two fingers while they are close together. Spread fingers apart as quickly as possible. Repeat exercise with each pair of fingers. Suggested Repetitions: 3

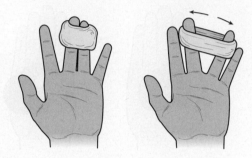

Hand exercises are reprinted with permission of **SportsHealth.**

Power Putty is available in four levels of rigidity: soft, soft/medium, medium/firm, and hard.

Power Putty can be purchased in sport stores or directly from: **SportsHealth,** 527 West Windsor Road, Glendale, California 91204 USA, (818) 240-7170.

http://www.powerputty.com

Section 4
Skill Application

PRACTICAL FOCUS

Evaluate the modified pen grasp in photographs 1 to 9 below. Indicate if each grasp is correct or incorrect. For each incorrect grasp element describe (1) what is incorrect about the finger placement and (2) what problems might result from the incorrect finger placement.

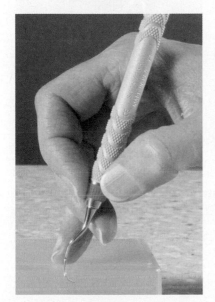

Photo 1

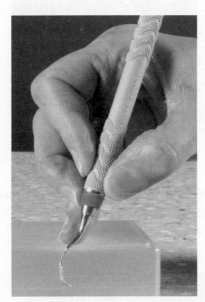

Photo 2

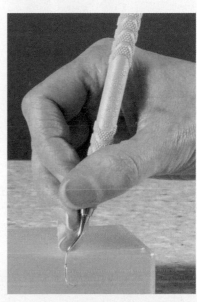

Photo 3

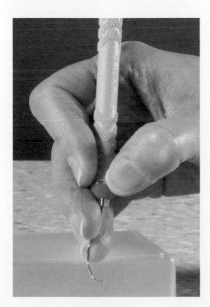

Photo 4

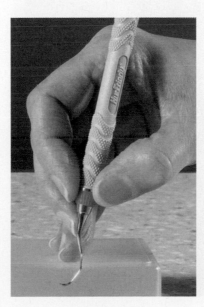

Photo 5

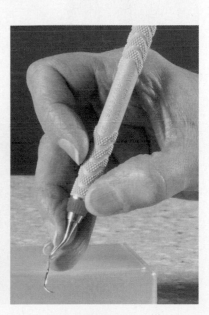

Photo 6

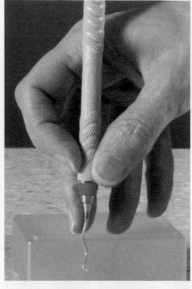

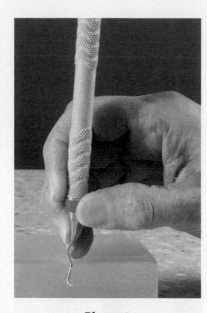

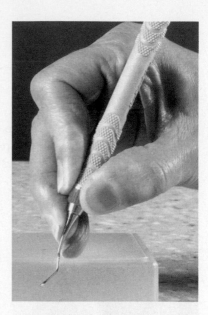

Photo 7   **Photo 8**   **Photo 9**

Examine the gloved hands pictured in photograph 10 below. Evaluate the glove fit for the right and left hands.

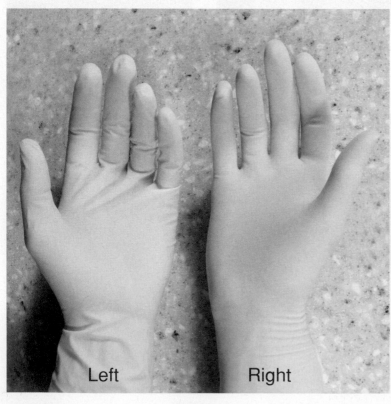

Left   Right

Photo 10

SKILL PRACTICE CHECKLIST MODULE 3 | INSTRUMENT GRASP

Module 3 has a skill practice checklist rather than a Skill Evaluation. Use the Checklist to help you assess your ability to grasp an instrument outside the mouth. Your ability to use a modified pen grasp in the mouth will be evaluated in Modules 4, 5, and 6.

Student: _____   1 = Grasp with mirror hand

Instructor: _____   2 = Grasp with instrument hand

Date: _____

DIRECTIONS: For each grasp, the student uses **Column S** and the instructor uses **Column E.** For each grasp, indicate the preliminary skill level as: **S** (satisfactory), **I** (improvement needed), or **U** (unsatisfactory).

	Grasp 1		Grasp 2	
CRITERIA:	S	E	S	E
Identifies handle, shank, and working-end(s) of mirror or instrument				
Describes the function each finger serves in the grasp				
Describes criteria for proper glove fit				
Holds handle with pad tips of index finger and thumb				
Thumb and index finger positioned opposite one another on handle				
Thumb and index finger do not touch or overlap				
Pad of middle finger rests lightly on shank				
Pad of middle finger touches the ring finger				
Thumb, index, and middle fingers are bent and relaxed (form "C" shape)				
Ring finger is straight and supports weight of hand				
Instrument handle rests against hand				
Grasp is relaxed (no blanching of fingers)				

SKILL PRACTICE CHECKLIST MODULE 3 | INSTRUMENT GRASP

Student: _____

EVALUATOR COMMENTS

_____
_____
_____
_____
_____
_____
_____
_____
_____
_____
_____
_____
_____
_____
_____
_____
_____

Box for sketches pertaining to written comments.

Mirror and Finger Rests in Anterior Sextants

Module Overview

This module describes techniques for using a dental mirror and finger rests in the anterior treatment areas. It begins with an introduction to the dental mirror and its uses. Covered next is information on recommended wrist position and hand placement during instrumentation. The third section of the module presents information on fulcrums and finger rests. A step-by-step technique practice for using a mirror and finger rests in the anterior treatment sextants is found in Sections 5 and 6.

Module Outline

Key Terms

Dental mirror	Indirect illumination	Fulcrum	Extraoral fulcrum
Indirect vision	Transillumination	Support beam	Advanced fulcrum
Retraction	Neutral wrist position	Intraoral fulcrum	

Learning Objectives

1. Name and describe three common types of dental mirrors.

2. Demonstrate use of the mirror for indirect vision, retraction, indirect illumination, and transillumination.

3. Demonstrate an extraoral and intraoral finger rest.

4. Position equipment so that it enhances neutral positioning.

5. Access the anterior teeth with optimum vision while maintaining neutral positioning.

6. Demonstrate correct mirror use, grasp, and finger rest in each of the anterior sextants while maintaining neutral positioning of your wrist.

7. Recognize incorrect mirror use, grasp, or finger rest, and describe how to correct the problem(s).

8. Understand the relationship between proper stabilization of the dominant hand during instrumentation and the prevention of (1) musculoskeletal problems in the clinician's hands and (2) injury to the patient.

9. Understand the relationship between the large motor skills, such as positioning, and small motor skills, such as finger rests. Recognize the importance of initiating these skills in a step-by-step manner.

Section 1
The Dental Mirror

TYPES OF DENTAL MIRRORS

The three common types of dental mirrors are the front surface mirror, the concave mirror, and the plane mirror. The plane mirror is also known as a flat surface mirror. The characteristics of each type of dental mirror are listed in Table 4-1.

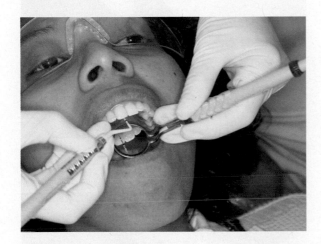

Dental Mirror or Mouth Mirror. The working-end of a dental mirror has a reflecting mirrored surface used to view tooth surfaces that cannot be seen directly.

TABLE 4-1.	Types of Mirror Surfaces
Type	**Characteristics**
Front Surface	Reflecting surface is on the front surface of the glass
	Produces a clear mirror image with no distortion
	Most commonly used type because of good image quality
	Reflecting surface of mirror is easily scratched
Concave	Reflecting surface is on the front surface of the mirror lens
	Produces a magnified image (image is enlarged)
	Not recommended because the magnification distorts the image
Plane (Flat Surface)	Reflecting surface is on the back surface of the mirror lens
	Produces a double image (ghost image)
	Not recommended because double image is distracting

USES OF DENTAL MIRROR

The dental mirror is used in four ways during instrumentation: (1) indirect vision, (2) retraction, (3) indirect illumination, and (4) transillumination. Box 4-1 lists proper use of the dental mirror.

Indirect Vision. Indirect vision is the use of a dental mirror to view a tooth surface or intraoral structure that cannot be seen directly.

In this example of indirect vision, a dental mirror is used to view the lingual surfaces of the maxillary premolar. Note that you can see the dental instrument in the mirror.

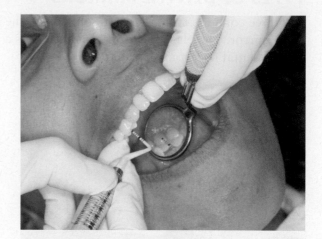

Retraction. Retraction is the use of the mirror head to hold the patient's cheek, lip, or tongue so that the clinician can view tooth surfaces that are otherwise hidden from view by these soft tissue structures. The clinician's index finger or thumb is also used for retraction, especially to retract the patient's lips.

In this example of retraction, a dental mirror is used to retract the tongue away from the lingual surfaces of the mandibular teeth.

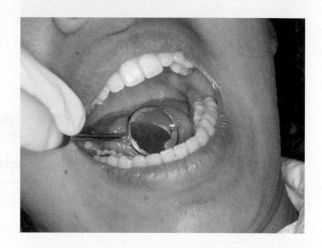

Retraction. In this second example of retraction, the index finger is used to retract the lip away from the facial aspect of anterior teeth. The patient will be more comfortable if you use your finger or thumb, rather than the mirror, for retraction of the lip.

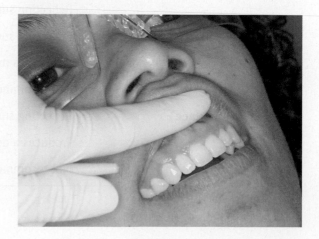

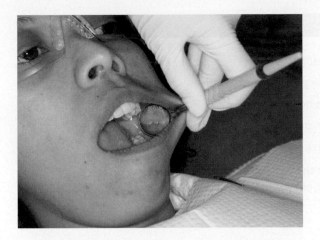

Retraction. In this third example of retraction, a dental mirror is used to retract the buccal mucosa away from the facial surfaces of the maxillary left posterior teeth. In this instance, the mirror is used both for retraction and to view the tooth surfaces indirectly.

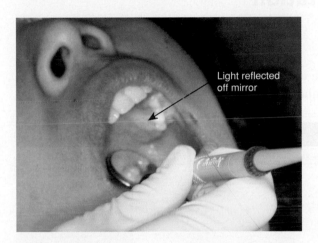

Light reflected off mirror

Indirect Illumination. Indirect illumination is the use of the mirror surface to reflect light onto a tooth surface in a dark area of the mouth.

In this example of indirect illumination, a mirror is being used to direct additional light onto the lingual surfaces of the maxillary left molars.

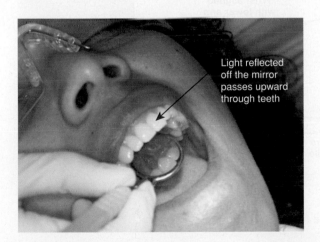

Light reflected off the mirror passes upward through teeth

Transillumination. Transillumination is the technique of directing light off of the mirror surface and through the anterior teeth. [*Trans* = through + *Illumination* = lighting up]. As light is reflected off the mirror surface, the light beams pass through the teeth.

Technique practice for transillumination is found on page 75. You should complete Section 3 of this module before attempting transillumination.

Box 4-1. Mirror Use

Use one of the following techniques to stop fogging of the reflecting surface:

- Warm the reflecting surface against the patient's buccal mucosa
- Ask the patient to breathe through the nose
- Wipe the reflecting surface with a commercial defogging solution
- Wipe the reflecting surface with a gauze square moistened with mouthwash

Avoid hitting the mirror head against the patient's teeth or resting the outer rim of the mirror head against the patient's gingival tissues.

Section 2
Wrist Position for Instrumentation

NEUTRAL WRIST POSITION

Neutral wrist position is the ideal positioning of the wrist while performing work activities and is associated with decreased risk of musculoskeletal injury (Box 4-2).

Box 4-2. Neutral Hand Position

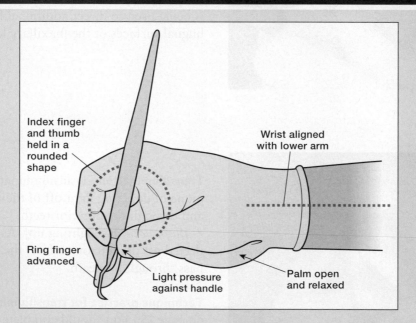

Index finger and thumb held in a rounded shape

Wrist aligned with lower arm

Ring finger advanced

Light pressure against handle

Palm open and relaxed

- Wrist aligned with the long axis of the lower arm
- Little finger-side of the palm rotated slightly downward
- Palm open and relaxed
- Thumb, middle, and index fingers held in a rounded shape
- Light finger pressure against the instrument handle
- Ring finger advanced ahead of other fingers in the grasp

GUIDELINES FOR NEUTRAL WRIST POSITION

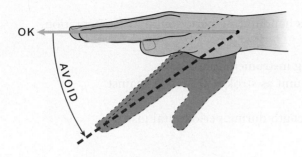

OK:

Wrist aligned with the long axis of the forearm

AVOID:

Bending the wrist and hand down toward the palm (flexion)

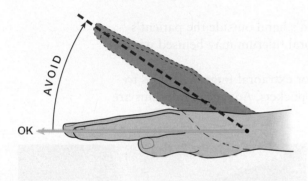

OK:

Wrist in alignment with the forearm

AVOID:

Bending the wrist and hand up and back (extension)

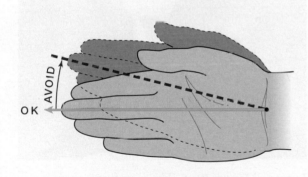

OK:

Wrist aligned with long axis of forearm

AVOID:

Bending the wrist toward the thumb (radial deviation)

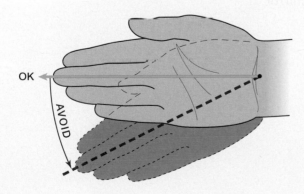

OK:

Wrist in alignment with the long axis of the forearm

AVOID:

Bending the wrist toward the little finger (ulnar deviation)

Section 3
The Fulcrum

Fulcrum—a finger rest used to stabilize the clinician's hand during periodontal instrumentation.

1. Functions of the Fulcrum.
   a. Serves as a "*support beam*" for the hand during instrumentation.
   b. Enables the hand and instrument to move as a unit as strokes are made against the tooth.
   c. Allows precise control of stroke pressure and length during periodontal instrumentation.
2. Types of Fulcrums.
   a. Intraoral fulcrum—stabilization of the clinician's dominant hand by placing the pad of the ring finger on a tooth near to the tooth being instrumented (Table 4-2).
   b. Extraoral fulcrum—stabilization of the clinician's hand outside the patient's mouth, usually on the chin or cheek. An extraoral fulcrum may be used with a mirror (Box 4-5).
   c. Advanced fulcrum—variations of an intraoral or extraoral finger rest used to gain access to root surfaces within periodontal pockets. Advanced fulcrums are discussed in Module 23.

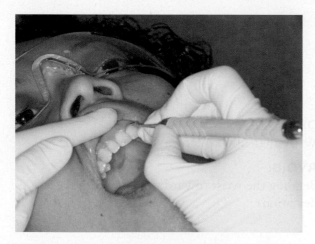

Intraoral Finger Rest. The pad of the ring finger is placed on a tooth near the tooth being instrumented.

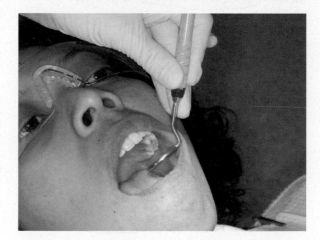

Extraoral Finger Rest. The ring finger rests on the patient's chin or cheek to stabilize the mirror.

INTRAORAL FULCRUM

Box 4-3. Characteristics of Intraoral Fulcrum

- Provides stable support for the hand.
- Enables the hand and instrument to move as a unit.
- Facilitates precise stroke pressure against the tooth surface.
- Decreases the likelihood of injury to the patient or clinician if the patient moves unexpectedly during instrumentation.

TABLE 4-2.   Summary Sheet: Technique for Intraoral Fulcrum

	Technique
Grasp	Hold the instrument in a modified pen grasp.
Fulcrum	Keep ring finger straight, with the tip of the finger supporting the weight of the hand.
Location	Position the finger rest near the tooth being instrumented • Depending on the tooth being instrumented and the size of your hand, the finger rest may be 1 to 4 teeth away from the tooth on which you are working. • A finger rest is always established out of the line of fire. • The rest is never established directly above the tooth surface being worked on. Staying out of the line of fire lessens the likelihood of instrument sticks.
Rest	Place the finger rest on the same arch as the tooth being instrumented. • Rest the fingertip of the fulcrum finger on an incisal (or occlusal) surface or on the occlusofacial or occlusolingual line angle of a tooth. • The teeth are saliva-covered, so you will be more likely to slip if you establish a finger rest on the facial or lingual surface. • Avoid resting on a mobile tooth or one with a large carious lesion.

FLOW CHART: SEQUENCE FOR ESTABLISHING A FINGER REST

For successful periodontal instrumentation, it is important to proceed in a step-by-step manner. Remember: If your *large motor skills* are incorrect (positioning of clinician, patient, and equipment), it is impossible for your *small motor skills* to be correct (mirror and fulcrum).

A useful saying to help you remember the step-by-step approach is "Me, My Patient, My Light, My Nondominant Hand, My Dominant Hand."

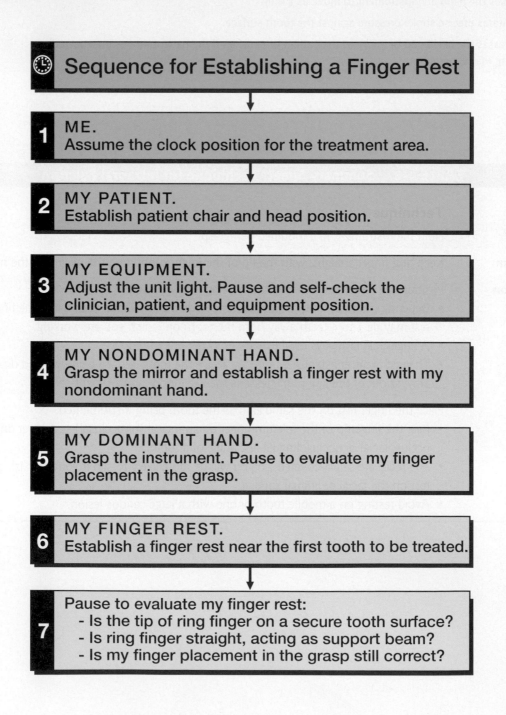

Sequence for Establishing a Finger Rest

1 ME.
Assume the clock position for the treatment area.

2 MY PATIENT.
Establish patient chair and head position.

3 MY EQUIPMENT.
Adjust the unit light. Pause and self-check the clinician, patient, and equipment position.

4 MY NONDOMINANT HAND.
Grasp the mirror and establish a finger rest with my nondominant hand.

5 MY DOMINANT HAND.
Grasp the instrument. Pause to evaluate my finger placement in the grasp.

6 MY FINGER REST.
Establish a finger rest near the first tooth to be treated.

7 Pause to evaluate my finger rest:
- Is the tip of ring finger on a secure tooth surface?
- Is ring finger straight, acting as support beam?
- Is my finger placement in the grasp still correct?

Section 4
Technique Practice for Transillumination

When transilluminating a tooth, *the mirror is used to reflect light through anterior teeth.* Transillumination is effective only with anterior teeth because they are thin enough to allow light to pass through. *A carious lesion of an anterior tooth appears as a shadow when an anterior tooth is transilluminated.*

PROCEDURE FOR TRANSILLUMINATION

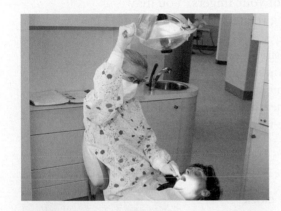

1. **Light Position.** Position the unit light directly over the oral cavity so that the light beam is perpendicular to the facial surfaces of the anterior teeth.

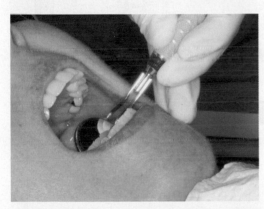

2. **Position Mouth Mirror.** Position yourself in the 12:00. Hold the mirror behind the central incisors so that the reflecting surface is parallel to the lingual surfaces.

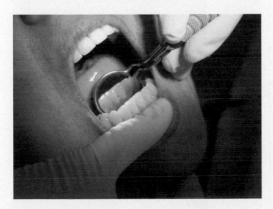

3. **View Transilluminated Anterior Teeth.** If you have correctly positioned the light and the mirror, the anterior teeth will appear to "glow". Remember, in this case, you are looking *directly at the teeth not in the mirror.*

   When practicing on a classmate, you probably will not see shadows on the teeth since he or she, most likely, does not have untreated interproximal decay.

RIGHT- and LEFT-Handed Sections. The Right-Handed section begins on the next page. Left-Handed clinicians should turn to page 89.

Section 5
Skills for the RIGHT-Handed Clinician

DIRECTIONS FOR TECHNIQUE PRACTICE

1. The photographs depict the use of a mirror and finger rests in the anterior treatment areas. Some photographs were taken using a patient. Others were taken using a manikin and without gloves so that you can easily see the finger placement in the grasp.

2. The photographs provide a *general guideline* for finger rests; however, the location of your own finger rest depends on the size and length of your fingers. You may need to fulcrum closer to or farther from the tooth being treated than is shown in the photograph.

3. Focus your attention on mastering mirror use, wrist position, and the finger rests. Use the following instruments in this module: For your nondominant (mirror) hand—Use a dental mirror. For your dominant (instrument) hand—(a) Remove the mirror head from one of your dental mirrors and use the mirror handle as if it were a periodontal instrument or (b) use a periodontal probe to represent the periodontal instrument in this module.

Icon Symbols

Icons appear in the book to assist you with identifying the clock position and treatment area.

 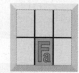

HANDLE POSITION FOR MANDIBULAR ANTERIOR TREATMENT AREAS

Box 4-4. Handle Position for Mandibular Anterior Teeth

1. Hold the hand in a palm down position.

2. Rest the handle against the index finger somewhere in the green shaded area.

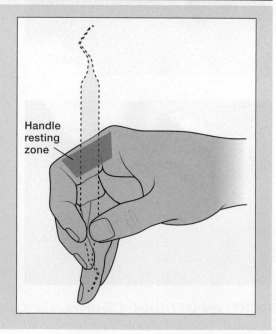

Handle resting zone

TECHNIQUE PRACTICE: MANDIBULAR ANTERIOR TEETH
Mandibular Anteriors, Facial Aspect: Surfaces Toward

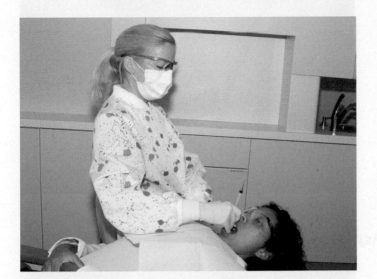

Position Overview

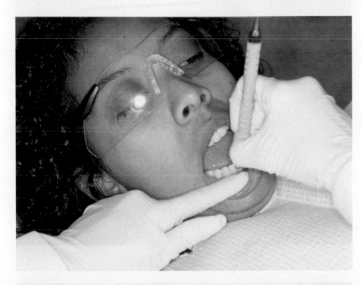

Retraction

Retract the lip with the index finger or thumb of your left hand.

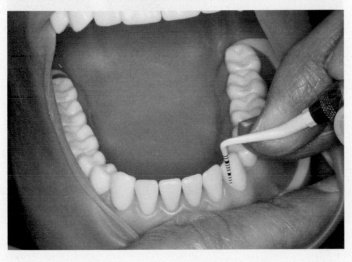

Task 1—Mesial Surface of the Left Canine

Finger rest on an occlusofacial line angle.

Task 2—Distal Surface of Right Canine

Finger rest on an incisal edge.

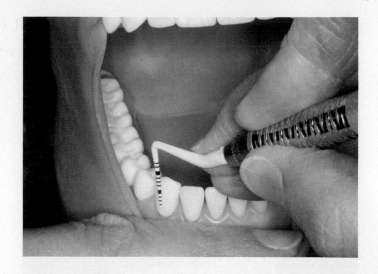

Mandibular Anteriors, Lingual Aspect: Surfaces Toward

Position Overview

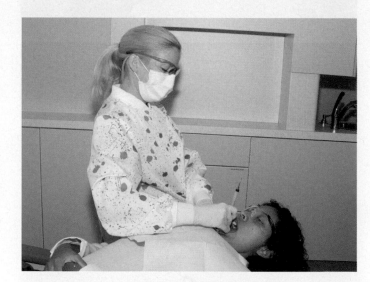

Mirror

Use the mirror head to push the tongue away gently so the lingual surfaces of the anterior teeth can be seen in the reflecting surface of the mirror.

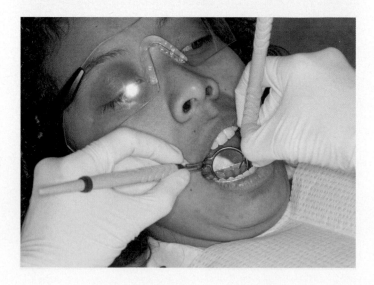

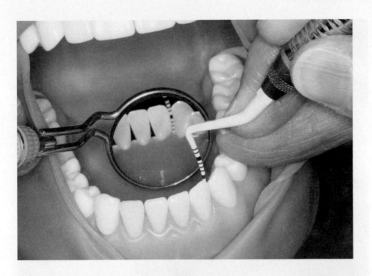

Task 1—Mesial Surface of the Left Canine

Finger rest on an occlusofacial line angle.

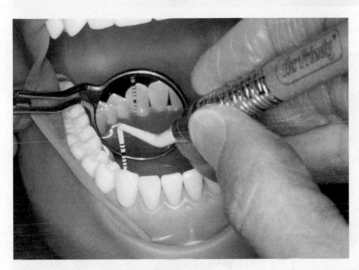

Task 2—Distal Surface of the Right Canine

Finger rest on an incisal edge.

Mandibular Anteriors, Facial Aspect: Surfaces Away

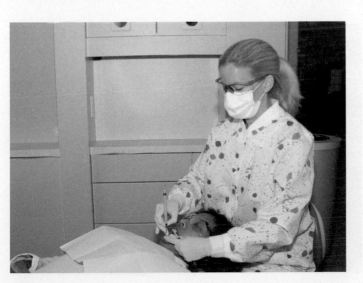

Position Overview

Retraction

Retract the lip with your index finger or thumb.

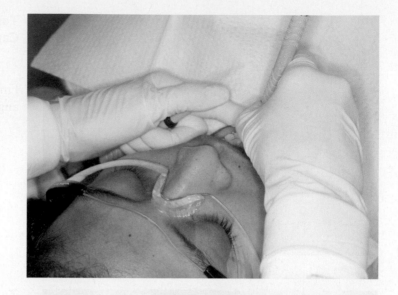

Task 1—Mesial Surface of the Right Canine

Finger rest on an occlusofacial line angle.

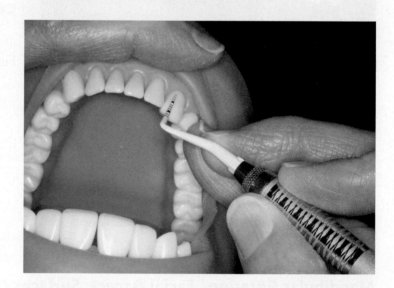

Task 2—Distal Surface of the Left Canine

Finger rest on an incisal edge.

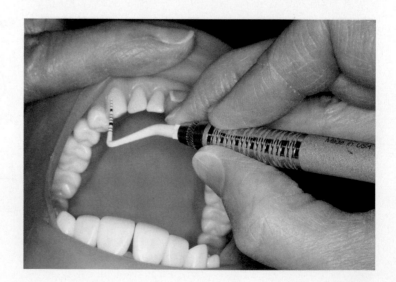

Mandibular Anteriors, Lingual Aspect: Surfaces Away

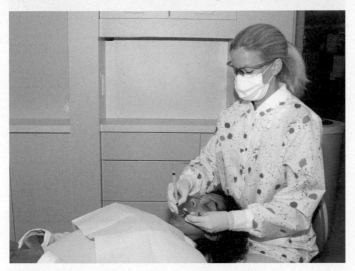

Position Overview

Mirror

Use the mirror head to push the tongue back gently so that the lingual surfaces of the teeth can be seen.

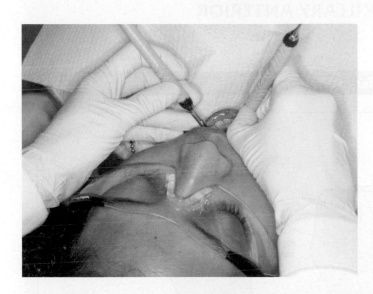

Task 1—Mesial Surface of the Right Canine

Finger rest on an occlusofacial line angle.

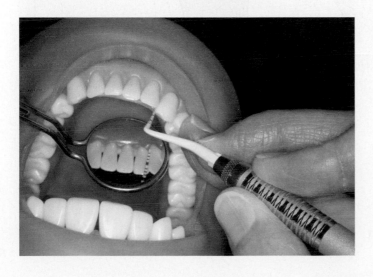

RIGHT-Handed Clinician

Task 2—Distal Surface of the Left Canine

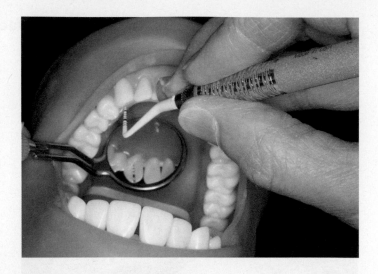

Finger rest on an incisal edge.

HANDLE POSITION FOR MAXILLARY ANTERIOR TREATMENT AREAS

Box 4-5. Handle Position for Maxillary Anterior Teeth

1. Hold the hand in a palm-up position.
2. Rest the handle against the index finger somewhere in the green shaded area.

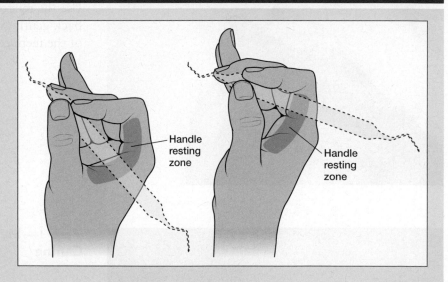

Handle resting zone

Handle resting zone

TECHNIQUE PRACTICE: MAXILLARY ANTERIOR TEETH
Maxillary Anteriors, Facial Aspect: Surfaces Toward

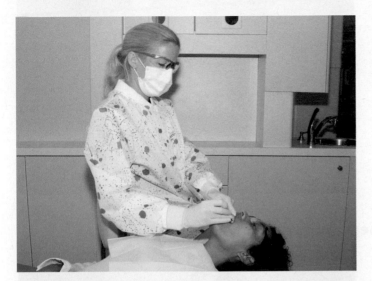

Position Overview

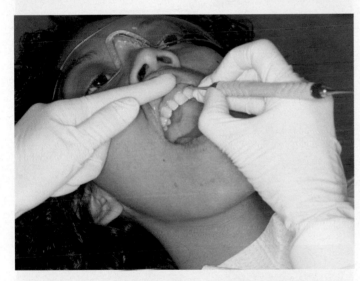

Retraction

Retract the lip with the index finger or thumb of your left hand.

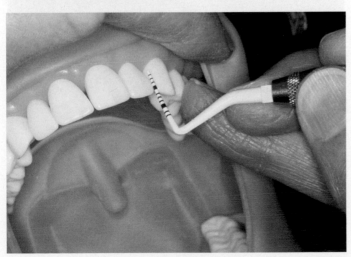

Task 1—Mesial Surface of the Left Canine

Finger rest on an occlusofacial line angle.

Task 2—Distal Surface of Right Canine

Finger rest on an incisal edge.

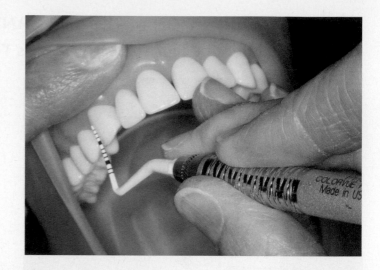

Maxillary Anteriors, Lingual Aspect: Surfaces Toward

Position Overview

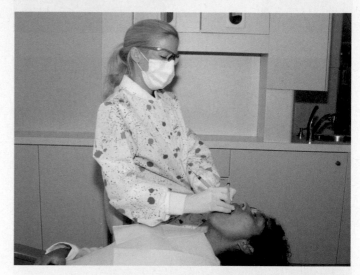

Mirror

Position the mirror head so the lingual surfaces of the anterior teeth can be seen in the reflecting surface of the mirror.

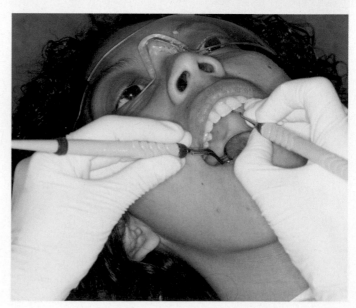

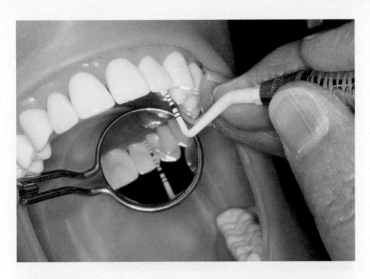

Task 1—Mesial Surface of the Left Canine

Finger rest on an occlusofacial line angle.

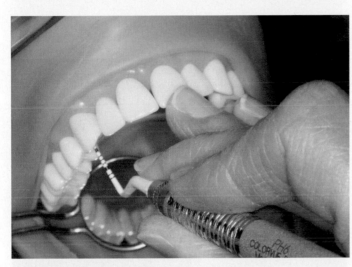

Task 2—Distal Surface of the Right Canine

Finger rest on an incisal edge.

Maxillary Anteriors, Facial Aspect: Surfaces Away

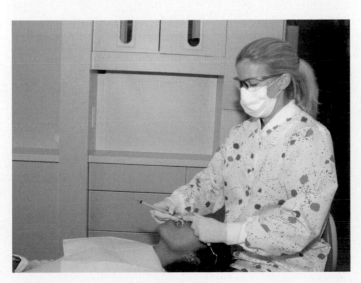

Position Overview

Retraction

Retract the lip with your index finger or thumb.

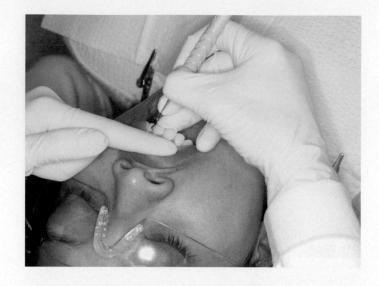

Task 1—Mesial Surface of the Right Canine

Finger rest on an occlusal surface. Place the instrument tip on the surface away from your nondominant hand.

Technique hint: Your dominant hand is positioned correctly if you can see the underside of your middle and ring fingers.

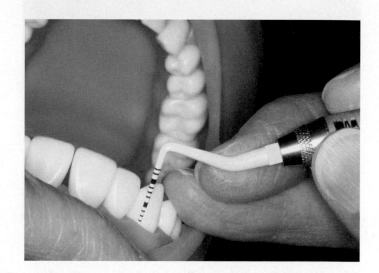

Task 2—Distal Surface of the Left Canine

Finger rest on an incisal edge.

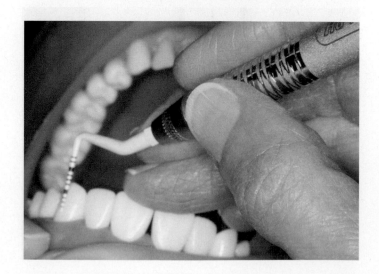

Maxillary Anterior Sextant, Lingual Aspect: Surfaces Away

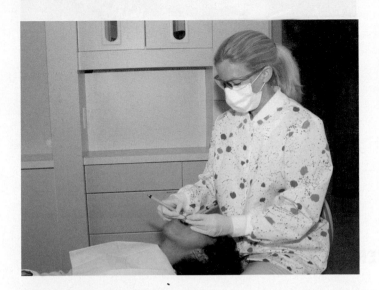

Position Overview

Mirror

Position the mirror head so that the lingual surfaces of the teeth can be seen.

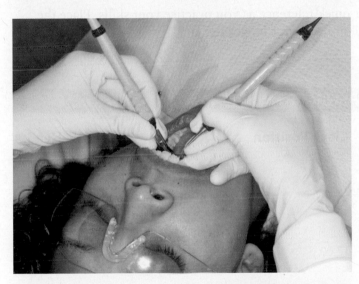

Task 1—Mesial Surface of the Right Canine

Finger rest on an occlusal surface.

Technique hint: Your dominant hand is positioned correctly if you can see the underside of your middle and ring fingers.

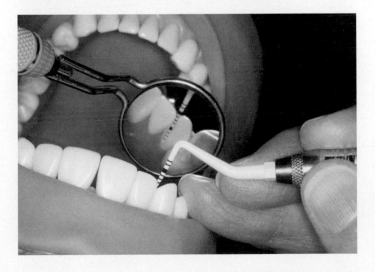

Task 2—Distal Surface of the Left Canine

Finger rest on an incisal edge.

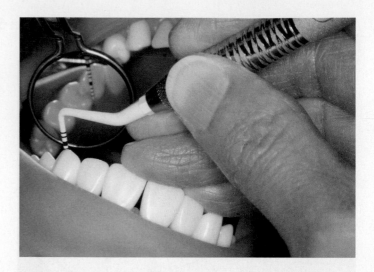

REFERENCE SHEET FOR ANTERIOR TREATMENT AREAS FOR THE RIGHT-HANDED CLINICIAN

Photocopy this reference sheet and use it for quick reference as you practice your skills. Place the photocopied reference sheet in a plastic page protector for longer use.

TABLE 4-3. Anterior Treatment Areas		
Treatment Area	**Clock Position**	**Patient's Head**
Mandibular Teeth		
Facial Surfaces Toward	8–9:00	
Lingual Surfaces Toward		Slightly toward Chin DOWN
Facial Surfaces Away	12:00	
Lingual Surfaces Away		
Maxillary Teeth		
Facial Surfaces Toward	8–9:00	
Lingual Surfaces Toward		Slightly toward Chin UP
Facial Surfaces Away	12:00	
Lingual Surfaces Away		

NOTE: This ends the section for RIGHT-Handed Clinicians. Turn to page 102 for the Skill Application section of this module.

RIGHT-Handed Clinician

Section 6
Skills for the LEFT-Handed Clinician

DIRECTIONS FOR TECHNIQUE PRACTICE

1. The photographs depict the use of a mirror and finger rests in the anterior treatment areas. Some photographs were taken using a patient. Others were taken using a manikin and without gloves so that you can easily see the finger placement in the grasp.
2. The photographs provide a *general guideline* for finger rests; however, the location of your own finger rest depends on the size and length of your fingers. You may need to fulcrum closer to or farther from the tooth being treated than that which is shown in the photograph.
3. Focus your attention on mastering mirror use, wrist position, and the finger rests. Use the following instruments in this module: For your nondominant (mirror) hand—Use a dental mirror. For your dominant (instrument) hand—(a) Remove the mirror head from one of your dental mirrors and use the mirror handle as if it were a periodontal instrument or (b) use a periodontal probe to represent the periodontal instrument in this module.
4. Icon symbols appear throughout the book to assist you in identifying the clinician clock position and treatment area.

HANDLE POSITION FOR MANDIBULAR ANTERIOR TREATMENT AREAS

Box 4-6. Handle Position for Mandibular Anterior Teeth

1. Hold the hand in a palm-down position.
2. Rest the handle against the index finger somewhere in the green shaded area.

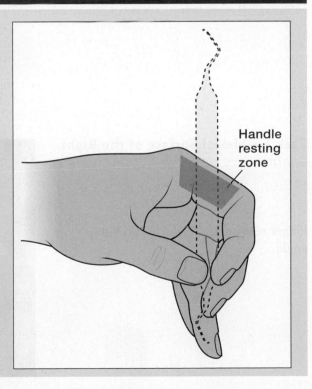

Handle resting zone

TECHNIQUE PRACTICE: MANDIBULAR ANTERIOR TEETH
Mandibular Anteriors, Facial Aspect: Surfaces Toward
Position Overview

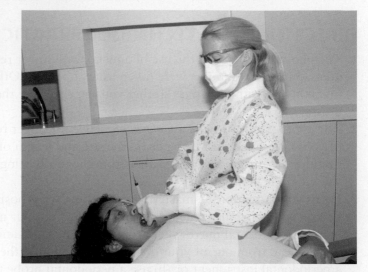

Retraction

Retract the lip with the index finger or thumb of your right hand.

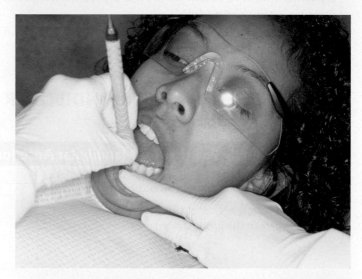

Task 1—Mesial Surface of the Right Canine

Finger rest on an occlusofacial line angle.

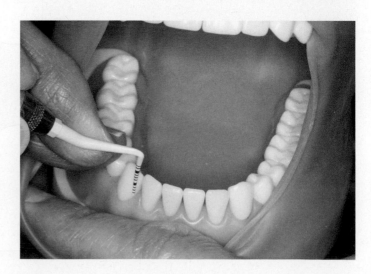

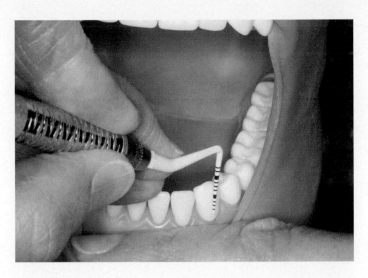

Task 2—Distal Surface of Left Canine

Finger rest on an incisal edge.

Mandibular Anteriors, Lingual Aspect: Surfaces Toward

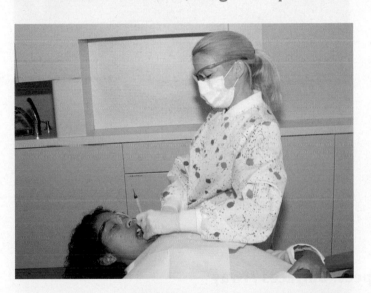

Position Overview

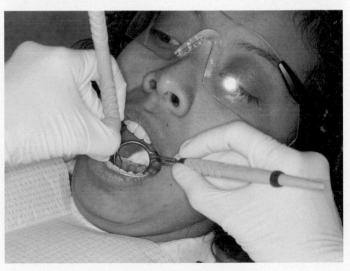

Mirror

Use the mirror head to push the tongue away gently so the lingual surfaces of the anterior teeth can be seen in the reflecting surface of the mirror.

Task 1—Mesial Surface of the Right Canine

Finger rest on an occlusofacial line angle.

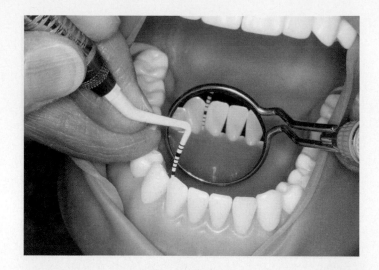

Task 2—Distal Surface of the Left Canine

Finger rest on an incisal edge.

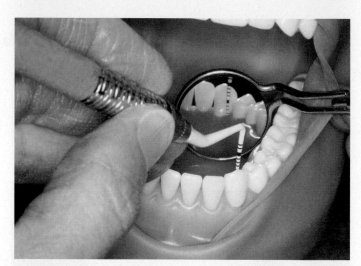

Mandibular Anteriors, Facial Aspect: Surfaces Away

Position Overview

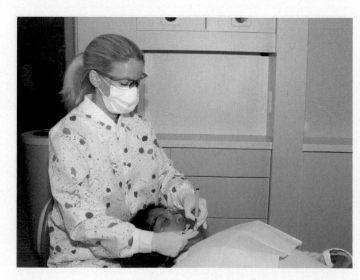

Retraction

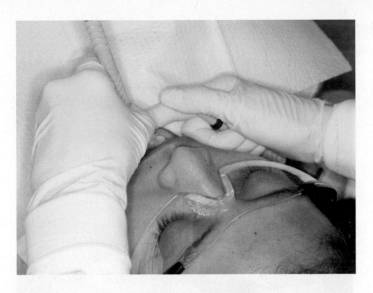

Retract the lip with your index finger or thumb.

Task 1—Mesial Surface of the Left Canine

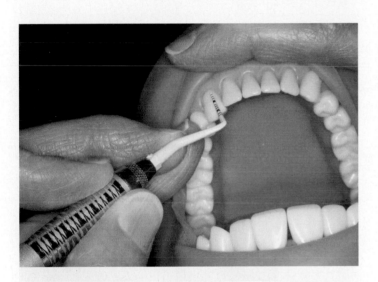

Finger rest on an occlusofacial line angle.

Task 2—Distal Surface of the Right Canine

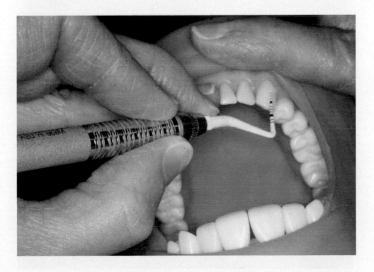

Finger rest on an incisal edge.

Mandibular Anteriors, Lingual Aspect: Surfaces Away

Position Overview

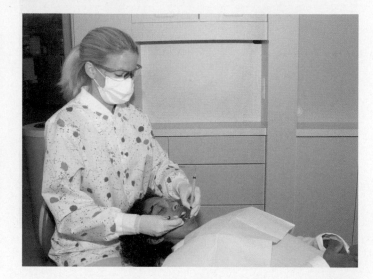

Mirror

Use the mirror head to push the tongue back gently so that the lingual surfaces of the teeth can be seen.

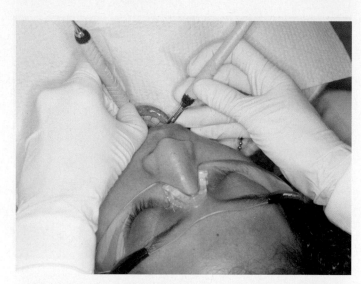

Task 1—Mesial Surface of the Left Canine

Finger rest on an occlusofacial line angle.

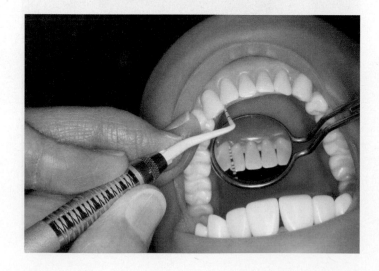

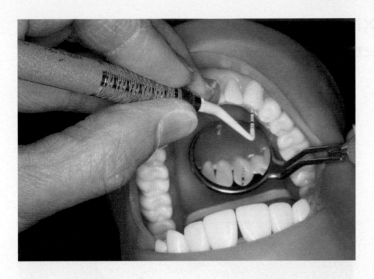

Task 2—Distal Surface of the Right Canine

Finger rest on an incisal edge.

HANDLE POSITION FOR MAXILLARY ANTERIOR TREATMENT AREAS

Box 4-7. Handle Position for Maxillary Anterior Teeth

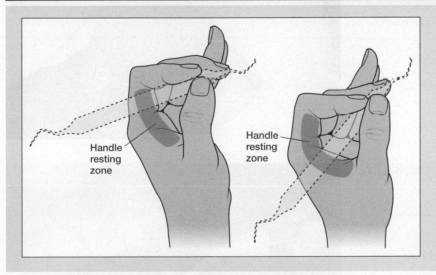

1. Hold the hand in a palm-up position.

2. Rest the handle against the index finger somewhere in the green shaded area.

TECHNIQUE PRACTICE: MAXILLARY ANTERIOR TEETH
Maxillary Anteriors, Facial Aspect: Surfaces Toward
Position Overview

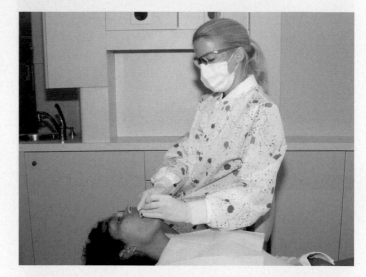

LEFT-Handed Clinician

Retraction

Retract the lip with the index finger or thumb of your right hand.

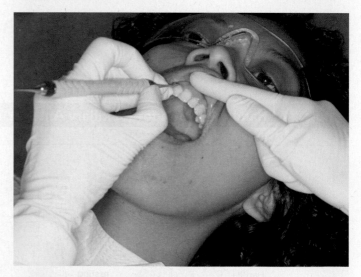

Task I—Mesial Surface of the Right Canine

Finger rest on an occlusofacial line angle.

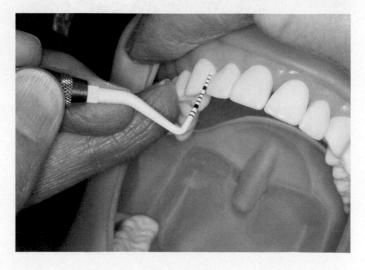

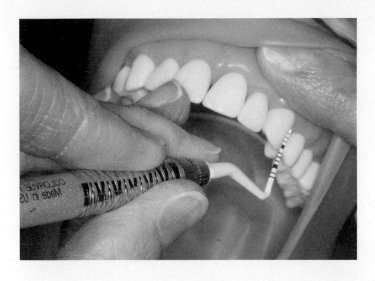

Task 2—Distal Surface of Left Canine

Finger rest on an incisal edge.

Maxillary Anteriors, Lingual Aspect: Surfaces Toward

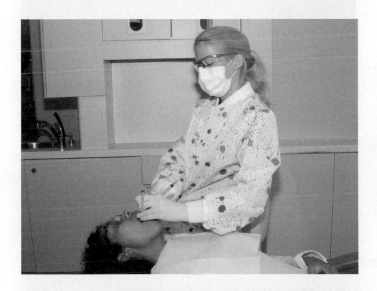

Position Overview

Mirror

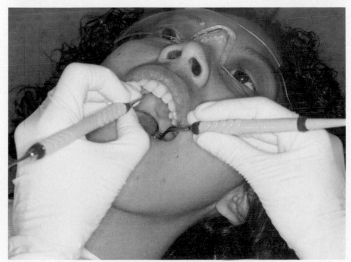

Position the mirror head so the lingual surfaces of the anterior teeth can be seen in the reflecting surface of the mirror.

Task 1—Mesial Surface of the Right Canine

Finger rest on an occlusofacial line angle.

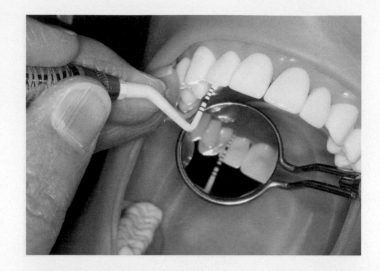

Task 2—Distal Surface of the Left Canine

Finger rest on an incisal edge.

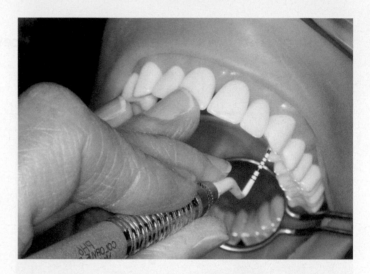

Maxillary Anteriors, Facial Aspect: Surfaces Away

Position Overview

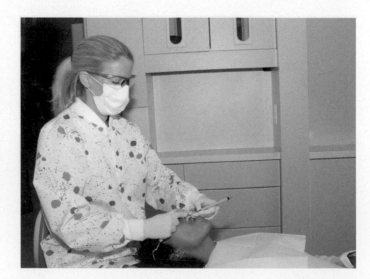

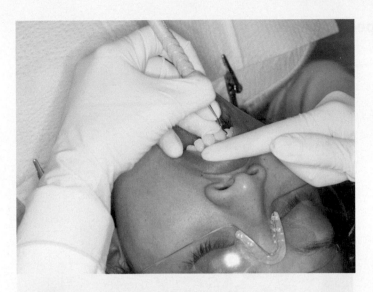

Retraction

Retract the lip with your index finger or thumb.

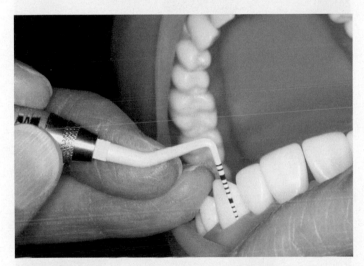

Task 1—Mesial Surface of the Left Canine

Finger rest on an occlusal surface.

Technique hint: Your dominant hand is positioned correctly if you can see the underside of your middle and ring fingers.

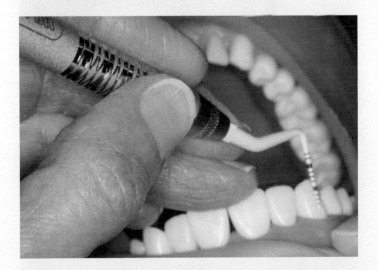

Task 2—Distal Surface of the Right Canine

Finger rest on an incisal edge.

LEFT-Handed Clinician

Maxillary Anteriors, Lingual Aspect: Surfaces

Position Overview

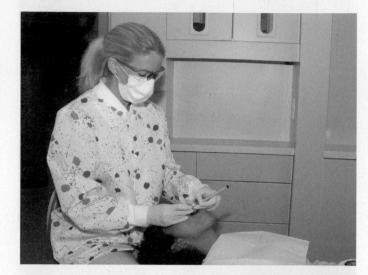

Mirror
Position the mirror head so that the lingual surfaces of the teeth can be seen.

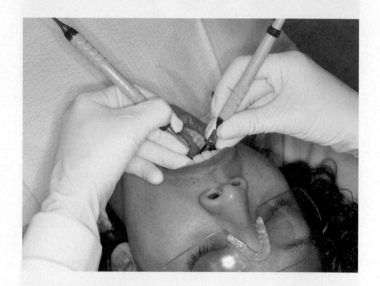

Task 1—Mesial Surface of the Left Canine

Finger rest on an occlusal surface.

Technique hint: Your dominant hand is positioned correctly if you can see the underside of your middle and ring fingers.

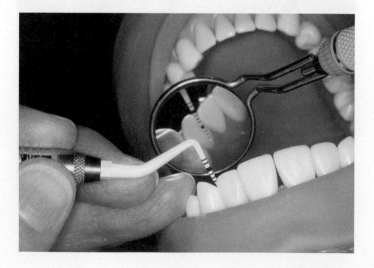

SKILL EVALUATION MODULE 4 — MIRROR AND FINGER RESTS IN ANTERIOR SEXTANTS

Student: _____

Evaluator: _____

Date: _____

Area 1 = mandibular anteriors, facial aspect
Area 2 = mandibular anteriors, lingual aspect
Area 3 = maxillary anteriors, facial aspect
Area 4 = maxillary anteriors, lingual aspect

DIRECTIONS FOR STUDENT: Use **Column S.** Evaluate your skill level as: **S** (satisfactory) or **U** (unsatisfactory).

DIRECTIONS FOR EVALUATOR: Use **Column E.** Indicate: **S** (satisfactory) or **U** (unsatisfactory). Each **S** equals 1 point, each **U** equals 0 points.

CRITERIA:	Area 1		Area 2		Area 3		Area 4	
	S	E	S	E	S	E	S	E
Position:								
Positioned correctly on clinician stool								
Positioned correctly in relation to patient, equipment, and treatment area								
Establishes correct patient head position								
Dental Mirror:								
Uses correct grasp with mirror								
Establishes secure rest with mirror								
Ensures patient comfort by not hitting teeth or resting the mirror rim against gingiva								
Uses mirror for retraction/indirect vision or finger for retraction of lip								
Modified Pen Grasp with Dominant Hand:								
Holds handle with pads of index finger and thumb								
Thumb and index finger positioned opposite one another on handle; fingers not touching or overlapped								
Pad of middle finger rests lightly on shank; touches the ring finger								
Thumb, index, and middle fingers held in a rounded shape (not flattened against the instrument handle)								
Instrument handle rests against index finger or "V" of the hand								
Grasp is relaxed (no blanching of fingers)								
Basic Intraoral Fulcrum:								
Ring finger is straight and supports weight of hand								
Fulcrums on same arch, near tooth being instrumented								
OPTIONAL GRADE PERCENTAGE CALCULATION Total **S**'s in each E column.								

Sum of **S**'s _____ divided by Total Points Possible (**60**) equals the Percentage Grade _____ **%**

SKILL EVALUATION MODULE 4   MIRROR AND FINGER RESTS IN ANTERIOR SEXTANTS

Student: _____

EVALUATOR COMMENTS

_____
_____
_____
_____
_____
_____
_____
_____
_____
_____
_____
_____
_____
_____
_____
_____
_____
_____

Box for sketches pertaining to written comments.

Mirror and Finger Rests in Mandibular Posterior Sextants

Module Overview

This module describes techniques for using a dental mirror and finger rests in the mandibular posterior treatment areas. It begins with a technique practice on using the dental mirror for retraction of the cheek. A step-by-step technique practice is found in Sections 2 and 3.

Module Outline

KEY TERMS

Review these terms from Module 4:

Neutral wrist position

Fulcrum

Support beam

Finger rest

Extraoral fulcrum

Intraoral fulcrum

LEARNING OBJECTIVES

1. Maintain neutral positioning when practicing finger rests in the mandibular posterior sextants.

2. Position equipment so that it enhances neutral positioning.

3. Access the mandibular posterior teeth with optimum vision while maintaining neutral positioning.

4. Demonstrate correct mirror use, grasp, and finger rest in each of the mandibular posterior sextants while maintaining neutral positioning of your wrist.

5. Recognize incorrect mirror use, grasp, or finger rest, and describe how to correct the problem(s).

6. Understand the relationship between proper stabilization of the dominant hand during instrumentation and the prevention of (1) musculoskeletal problems in the clinician's hands and (2) injury to the patient.

7. Understand the relationship between the large motor skills, such as positioning, and small motor skills, such as finger rests. Recognize the importance of initiating these skills in a step-by-step manner.

Section 1
Introduction to Mirror Skills

TECHNIQUE PRACTICE: USING THE MIRROR FOR RETRACTION

Retracting the buccal mucosa away from the facial surfaces of the posterior teeth can be a challenging task, especially if your patient tenses his or her cheek muscles. It is a good idea to practice this technique before attempting the posterior finger rests.

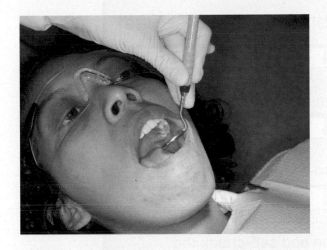

1. RIGHT-Handed: Assume the clock position for the facial aspect of the mandibular left posteriors. LEFT-Handed: Assume the clock position for the facial aspect of the mandibular right posteriors.
2. Grasp the mirror in your nondominant hand.
3. Place the mirror head between the dental arches with the reflecting surface parallel to the maxillary occlusal surfaces ("Frisbee-style").
4. Slide the mirror back until it is in line with the second molar.

(Photographs show a RIGHT-Handed clinician.)

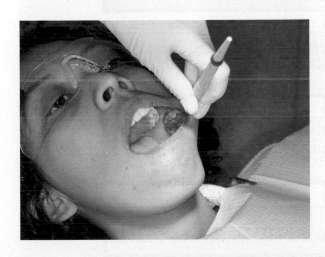

5. Position the mirror by turning the mirror handle until the mirror head is parallel to the buccal mucosa. The back of the mirror head is against the buccal mucosa, and the mirror's reflecting surface is facing the facial surfaces of the teeth.
6. Establish a finger rest on the side of the patient's cheek.
7. Use your arm muscles for retraction. Pulling with only your finger muscles is a difficult and tiring way to retract the cheek.

Note: Do NOT use the instrument shank for retraction. Retracting in this manner will be uncomfortable for your patient.

RIGHT- AND LEFT-HANDED SECTIONS: The Right-Handed section begins on the next page. Left-Handed clinicians should turn to page 116.

Section 2
Skills for the RIGHT-Handed Clinician

FLOW CHART: SEQUENCE FOR ESTABLISHING A FINGER REST

As discussed in the previous module, it is important to proceed in a step-by-step manner. Remember: "Me, My Patient, My Light, My Nondominant Hand, My Dominant Hand."

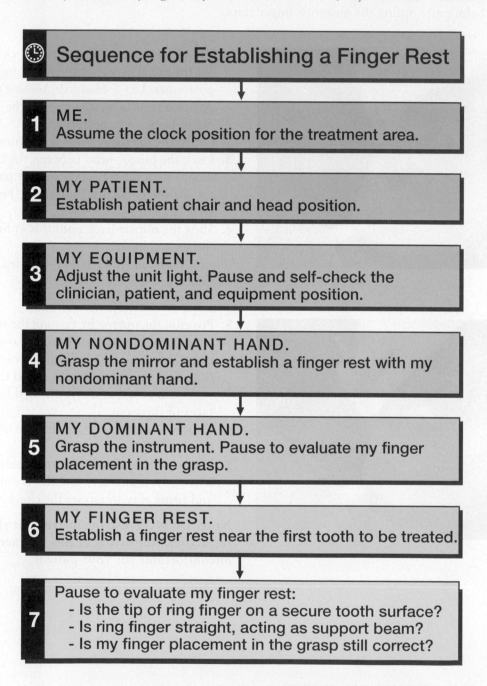

🕐 Sequence for Establishing a Finger Rest

1 ME.
Assume the clock position for the treatment area.

2 MY PATIENT.
Establish patient chair and head position.

3 MY EQUIPMENT.
Adjust the unit light. Pause and self-check the clinician, patient, and equipment position.

4 MY NONDOMINANT HAND.
Grasp the mirror and establish a finger rest with my nondominant hand.

5 MY DOMINANT HAND.
Grasp the instrument. Pause to evaluate my finger placement in the grasp.

6 MY FINGER REST.
Establish a finger rest near the first tooth to be treated.

7 Pause to evaluate my finger rest:
- Is the tip of ring finger on a secure tooth surface?
- Is ring finger straight, acting as support beam?
- Is my finger placement in the grasp still correct?

DIRECTIONS FOR SKILL PRACTICE

1. The photographs depict the use of a mirror and finger rests in the mandibular posterior sextants. Some photographs were taken using a patient. Others were taken using a manikin and without gloves so that you can easily see the finger placement in the grasp.

2. The photographs provide a *general guideline* for finger rests; however, the location of your own finger rest depends on the size and length of your fingers. You may need to fulcrum closer to or farther from the tooth being treated than that which is shown in the photograph.

3. Focus your attention on mastering mirror use, wrist position, and finger rests. Use the following instruments in this module: For your nondominant (mirror) hand— Use a dental mirror. For your dominant (instrument) hand—(a) Remove the mirror head from one of your dental mirrors and use the mirror handle as if it were a periodontal instrument or (b) use a periodontal probe to represent the periodontal instrument in this Module.

HANDLE POSITION FOR MANDIBULAR POSTERIOR TEETH

Box 5-1. Handle Position for Mandibular Posterior Teeth

1. Hold the hand in a palm-down position.

2. Rest the handle against the index finger somewhere in the green shaded area.

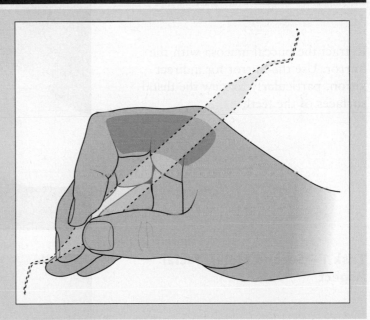

RIGHT-Handed Clinician

TECHNIQUE PRACTICE: MANDIBULAR POSTERIOR SEXTANTS

Mandibular Right Posterior Sextant, Facial Aspect

Position Overview

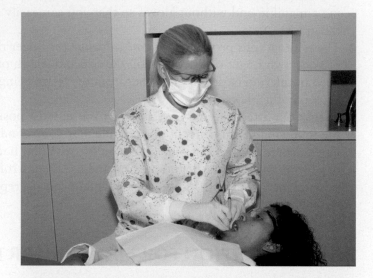

Retraction

Retract the buccal mucosa with the mirror. Use the mirror for indirect vision, particularly to view the distal surfaces of the teeth.

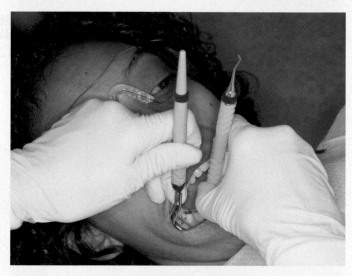

Task 1—Second Molar, Facial Aspect

Finger rest on an occlusal surface.

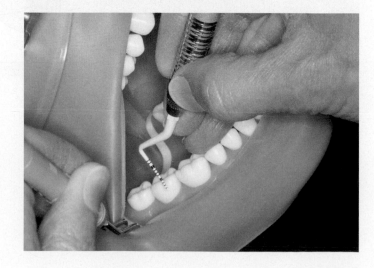

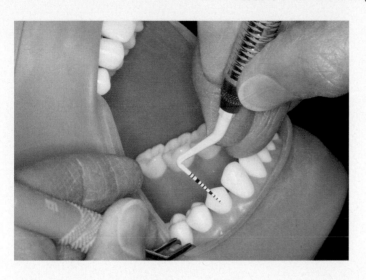

Task 2—First Premolar, Facial Aspect
Finger rest on an incisal surface of one of the mandibular anteriors.

Mandibular Left Posterior Sextant, Lingual Aspect

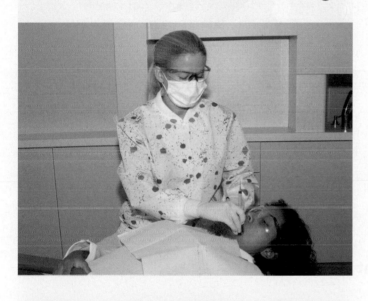

Position Overview

Mirror

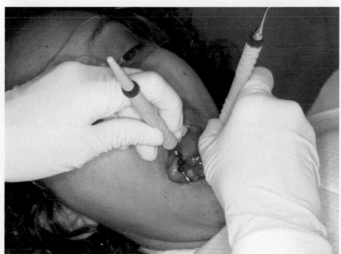

Use the mirror to gently pull the tongue away from the teeth, toward the midline of the mouth. Once in position, the mirror is also used for indirect vision of the tooth surfaces.

RIGHT-Handed Clinician

Task I—Second Molar, Lingual Aspect

Finger rest on an occlusofacial line angle.

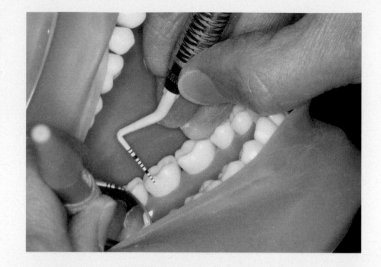

Task 2—First Premolar, Lingual Aspect

Finger rest on an incisal edge of one of the mandibular anterior teeth.

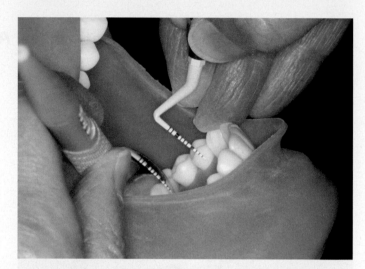

Mandibular Left Posterior Sextant, Facial Aspect

Position Overview

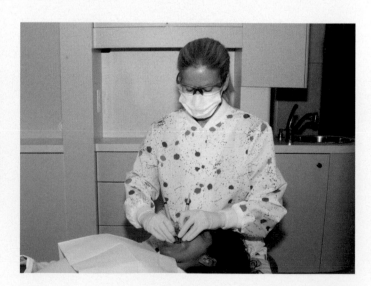

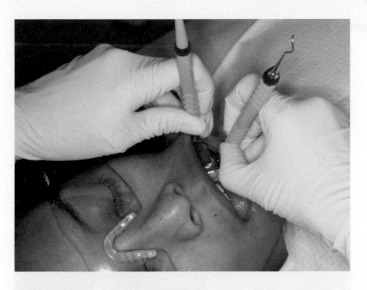

Retraction

Use the mirror to retract the buccal mucosa down and away from the teeth.

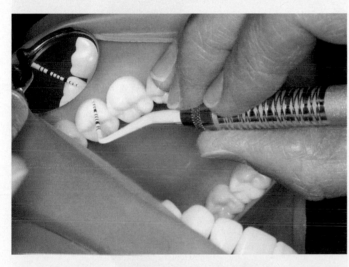

Task 1—Second Molar, Facial Aspect

Finger rest on an occlusofacial line angle.

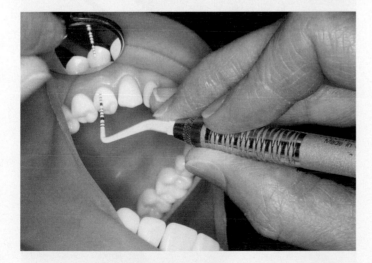

Task 2—First Premolar, Facial Aspect

Finger rest on an incisal edge of an anterior tooth.

Mandibular Right Posterior Sextant, Lingual Aspect

Position Overview

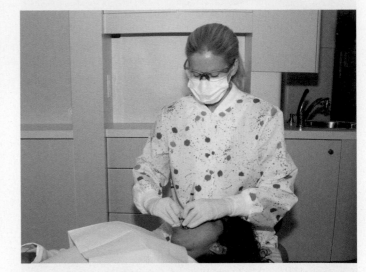

Mirror

Use the mirror head to push the tongue back gently so that the lingual surfaces of the teeth can be seen. Once in position, the mirror is also used for indirect vision.

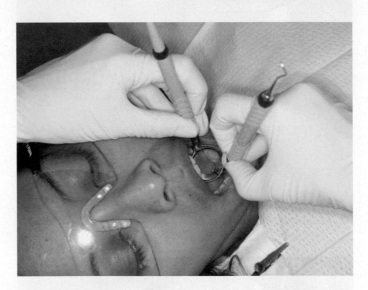

Task 1—Second Molar, Lingual Aspect

Finger rest on an occlusal surface.

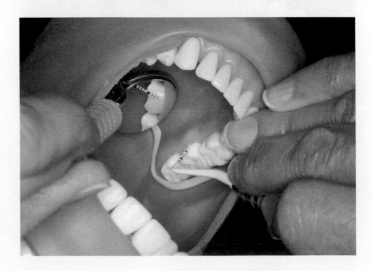

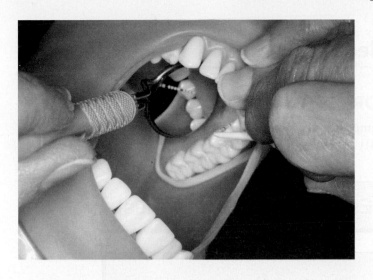

Task 2—First Premolar, Lingual Aspect

Finger rest on an incisal edge of an anterior tooth.

REFERENCE SHEET FOR MANDIBULAR POSTERIOR SEXTANTS (RIGHT-HANDED CLINICIAN)

Photocopy this reference sheet and use it for quick reference as you practice your skills. Place the photocopied reference sheet in a plastic page protector for longer use.

TABLE 5-1.	Mandibular Posterior Sextants	
Treatment Area	**Clock Position**	**Patient's Head**
Posterior Aspects Facing Toward	9:00	Straight or slightly away
(Right Posterior, Facial Aspect)		Chin DOWN
(Left Posterior, Lingual Aspect)		
Posterior Aspects Facing Away	10–11:00	Toward
(Right Posterior, Lingual Aspect)		Chin DOWN
(Left Posterior, Facial Aspect)		

RIGHT-Handed Clinician

NOTE: This ends the section for RIGHT-Handed Clinicians. Turn to page 124 for the Skill Application section of this module.

Section 3
Skills for the LEFT-Handed Clinician

FLOW CHART: SEQUENCE FOR ESTABLISHING A FINGER REST

As discussed in the previous module, it is important to proceed in a step-by-step manner. Remember: "Me, My Patient, My Light, My Nondominant Hand, My Dominant Hand."

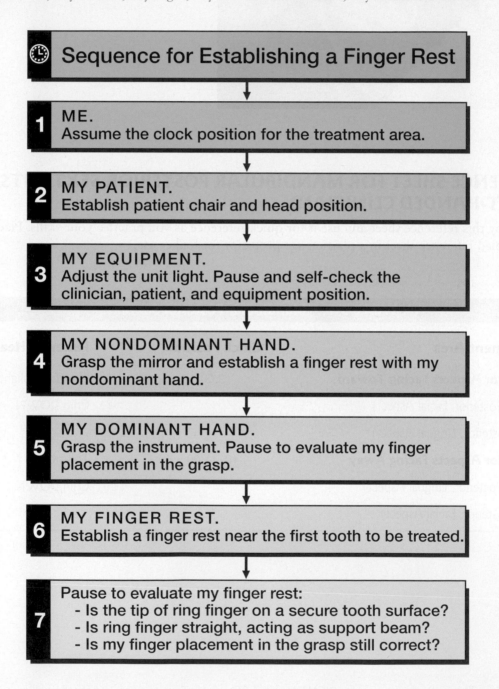

Sequence for Establishing a Finger Rest

1 ME.
Assume the clock position for the treatment area.

2 MY PATIENT.
Establish patient chair and head position.

3 MY EQUIPMENT.
Adjust the unit light. Pause and self-check the clinician, patient, and equipment position.

4 MY NONDOMINANT HAND.
Grasp the mirror and establish a finger rest with my nondominant hand.

5 MY DOMINANT HAND.
Grasp the instrument. Pause to evaluate my finger placement in the grasp.

6 MY FINGER REST.
Establish a finger rest near the first tooth to be treated.

7 Pause to evaluate my finger rest:
- Is the tip of ring finger on a secure tooth surface?
- Is ring finger straight, acting as support beam?
- Is my finger placement in the grasp still correct?

DIRECTIONS FOR SKILL PRACTICE

1. The photographs depict the use of a mirror and finger rests in the mandibular posterior sextants. Some photographs were taken using a patient. Others were taken using a manikin and without gloves so that you can easily see the finger placement in the grasp.

2. The photographs provide a *general guideline* for finger rests; however, the location of your own finger rest depends on the size and length of your fingers. You may need to fulcrum closer to or farther from the tooth being treated than that which is shown in the photograph.

3. Focus your attention on mastering mirror use, wrist position, and the finger rests. Use the following instruments in this module: For your nondominant (mirror) hand—Use a dental mirror. For your dominant (instrument) hand—(a) Remove the mirror head from one of your dental mirrors and use the mirror handle as if it were a periodontal instrument or (b) use a periodontal probe to represent the periodontal instrument in this module.

HANDLE POSITION FOR MANDIBULAR POSTERIOR TEETH

Box 5-2. Handle Position for Mandibular Posterior Teeth

1. Hold the hand in a palm-down position.
2. Rest the handle against the index finger somewhere in the green shaded area.

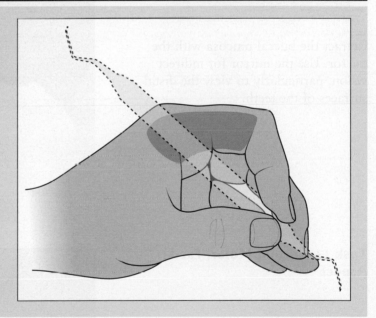

LEFT-Handed Clinician

TECHNIQUE PRACTICE: MANDIBULAR POSTERIOR SEXTANTS

Mandibular Left Posterior Sextant, Facial Aspect

Position Overview

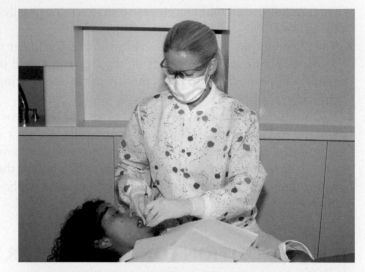

Retraction

Retract the buccal mucosa with the mirror. Use the mirror for indirect vision, particularly to view the distal surfaces of the teeth.

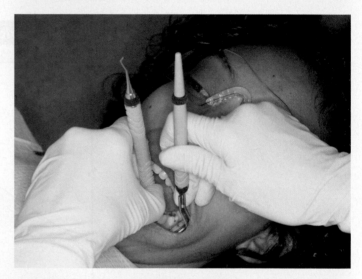

Task 1—Second Molar, Facial Aspect

Finger rest on an occlusal surface.

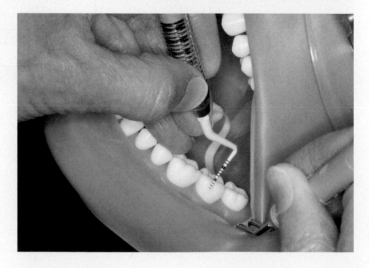

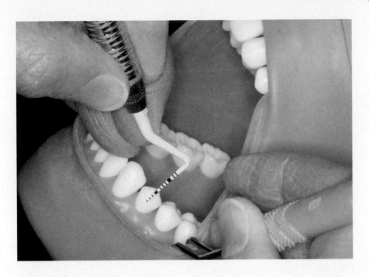

Task 2—First Premolar, Facial Aspect

Finger rest on an incisal surface of one of the mandibular anteriors.

Mandibular Right Posterior Sextant, Lingual Aspect

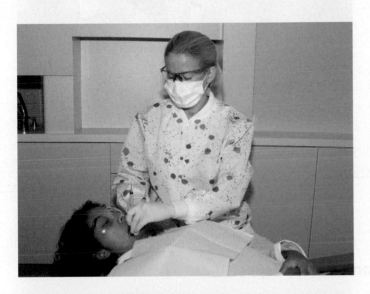

Position Overview

Mirror

Use the mirror to gently pull the tongue away from the teeth, toward the midline of the mouth. Once in position, the mirror is also used for indirect vision of the tooth surfaces.

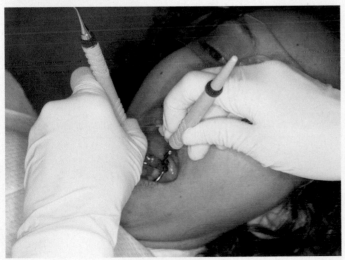

LEFT-Handed Clinician

Task 1—Second Molar, Lingual Aspect

Finger rest on an occlusofacial line angle.

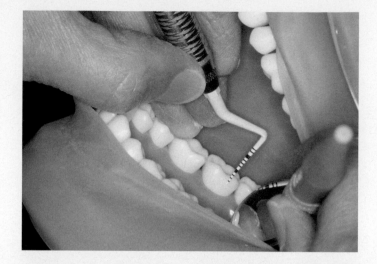

Task 2—First Premolar, Lingual Aspect

Finger rest on an incisal edge of one of the mandibular anterior teeth.

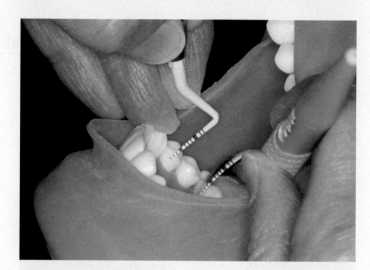

Mandibular Right Posterior Sextant, Facial Aspect

Position Overview

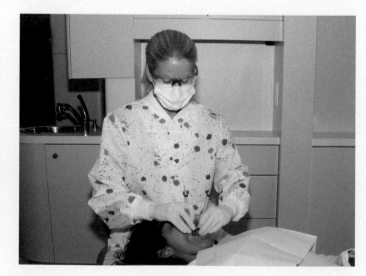

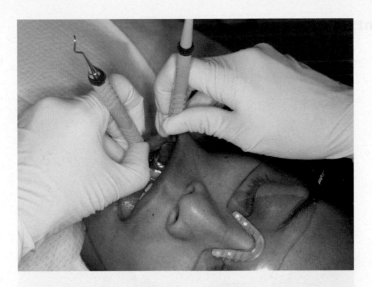

Retraction

Use the mirror to retract the buccal mucosa down and away from the teeth.

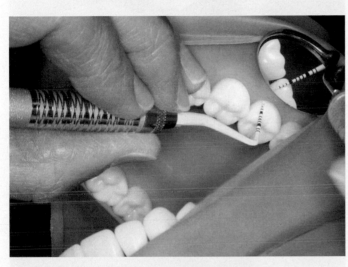

Task 1—Second Molar, Facial Aspect

Finger rest on an occlusofacial line angle.

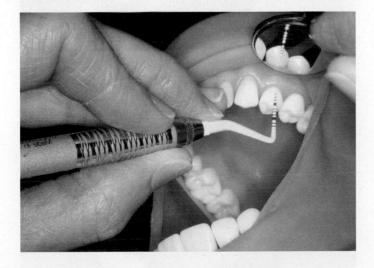

Task 2—First Premolar, Facial Aspect

Finger rest on an incisal edge of an anterior tooth.

Mandibular Left Posterior Sextant, Lingual Aspect

Position Overview

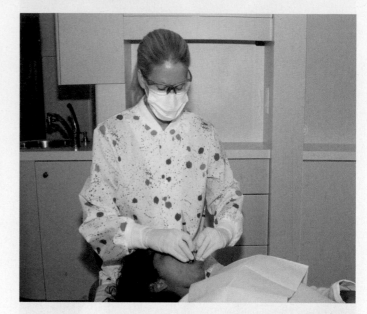

Mirror

Use the mirror head to push the tongue back gently so that the lingual surfaces of the teeth can be seen. Once in position, the mirror is also used for indirect vision.

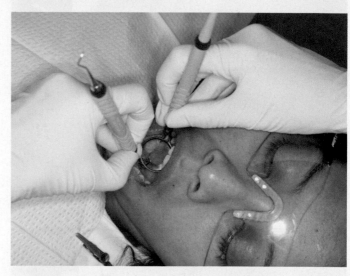

Task 1—Second Molar, Lingual Aspect
Finger rest on an occlusal surface.

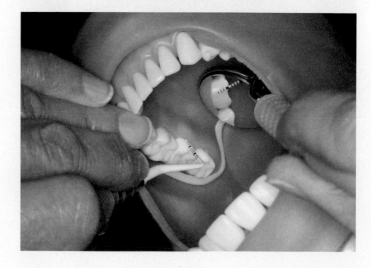

LEFT-Handed Clinician

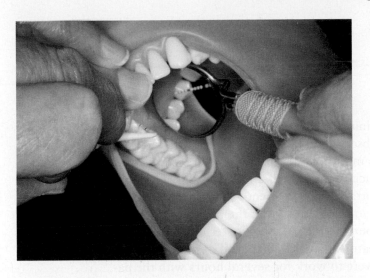

Task 2—First Premolar, Lingual Aspect

Finger rest on an incisal edge of an anterior tooth.

REFERENCE SHEET FOR MANDIBULAR POSTERIOR SEXTANTS (LEFT-HANDED CLINICIAN)

Photocopy this reference sheet and use it for quick reference as you practice your skills. Place the photocopied reference sheet in a plastic page protector for longer use.

TABLE 5-2.	Mandibular Posterior Sextants	
Treatment Area	**Clock Position**	**Patient's Head**
Posterior Aspects Facing Toward	3:00	Straight or slightly away
(Left Posterior, Facial Aspect)		Chin DOWN
(Right Posterior, Lingual Aspect)		
Posterior Aspects Facing Away	2–1:00	Toward
(Left Posterior, Lingual Aspect)		Chin DOWN
(Right Posterior, Facial Aspect)		

LEFT-Handed Clinician

Section 4
Skill Application

PRACTICAL FOCUS

1. A second-year student has been complaining of back and shoulder pain after each clinic period of treating patients. You observe him in clinic and notice that he is positioning his patient too high, so that he must hold his elbows up to reach the patient's mouth. Unfortunately, many clinicians do not self-check their large motor skills (thinking these skills to be unimportant). To experience the importance of large motor skills for yourself, position your patient so that the tip of the patient's mouth is level with the mid-region of your chest (base of your sternum). Establish a finger rest in each of the mandibular treatment areas. What kind of muscle strain do you think you might experience if you were to work for several hours with the patient positioned in this manner?

2. Your course assignment is to visit a local dental office and photograph a clinician at work on the mandibular posterior teeth. Your photographs are shown below. (1) Evaluate each photograph for position, grasp, and finger rest. (2) For each incorrect element, describe (a) how the problem could be corrected and (b) the musculoskeletal problems that could result from each positioning problem.

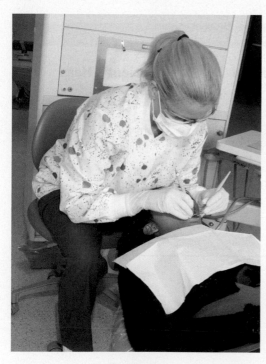

Photo 1

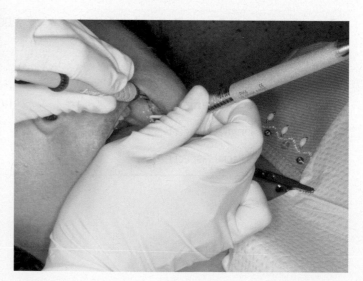

Photo 2

SKILL EVALUATION MODULE 5	MIRROR AND RESTS IN MANDIBULAR POSTERIOR SEXTANTS

Student: _____

Evaluator: _____

Date: _____

Area 1 = right posterior sextant, facial aspect
Area 2 = right posterior sextant, lingual aspect
Area 3 = left posterior sextant, facial aspect
Area 4 = left posterior sextant, lingual aspect

DIRECTIONS FOR STUDENT: Use **Column S.** Evaluate your skill level as: **S** (satisfactory) or **U** (unsatisfactory).

DIRECTIONS FOR EVALUATOR: Use **Column E.** Indicate: **S** (satisfactory) or **U** (unsatisfactory). Each **S** equals 1 point, each **U** equals 0 points.

CRITERIA:	Area 1		Area 2		Area 3		Area 4	
	S	E	S	E	S	E	S	E
Position:								
Positioned correctly on clinician stool								
Positioned correctly in relation to patient, equipment, and treatment area								
Establishes correct patient head position								
Dental Mirror:								
Uses correct grasp with mirror								
Establishes secure rest with mirror								
Assures patient comfort by not hitting teeth or using the mirror shank for retraction								
Uses the mirror correctly for retraction and/or indirect vision								
Modified Pen Grasp with Dominant Hand:								
Holds handle with pads of index finger and thumb								
Thumb and index finger positioned opposite one another on handle; fingers not touching or overlapped								
Pad of middle finger rests lightly on shank; touches the ring finger								
Thumb, index, and middle fingers held in a rounded shape (not flattened against the instrument handle)								
Instrument handle rests against index finger between 2nd and 3rd knuckle								
Grasp is relaxed (no blanching of fingers)								
Basic Intraoral Fulcrum:								
Ring finger is straight and supports weight of hand								
Fulcrums on same arch, near tooth being instrumented								
OPTIONAL GRADE PERCENTAGE CALCULATION Total **S**'s in each E column.								

Sum of **S**'s _____ divided by Total Points Possible (**60**) equals the Percentage Grade _____%

SKILL EVALUATION MODULE 5   MIRROR AND RESTS IN MANDIBULAR POSTERIOR SEXTANTS

Student: _____

EVALUATOR COMMENTS

_____

_____

_____

_____

_____

_____

_____

_____

_____

_____

_____

_____

_____

_____

_____

_____

Box for sketches pertaining to written comments.

Mirror and Finger Rests in Maxillary Posterior Sextants

Module Overview

This module describes techniques for using a dental mirror and finger rests in the maxillary posterior treatment areas. A step-by-step technique practice is found in Sections 1 and 2.

Module Outline

Key Terms

Review these terms from Module 4:

Neutral wrist position	Support beam	Extraoral fulcrum	Intraoral fulcrum
Fulcrum	Finger rest		

Learning Objectives

1. Maintain neutral positioning when practicing finger rests in the maxillary posterior sextants.

2. Position equipment so that it enhances neutral positioning.

3. Access the maxillary posterior teeth with optimum vision while maintaining neutral positioning.

4. Demonstrate correct mirror use, grasp, and finger rest in each of the maxillary posterior sextants while maintaining neutral positioning of your wrist.

5. Recognize incorrect mirror use, grasp, or finger rest and describe how to correct the problem(s).

6. Understand the relationship between proper stabilization of the dominant hand during instrumentation and the prevention of (1) musculoskeletal problems in the clinician's hands and (2) injury to the patient.

7. Understand the relationship between the large motor skills, such as positioning, and small motor skills, such as finger rests. Recognize the importance of initiating these skills in a step-by-step manner.

Section 1
Skills for the RIGHT-Handed Clinician

DIRECTIONS FOR SKILL PRACTICE

1. The photographs depict the use of a mirror and finger rests in the maxillary posterior sextants. Some photographs were taken using a patient. Others were taken using a manikin and without gloves so that you can easily see the finger placement in the grasp.

2. The photographs provide a *general guideline* for finger rests; however, the location of your own finger rest depends on the size and length of your fingers. You may need to fulcrum closer to or farther from the tooth being treated than that which is shown in the photograph.

3. Focus your attention on mastering mirror use, wrist position, and the finger rests. Use the following instruments in this module: For your nondominant (mirror) hand—Use a dental mirror. For your dominant (instrument) hand—(a) Remove the mirror head from one of your dental mirrors and use the mirror handle as if it were a periodontal instrument or (b) use a periodontal probe to represent the periodontal instrument in this module.

HANDLE POSITION FOR MAXILLARY POSTERIOR TEETH

Box 6-1. Handle Position for Maxillary Posterior Teeth

1. Hold the hand in a palm-up position.

2. Rest the handle against the index finger somewhere in the green shaded area.

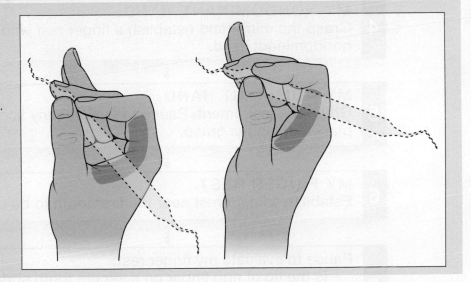

FLOW CHART: SEQUENCE FOR ESTABLISHING A FINGER REST

Remember to perform each skill in a step-by-step manner. Your *small motor skills*, such as the grasp and finger rest, cannot be correct if your *large motor skills* are incorrect. As you begin your practice for each treatment area think: "Me, My Patient, My Light, My Nondominant Hand, My Dominant Hand."

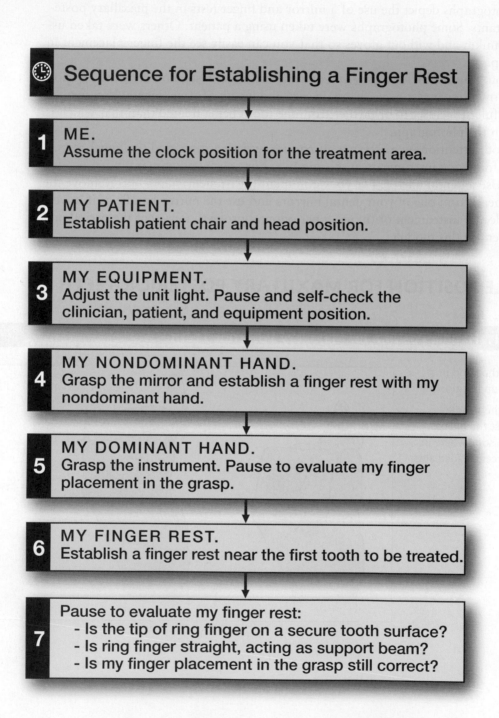

🕐 **Sequence for Establishing a Finger Rest**

1   ME.
Assume the clock position for the treatment area.

2   MY PATIENT.
Establish patient chair and head position.

3   MY EQUIPMENT.
Adjust the unit light. Pause and self-check the clinician, patient, and equipment position.

4   MY NONDOMINANT HAND.
Grasp the mirror and establish a finger rest with my nondominant hand.

5   MY DOMINANT HAND.
Grasp the instrument. Pause to evaluate my finger placement in the grasp.

6   MY FINGER REST.
Establish a finger rest near the first tooth to be treated.

7   Pause to evaluate my finger rest:
  - Is the tip of ring finger on a secure tooth surface?
  - Is ring finger straight, acting as support beam?
  - Is my finger placement in the grasp still correct?

TECHNIQUE PRACTICE: MAXILLARY POSTERIOR SEXTANTS
Maxillary Right Posterior Sextant, Facial Aspect
Position Overview

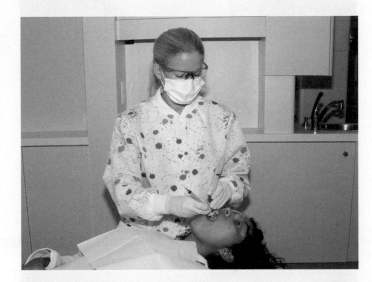

Retraction

Retract the buccal mucosa with the mirror. Use the mirror for indirect vision, particularly to view the distal surfaces of the teeth.

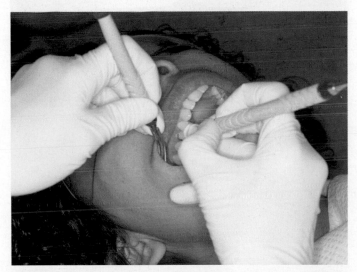

Task 1—Second Molar, Facial Aspect

Finger rest on an occlusal surface.

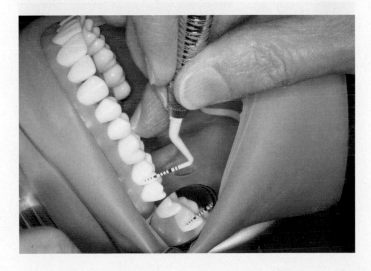

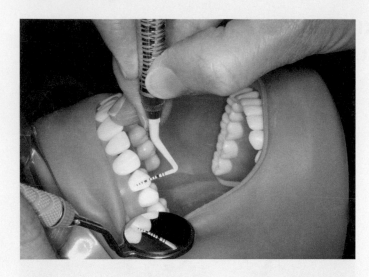

Task 2—First Premolar, Facial Aspect

Finger rest on an incisal surface of one of the maxillary anteriors.

Maxillary Left Posterior Sextant, Lingual Aspect

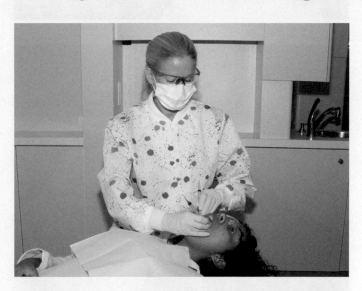

Position Overview

Mirror

Use the mirror to view the distal surfaces of the teeth.

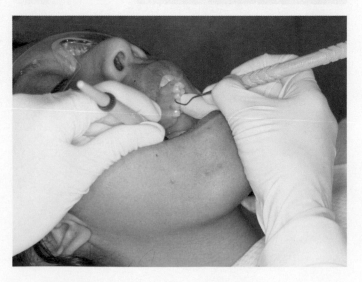

Task 1—Second Molar, Lingual Aspect

Finger rest on an occlusofacial line angle.

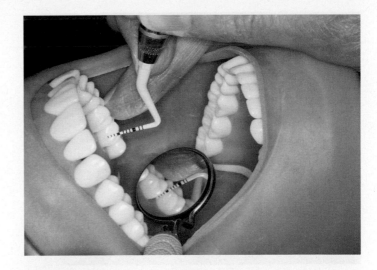

Task 2—First Premolar, Lingual Aspect

Finger rest on the occlusofacial line angle or an incisal edge.

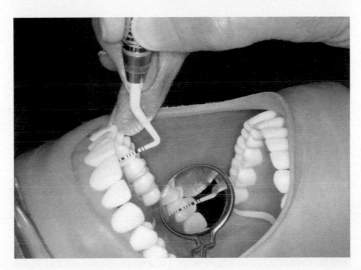

Maxillary Left Posterior Sextant, Facial Aspect

Position Overview

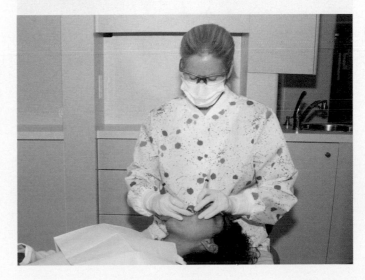

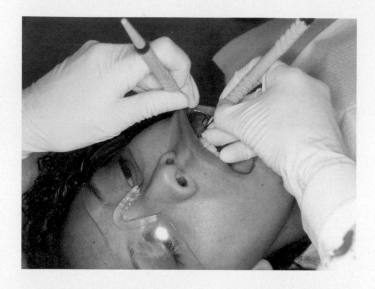

Retraction

Use the mirror to retract the buccal mucosa down and away from the teeth.

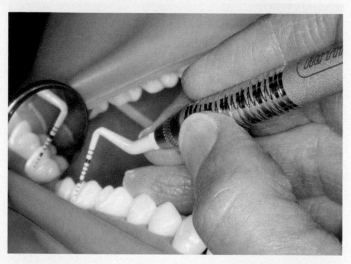

Task 1—Second Molar, Facial Aspect

Finger rest on an occlusal surface.

Technique hint: Your dominant hand is positioned correctly if you can see the underside of your middle and ring fingers.

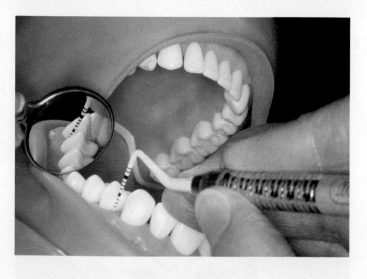

Task 2—First Premolar, Facial Aspect

Finger rest on an incisal edge of an anterior tooth.

Maxillary Right Posterior Sextant, Lingual Aspect

Position Overview

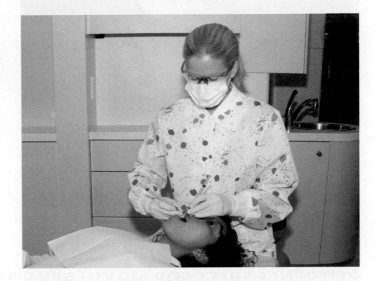

Mirror

Use the mirror for indirect vision.

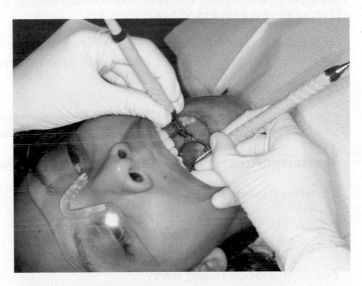

Task 1—Second Molar, Lingual Aspect

Finger rest on an occlusal surface.

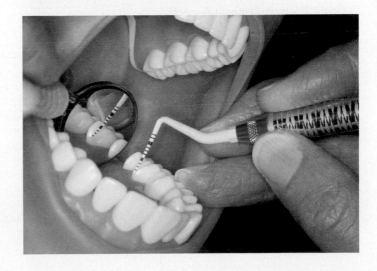

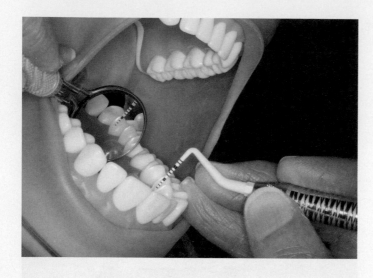

Task 2—First Premolar, Lingual Aspect

Finger rest on the occlusal surface or an incisal edge.

REFERENCE SHEET FOR MAXILLARY POSTERIOR SEXTANTS (RIGHT-HANDED CLINICIAN)

Photocopy this reference sheet and use it for quick reference as you practice your skills. Place the photocopied reference sheet in a plastic page protector for longer use.

TABLE 6-1. Maxillary Posterior Sextants		
Treatment Area	**Clock Position**	**Patient's Head**
Posterior Aspects Facing Toward	9:00	Straight or slightly away
(Right Posterior, Facial Aspect)		Chin UP
(Left Posterior, Lingual Aspect)		
Posterior Aspects Facing Away	10–11:00	Toward
(Right Posterior, Lingual Aspect)		Chin UP
(Left Posterior, Facial Aspect)		

NOTE: This ends the section for RIGHT-Handed Clinicians. Turn to page 145 for the Skill Application section of this module.

Section 2
Skills for the LEFT-Handed Clinician

DIRECTIONS FOR SKILL PRACTICE

1. The photographs depict the use of a mirror and finger rests in the maxillary posterior sextants. Some photographs were taken using a patient. Others were taken using a manikin and without gloves so that you can easily see the finger placement in the grasp.
2. The photographs provide a *general guideline* for finger rests; however, the location of your own finger rest depends on the size and length of your fingers. You may need to fulcrum closer to or farther from the tooth being treated than that which is shown in the photograph.
3. Focus your attention on mastering mirror use, wrist position, and the finger rests. Use the following instruments in this module: For your nondominant (mirror) hand—Use a dental mirror. For your dominant (instrument) hand—(a) Remove the mirror head from one of your dental mirrors and use the mirror handle as if it were a periodontal instrument or (b) use a periodontal probe to represent the periodontal instrument in this module.

HANDLE POSITION FOR MAXILLARY POSTERIOR TEETH

Box 6-2. Handle Position for Maxillary Posterior Teeth

1. Hold the hand in a palm-up position.

2. Rest the handle against the index finger somewhere in the green shaded area.

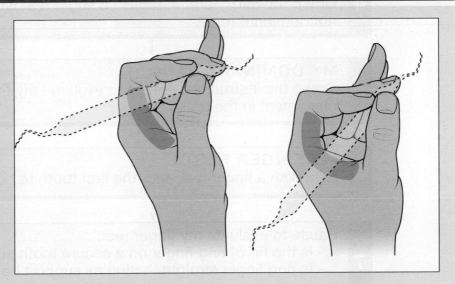

FLOW CHART: SEQUENCE FOR ESTABLISHING A FINGER REST

Remember to perform each skill in a step-by-step manner. Your *small motor skills,* such as the grasp and finger rest, cannot be correct if your *large motor skills* are incorrect. As you begin your practice for each treatment area think: "Me, My Patient, My Light, My Nondominant Hand, My Dominant Hand."

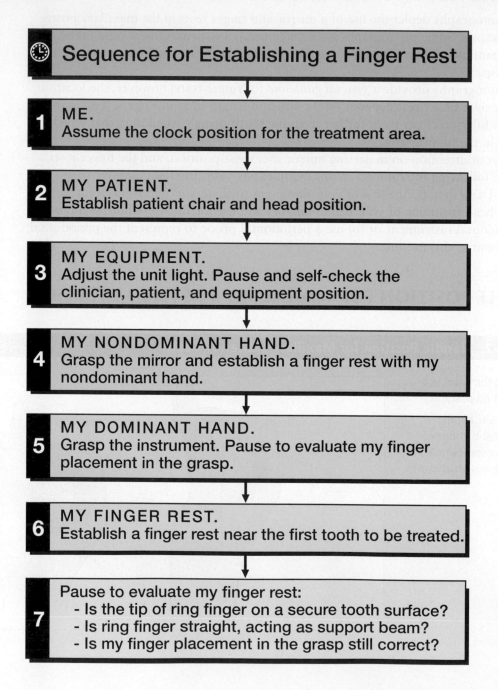

🕐 **Sequence for Establishing a Finger Rest**

1 **ME.**
Assume the clock position for the treatment area.

2 **MY PATIENT.**
Establish patient chair and head position.

3 **MY EQUIPMENT.**
Adjust the unit light. Pause and self-check the clinician, patient, and equipment position.

4 **MY NONDOMINANT HAND.**
Grasp the mirror and establish a finger rest with my nondominant hand.

5 **MY DOMINANT HAND.**
Grasp the instrument. Pause to evaluate my finger placement in the grasp.

6 **MY FINGER REST.**
Establish a finger rest near the first tooth to be treated.

7 Pause to evaluate my finger rest:
  - Is the tip of ring finger on a secure tooth surface?
  - Is ring finger straight, acting as support beam?
  - Is my finger placement in the grasp still correct?

LEFT-Handed Clinician

TECHNIQUE PRACTICE: MAXILLARY POSTERIOR SEXTANTS
Maxillary Left Posterior Sextant, Facial Aspect
Position Overview

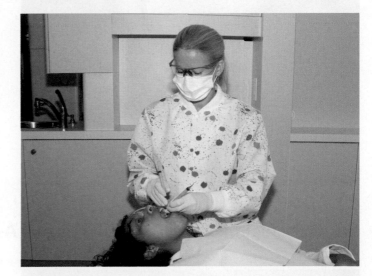

Retraction

Retract the buccal mucosa with the mirror. Use the mirror for indirect vision, particularly to view the distal surfaces of the teeth.

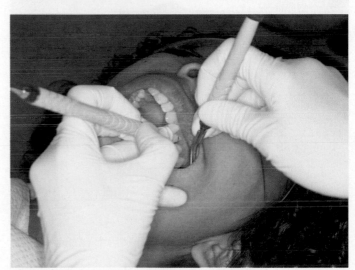

Task 1—Second Molar, Facial Aspect

Finger rest on an occlusal surface.

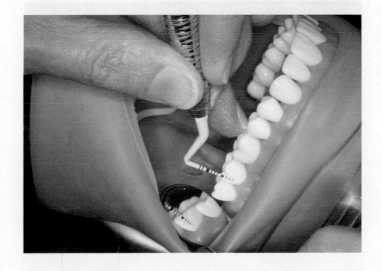

LEFT-Handed Clinician

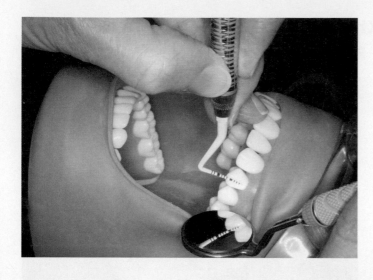

Task 2—First Premolar, Facial Aspect

Finger rest on an incisal surface of one of the maxillary anteriors.

Maxillary Right Posterior Sextant, Lingual Aspect

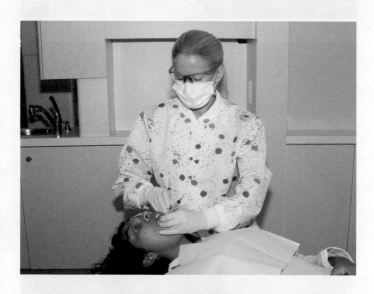

Position Overview

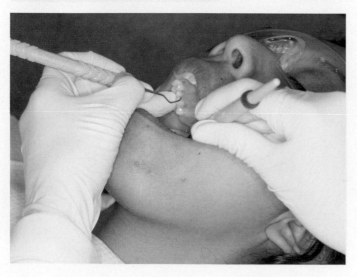

Mirror

Use the mirror to view the distal surfaces of the teeth.

Task 1—Second Molar, Lingual Aspect

Finger rest on an occlusofacial line angle.

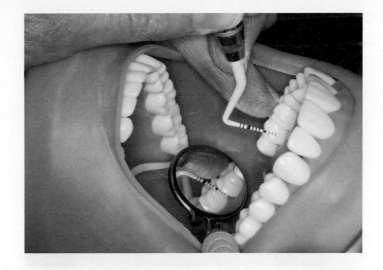

Task 2—First Premolar, Lingual Aspect

Finger rest on the occlusofacial line angle or an incisal edge.

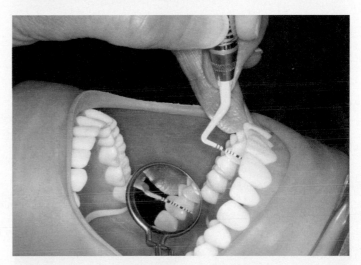

Maxillary Right Posterior Sextant, Facial Aspect

Position Overview

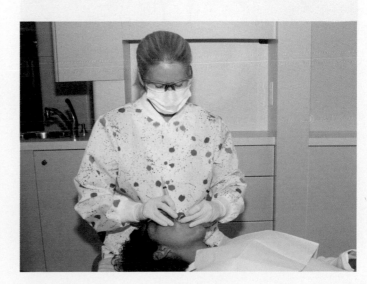

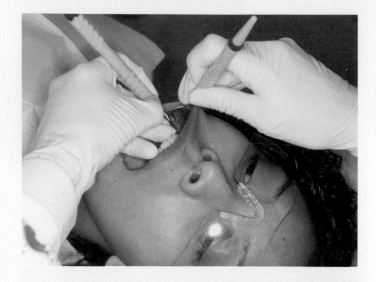

Retraction

Use the mirror to retract the buccal mucosa down and away from the teeth.

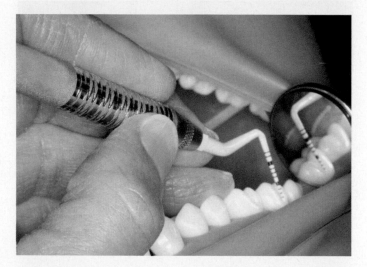

Task 1—Second Molar, Facial Aspect

Finger rest on an occlusal surface.

Technique hint: Your dominant hand is positioned correctly if you can see the underside of your middle and ring fingers.

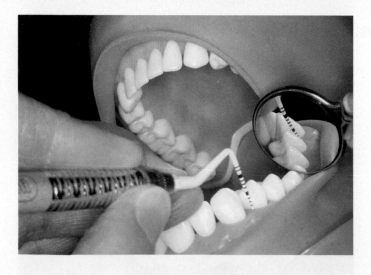

Task 2—First Premolar, Facial Aspect

Finger rest on an incisal edge of an anterior tooth.

Maxillary Left Posterior Sextant, Lingual Aspect

Position Overview

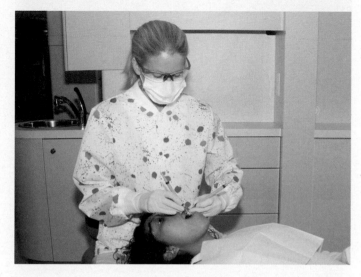

Mirror

Use the mirror for indirect vision.

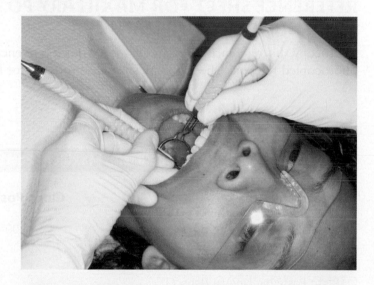

Task 1—Second Molar, Lingual Aspect

Finger rest on an occlusal surface.

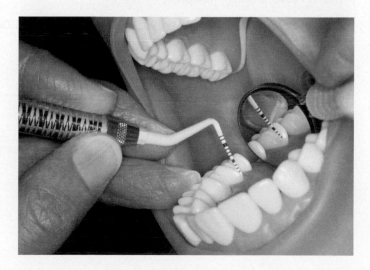

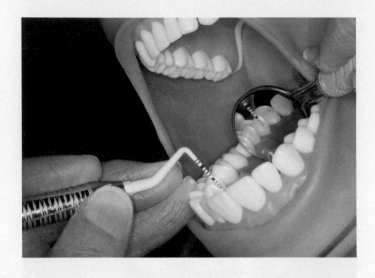

Task 2—First Premolar, Lingual Aspect

Finger rest on the occlusal surface or an incisal edge.

REFERENCE SHEET FOR MAXILLARY POSTERIOR SEXTANTS (LEFT-HANDED CLINICIAN)

Photocopy this reference sheet and use it for quick reference as you practice your skills. Place the photocopied reference sheet in a plastic page protector for longer use.

TABLE 6-2. Maxillary Posterior Sextants		
Treatment Area	**Clock Position**	**Patient's Head**
Posterior Aspects Facing Toward	3:00	Straight or slightly away
(Left Posterior, Facial Aspect)		Chin UP
(Right Posterior, Lingual Aspect)		
Posterior Aspects Facing Away	2–1:00	Toward
(Left Posterior, Lingual Aspect)		Chin UP
(Right Posterior, Facial Aspect)		

LEFT-Handed Clinician

Section 3
Skill Application

PRACTICAL FOCUS

Do you sometimes forget about neutral body position as you concentrate on the finger rests? Use this checklist to assess your habits. *A "YES" answer means that changes are indicated.*

Body Breakers Risk Assessment Checklist			
Structure	**Incorrect Body Mechanics**	**YES**	**NO**
Head	Tilted to one side?	☐	☐
	Tipped too far forward?	☐	☐
Shoulders	Lifted up toward ears?	☐	☐
	Tense?	☐	☐
	Hunched forward?	☐	☐
Upper Arms	Held more than 20 degrees away from body?	☐	☐
Elbows	Raised above waist level?	☐	☐
Wrists	Hand bent up? Down?	☐	☐
	Hand angled toward thumb? Toward little finger?	☐	☐
	Thumb-side of palm tipped down?	☐	☐
Hands	Gloves too tight?	☐	☐
	Fingers blanched in grasp?	☐	☐
	Fingers tense?	☐	☐
Back	Rounded back?	☐	☐
Hips	Perched forward on seat?	☐	☐
	All weight on one hip?	☐	☐
Legs	Under back of patient's chair?	☐	☐
	Thighs "cut" by edge of chair seat?	☐	☐
	Legs crossed?	☐	☐
Feet	Dangling?	☐	☐
	Ankles crossed?	☐	☐

1. Your course assignment is to visit a local dental office and photograph a clinician at work on the maxillary teeth. Your photographs are shown below. (1) Evaluate each photograph for position, grasp, and finger rest. (2) For each incorrect element describe (a) how the problem could be corrected and (b) the musculoskeletal problems that could result from each positioning problem.

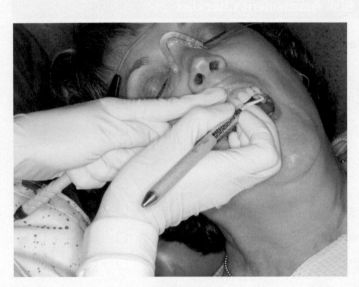 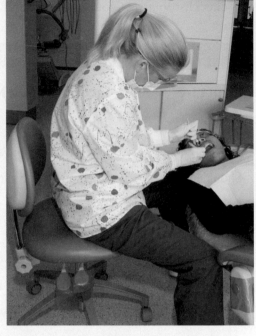

Photo 1   **Photo 2**

2. **Precise Instrument Control.** This activity simulates the skills you will need to use when placing the instrument's working-end on the various tooth surfaces while using indirect vision. It was designed by Margaret Starr, R.D.H., when she was a student learning instrumentation. Can you name several tooth surfaces that can best be seen with indirect vision?

   Materials and Equipment: Printed page from a textbook or magazine, a dental mirror, and a sharpened pencil.

   a. Lay the printed page flat on a desk or tabletop. Hold a dental mirror in your nondominant hand, and position it on the page. Angle the mirror head so that you are able to see several letters reflected in the mirror. How do the letters appear?

   b. Still looking in the mirror, locate a letter "e" in one of the words. Grasp the pencil in a modified pen grasp and touch the pencil point to the "e" *on the paper.*

   c. Move the mirror to a different location on the paper. Looking in the mirror, select a letter and touch it with the pencil point.

SKILL EVALUATION MODULE 6	MIRROR AND RESTS IN MAXILLARY POSTERIOR SEXTANTS

Student: _____

Evaluator: _____

Date: _____

Area 1 = right posterior sextant, facial aspect
Area 2 = right posterior sextant, lingual aspect
Area 3 = left posterior sextant, facial aspect
Area 4 = left posterior sextant, lingual aspect

DIRECTIONS FOR STUDENT: Use **Column S.** Evaluate your skill level as: **S** (satisfactory) or **U** (unsatisfactory).

DIRECTIONS FOR EVALUATOR: Use **Column E.** Indicate: **S** (satisfactory) or **U** (unsatisfactory). Each **S** equals 1 point, each **U** equals 0 points.

CRITERIA:	Area 1 S	E	Area 2 S	E	Area 3 S	E	Area 4 S	E
Position:								
Positioned correctly on clinician stool								
Positioned correctly in relation to patient, equipment, and treatment area								
Establishes correct patient head position								
Dental Mirror:								
Uses correct grasp with mirror								
Establishes secure rest with mirror								
Ensures patient comfort by not hitting teeth or using the mirror shank for retraction								
Uses the mirror correctly for retraction and/or indirect vision								
Modified Pen Grasp with Dominant Hand:								
Holds handle with pads of index finger and thumb								
Thumb and index finger positioned opposite one another on handle; fingers not touching or overlapped								
Pad of middle finger rests lightly on shank; touches the ring finger								
Thumb, index, and middle fingers held in a rounded shape (not flattened against the instrument handle)								
Instrument handle rests against index finger between the 2nd knuckle and the "V" of the hand								
Grasp is relaxed (no blanching of fingers)								
Basic Intraoral Fulcrum:								
Ring finger is straight and supports weight of hand								
Fulcrums on same arch, near tooth being instrumented								
OPTIONAL GRADE PERCENTAGE CALCULATION Total **S**'s in each E column.								

Sum of **S**'s _____ divided by Total Points Possible (**60**) equals the Percentage Grade _____%

| SKILL EVALUATION MODULE 6 | MIRROR AND RESTS IN MAXILLARY POSTERIOR SEXTANTS |

Student: _____

EVALUATOR COMMENTS

_____

_____

_____

_____

_____

_____

_____

_____

_____

_____

_____

_____

_____

_____

Box for sketches pertaining to written comments.

Instrument Design and Classification

Module Overview

This module introduces the various design characteristics of periodontal instruments. To select an appropriate instrument for a particular instrumentation task, the clinician must have a thorough understanding of the design features of the handles, shanks, and working-ends of periodontal instruments. With so many instruments on the market and new designs introduced regularly, it is impossible for any one clinician to recognize each instrument by name. Fortunately, a clinician who understands the principles of design and classification can easily determine the intended use of any unfamiliar instrument.

Module Outline

Practical Focus
Skill Evaluation Module 7: Instrument Design and Classification

Key Terms

Paired working-ends	Complex shank	Lower shank	Tip of working-end
Unpaired working- ends	Proximal surfaces	Terminal shank	Cross section
Design name	Rigid shank	Extended lower shank	Classifications
Design number	Flexible shank	Face	Periodontal probe
Knurling	Visual information	Back	Explorer
Balanced instrument	Tactile information	Lateral surfaces	Sickle scaler
Simple shank	Tactile sensitivity	Cutting edge	Curet
	Functional shank	Toe of working-end	Periodontal file

Learning Objectives

1. Identify each working-end of a periodontal instrument by its design name and number.

2. Recognize the design features of instrument handles and shanks, and discuss how these design features relate to the instrument's use. Describe the advantages and limitations of the various design features available for instrument handles and shanks.

3. Given a variety of periodontal instruments, sort the instruments into those with simple shank design and those with complex shank design.

4. Given a variety of periodontal instruments, identify the face, back, lateral surfaces, cutting edges, and toe or tip on each working-end.

5. Given a variety of periodontal instruments, determine the intended use of each instrument by evaluating its design features and classification.

6. Given any instrument, identify where and how it may be used on the dentition (i.e., assessment or calculus removal, anterior/posterior teeth, supragingival or subgingival use).

Section 1
Characteristics Common to All Periodontal Instruments

SINGLE- AND DOUBLE-ENDED INSTRUMENTS

1. Periodontal instruments are available in single-ended and double-ended configurations.
2. Single-ended instruments are less efficient to use because the clinician must stop more often to lay down one instrument and pick up another.
3. Double-ended instruments allow the clinician to simply flip the instrument to use the other working-end.
4. Most double-ended instruments have paired working-ends that are exact mirror images of each other. Some double-ended instruments have unpaired (dissimilar) working-ends. An example of a double-ended instrument with unpaired working-ends is an explorer and a probe combination.

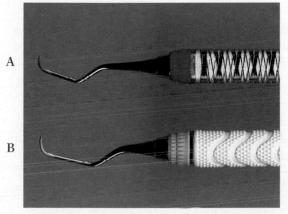
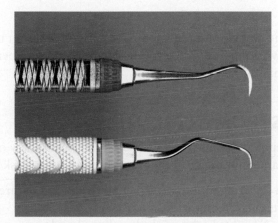

Unpaired and Paired Working-Ends. Instrument A has unpaired, dissimilar working-ends. Instrument B has paired, mirror image working-ends.

INSTRUMENT IDENTIFICATION

Each periodontal instrument is identified by a unique design name and number.

1. Design name—identifies the school or individual originally responsible for the design or development of an instrument or group of instruments. Instruments often are named after the designer or an academic institution. A well-known example is the design name "Gracey." In the late 1930s, Dr. Clayton H. Gracey designed the 14 original single-ended instruments in this series that bears his name.
2. Design number—a number designation that when combined with the design name provides an exact identification of the working-end. Using an instrument from the Gracey series as an example—Gracey 11—"Gracey" is the design name and "11" is the design number that identifies a specific instrument in this instrument series.
3. The design name and number are stamped on the handle of the instrument.

WORKING-END IDENTIFICATION

A double-ended instrument has two design numbers, one to identify each working-end of the instrument. For example, the original Gracey series of instruments includes 7 double-ended instruments, such as the Gracey 3/4, Gracey 5/6, Gracey 11/12, and Gracey 13/14.

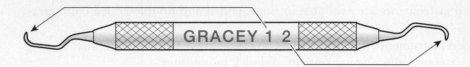

Name and Number Marked Along the Handle. In this case, each working-end is identified by the number closest to it.

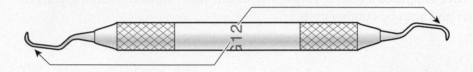

Name and Number Marked Across the Handle. In this case, the first number (on the left) identifies the working-end at the top and the second number identifies the working-end at the lower end of the handle.

INSTRUMENT HANDLES

Instrument handles are available in a wide variety of diameters and textures. Handle design is an important component in the prevention of musculoskeletal injury during instrumentation (Table 7-1).

1. In selecting an instrument handle, there are three characteristics to consider: (1) weight, (2) diameter, and (3) texture.
   a. Weight. Lightweight handles place less stress on the muscles of the hand and fingers.
   b. Diameter.
      1) Small-diameter handles (3/17 inch) are difficult to hold and tend to cause muscle cramping.
      2) Large-diameter handles (3/8 inch) are easier to hold and decrease muscle strain.
   c. Texture. Another term for texturing is knurling.
      1) Handles with no texturing decrease control of the instrument and increase muscle fatigue.
      2) Handles with bumpy texturing maximize control of the instrument and reduce muscle fatigue.
2. It may be helpful to select handles in a range of larger diameters, thus providing some variety for the muscles of your fingers.

TABLE 7-1. Handle Selection Criteria	
Recommended	**Avoid**
Large diameter (3/8 inch)	Small diameter (3/17 inch)
Lightweight, hollow handle	Heavy, solid metal handle
Bumpy texturing	Smooth or flat texturing

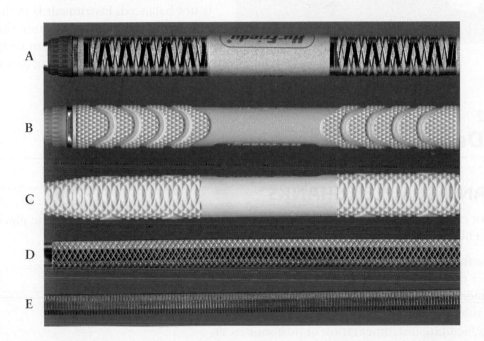

Design Characteristics of Instrument Handles. Instruments A, B, and C with large-diameter handles and bumpy texturing would be easy to hold and would reduce muscle fatigue. Instruments A and B have additional texturing on the tapered portion of the handle. This feature reduces muscle strain for short-fingered clinicians who must grip the tapered portion of the handle. Instrument D has a small-diameter handle and less pronounced texturing. Instrument E is not recommended because it has a small-diameter handle and very limited texturing.

INSTRUMENT BALANCE

Balanced instrument—a periodontal instrument that has working-ends that are aligned with the long axis of the handle.

1. During instrumentation, balance ensures that finger pressure applied against the handle is transferred to the working-end, resulting in pressure against the tooth.
2. An instrument that is not balanced is more difficult to use and stresses the muscles of the hand and arm.

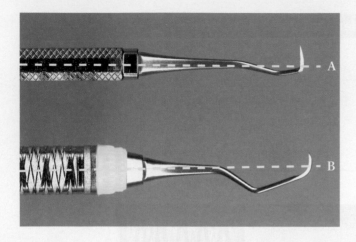

Determining Instrument Balance. An easy method of determining whether an instrument is balanced is to place the instrument on a line of a lined writing tablet. Align the midline of the handle with a line on the paper; the instrument is balanced if the working-ends are centered on the line.

In the photograph on the left, **instrument A** is not balanced. **Instrument B** in the photograph is balanced because the working-end is centered on an imaginary line running through the long axis of the handle.

Section 2
Shank Design

SIMPLE AND COMPLEX SHANKS

The shanks of most periodontal instruments are bent in one or more places to facilitate placement of the working-end against the tooth surface.

1. Simple shank design—a shank that is bent in one plane (front-to-back).
   a. Another term for a simple shank is a straight shank.
   b. Instruments with simple shanks are used primarily on anterior teeth.
2. Complex shank design—a shank that is bent in two planes (front-to-back and side-to-side) to facilitate instrumentation of posterior teeth.
   a. Another term for a complex shank is an angled or curved shank.
   b. The crowns of posterior teeth are rounded and overhang their roots. An instrument with a complex shank is needed to reach around the crown and onto the root surface.

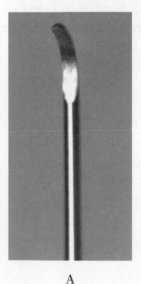 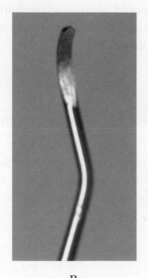

Simple and Complex Shank Design. To determine whether the shank is simple or complex, *hold the instrument so that the working-end tip or toe is facing you.*
Instrument A, when viewed from the front, the shank of this instrument appears to be straight. Therefore, this instrument has a simple shank design.
Instrument B, when viewed from the front, the shank of this instrument is bent from side to side. Therefore, this instrument has a complex shank design.

A   B

APPLICATION OF SIMPLE AND COMPLEX SHANKS

Simple Shank on an Anterior Tooth. The crowns of anterior teeth are wedge-shaped. A simple shank design is adequate to reach along the crown and onto the root surface.

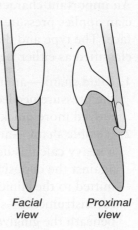

Facial view   Proximal view

Complex Shank on a Lingual Surface. The illustration shows a mandibular molar when viewed from the mesial aspect. The front-to-back shank bends allow the clinician to reach the lingual and facial surfaces of the root.

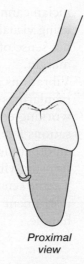

Proximal view

Complex Shank on a Proximal Surface. The illustration shows a mandibular molar when viewed from the facial aspect. The side-to-side bends allow the clinician to reach the proximal (mesial and distal) surfaces of the tooth.

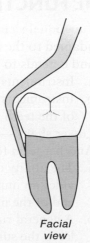

Facial view

Simple / complex : anterior / posterior

long / short : subgingival / supragingival

SHANK FLEXIBILITY

An important characteristic of an instrument shank is its strength. During instrumentation, the clinician applies pressure against the handle and shank to press the working-end against the tooth surface. The type and diameter of metal used in a shank determine its strength. Instrument shanks are classified as either rigid or flexible in design.

1. Rigid shank—an instrument shank that is larger in diameter and thus will withstand the pressure needed to remove heavy calculus deposits. A calculus deposit can be removed more quickly and with less effort if the instrument has a rigid shank.
2. Flexible shank—an instrument shank that is thinner in diameter. When used against a heavy calculus deposit, a flexible shank bends or flexes as pressure is applied against the deposit. Flexible shanks enhance the amount of tactile information transmitted to the clinician's fingers. For this reason, a flexible shank design is desirable for instruments—such as explorers—that are used to locate calculus deposits hidden beneath the gingival margin.
   a. Visual information is of limited use when working subgingivally because the clinician cannot see the working-end hidden beneath the gingival margin. Instead of using visual information, the clinician must rely on tactile information—his or her sense of touch—to locate the calculus deposits hidden beneath the gingival margin.
   b. Vibrations are created when the working-end quivers slightly as it moves over irregularities on the surface of the tooth. These vibrations are transmitted from the working-end, through the shank, and into the handle. This is similar to the sensations felt in the soles of the feet when roller blading over a section of gravel on an otherwise paved road surface. The rollers encounter the gravel patch and transmit vibrations to the soles of the feet.
   c. Tactile sensitivity is the clinician's ability to feel vibrations transmitted from the instrument working-end with his or her fingers as they rest on the shank and handle.

THE FUNCTIONAL SHANK AND THE LOWER SHANK

1. Functional shank—the portion of the shank that allows the working-end to be adapted to the tooth surface. The functional shank begins below the working-end and extends to the last bend in the shank nearest the handle.
   a. Instruments with short functional shanks are used on the crowns of the teeth.
   b. Instruments with long functional shanks are used on both the crowns and roots of the teeth (Table 7-2).
2. Lower shank—the portion of the functional shank nearest to the working-end. Another term for the lower shank is the **terminal shank**.
   a. The ability to identify the lower shank is important because the lower shank provides an important visual clue for the clinician in selecting the correct working-end of the instrument.
   b. A general rule for working-end selection is that the lower shank should be parallel to the surface to be instrumented.

Explorer & prob function is assessment
hold firm but light

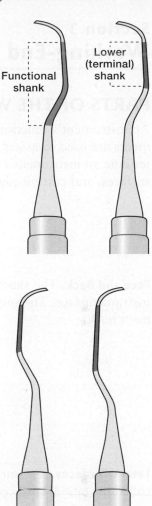

Functional and Lower Shanks. The functional shank begins below the working-end and extends to the last bend in the shank nearest the handle. The lower shank is the portion of the functional shank nearest to the working-end. The lower shank is also termed the terminal shank.

functional shank includes all turns and twists.

Extended Lower Shanks. Instrument **A** in this illustration has a standard lower shank. **Instrument B** has an extended lower shank. An extended lower shank is 3 mm longer than a standard lower shank. Instruments with extended lower shanks are ideal for working in deep periodontal pockets or when using advanced fulcruming techniques.

TABLE 7-2.	Shank Curvature and Functional Length Related to Instrument Use
Shank Design	**Use**
Simple shank with short functional length	Supragingival use on anterior teeth
Simple shank with long functional length	Subgingival use on anterior teeth
Complex shank with short functional length	Supragingival use on posterior teeth
Complex shank with long functional length	Subgingival use on posterior teeth

Know For Exam!

Section 3
Working-End Design

PARTS OF THE WORKING-END

An instrument's function is determined, primarily, by the design of its working-end. Some instruments are used to assess the teeth or soft tissues, others are used to remove calculus deposits. To determine an instrument's use, you must recognize the design characteristics of the face, back, lateral surfaces, and cutting edges of the working-end.

Face and Back. The shaded surface on this illustration is the instrument face. The surface opposite the face is the instrument back.

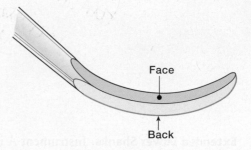

Lateral Surfaces. The surfaces on either side of the face are called the lateral surfaces of the instrument.

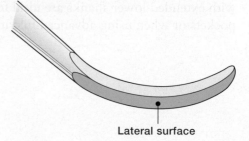

Cutting Edge. The cutting edge is a sharp edge formed where the face and lateral surfaces meet.

Reading third

Toe or Tip. These illustrations show a curet and a sickle scaler from a birds-eye view, looking down on the instrument face.

The cutting edges of a curet meet to form a rounded surface called a toe. The cutting edges of a sickle scaler meet in a point called a tip. *Usually* *Used above gumline*

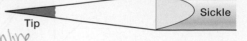

Subgingiva

THE WORKING-END IN CROSS SECTION

The cross section of a working-end is exposed by cutting through the working-end at right angles to its longest dimension. The cross section of a working-end determines whether it can be used subgingivally beneath the gingival margin or is restricted to supragingival use. At first, understanding cross sections may seem difficult, but looking at an everyday object should help you to understand this concept.

Creating a Cross Section. Imagine sawing a lead pencil into two parts by cutting it in the middle perpendicular to the long axis of the pencil. When the pencil has been cut, it is possible to view its shape in cross section.

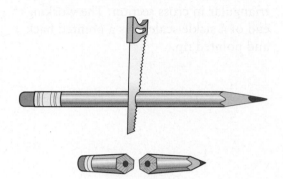

Viewing the Cross Section. The pencil is hexagonal in cross section. (A hexagon is a six-sided figure.)

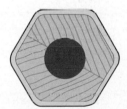

Instrument Working-Ends in Cross Section. In a similar manner, imagine cutting the working-ends of these instruments in half. After the cut is made, the cross sections of the working-ends are visible.

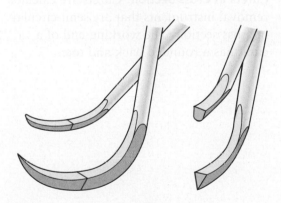

Shape of Working-Ends in Cross Section. The top instrument is semi-circular in cross section. The bottom instrument is triangular in cross section.

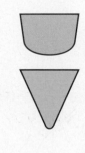

terminal shank will be parallel to long axis of tooth

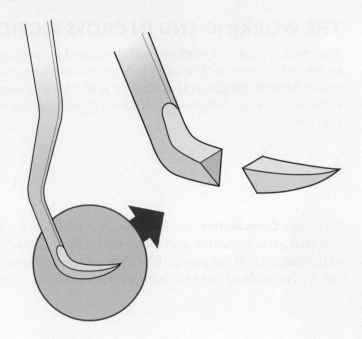

Sickle Scalers in Cross Section. Sickle scalers are calculus removal instruments that are triangular in cross section. The working-end of a sickle scaler has a pointed back and pointed tip.

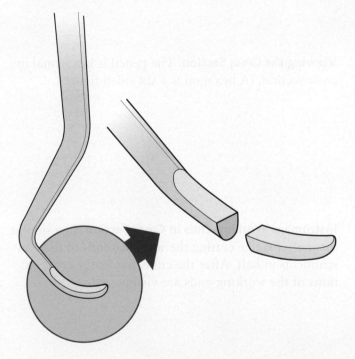

Curets in Cross Section. Curets are calculus removal instruments that are semi-circular in cross section. The working-end of a curet has a rounded back and toe.

Section 4
Introduction to Instrument Classification

Periodontal instruments are divided into types, or classifications, based on the specific design characteristics of the working-ends. This section presents a basic introduction to instrument classification; detailed information about each of the different instrumentation classifications is presented in later modules. Nonsurgical, hand-activated periodontal instruments are classified as periodontal probes, explorers, sickle scalers, periodontal files, curets, hoes, or chisels. Hoes and chisels are rarely used; mechanized instruments have largely replaced their function.

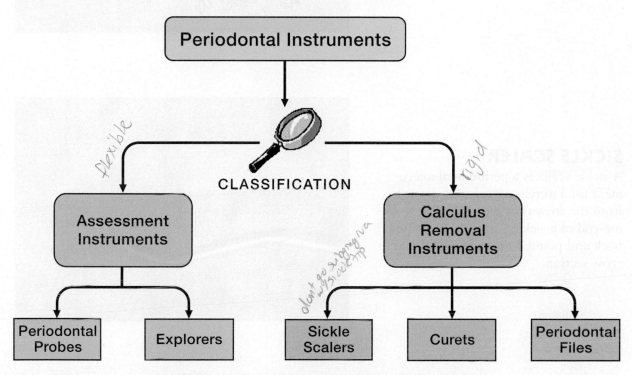

Classification of Hand-Activated Periodontal Instruments

PERIODONTAL PROBE
The periodontal probe is a slender assessment instrument used to evaluate the health of the periodontal tissues. Probes have blunt, rod-shaped working-ends that are circular or rectangular in cross section.

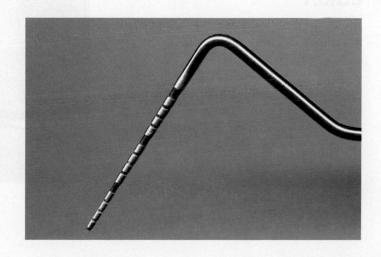

EXPLORER

An explorer is an assessment instrument used to locate calculate deposits, tooth surface irregularities, defective margins on restorations, and carious lesions. Explorers have flexible shanks and are circular in cross section.

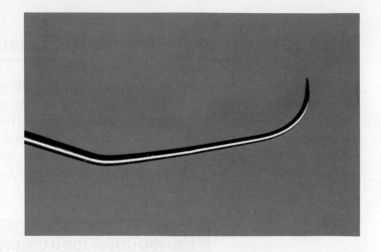

SICKLE SCALER

A sickle scaler is a periodontal instrument used to remove calculus deposits from the crowns of the teeth. The working-end of a sickle scaler has a pointed back and pointed tip and is triangular in cross section.

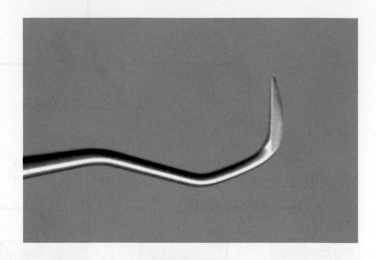

CURET

A curet is a periodontal instrument used to remove calculus deposits from the crowns and roots of the teeth. The working-end of a curet has a rounded back and rounded toe and is semi-circular in cross section. Two curet sub-types are the universal curet and area-specific curet.

2 cutting edges

only one cutting edge

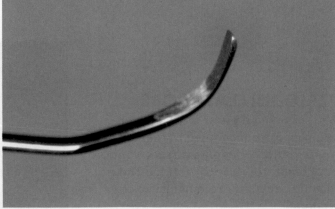

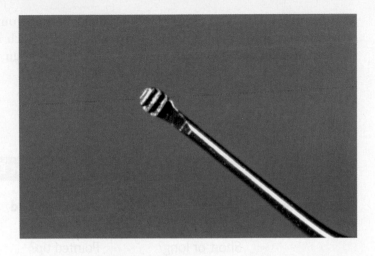

PERIODONTAL FILES

A **periodontal file** is an instrument used to crush large calculus deposits. Each working-end of a periodontal file has several cutting edges.

Section 5
Skill Application

PRACTICAL FOCUS

1. Use nail polish to identify the design elements of several periodontal instruments.

Equipment: Ask your instructor to help you assemble the following instruments—a sickle scaler, a universal curet, and an area-specific curet.

Materials: Four bottles of nail polish in different colors and nail polish remover or orange solvent (to remove nail polish from your instruments at the completion of this activity).

a. Paint the lateral surfaces of each working-end with one color of nail polish.

b. Use a contrasting color of polish to paint the face of each instrument.

c. Paint the functional shank on each instrument. Compare the functional shank lengths on the various instruments.

d. Use a contrasting color of polish to paint the lower shank on each instrument.

e. Ask an instructor to check your work.

2. Assemble a variety of periodontal instruments from your instrument kit, including assessment and calculus removal instruments. For each instrument, determine its classification and intended use by evaluating the design features of the shank and working-end. Enter the information in Table 7-3.

TABLE 7-3. Evaluation of Instrument Design and Classification				
Instrument	**Shank** Simple or complex? Short or long?	**Working-End** Rounded toe? Pointed tip?	**Classification**	**Instrument Use** Assessment? Calculus removal?
A				
B				
C				
D				
E				
F				
G				
H				
I				
J				
K				
L				
M				
N				

SKILL EVALUATION MODULE 7   INSTRUMENT DESIGN AND CLASSIFICATION

Student: _____

Evaluator: _____

Date: _____

Instrument 1 = _____

Instrument 2 = _____

Instrument 3 = _____

Instrument 4 = _____

Instrument 5 = _____

DIRECTIONS FOR STUDENT: Use **Column S.** Evaluate your skill level as: **S** (satisfactory) or **U** (unsatisfactory).

DIRECTIONS FOR EVALUATOR: Use **Column E.** Indicate: **S** (satisfactory) or **U** (unsatisfactory). Each **S** equals 1 point, each **U** equals 0 points.

CRITERIA:	1 S	1 E	2 S	2 E	3 S	3 E	4 S	4 E	5 S	5 E
Instrument										
Identifies each working-end by its design name and number										
Determines whether the instrument is balanced										
Working-End										
Identifies the classification of each working-end										
Identifies parts of the working-end (face, back, lateral surfaces, tip or toe, cutting edges)										
States the shape of the working-end in cross section										
Shank										
Identifies the functional shank										
Identifies the lower shank										
Identifies the shank as simple or complex										
OPTIONAL GRADE PERCENTAGE CALCULATION Total **S**'s in each E column.										

Sum of **S**'s _____ divided by Total Points Possible (**40**) equals the Percentage Grade _____%

SKILL EVALUATION MODULE 7 | INSTRUMENT DESIGN AND CLASSIFICATION

Student: _____

EVALUATOR COMMENTS

_____

_____

_____

_____

_____

_____

_____

_____

_____

_____

_____

_____

_____

_____

_____

_____

_____

_____

Box for sketches pertaining to written comments.

Adaptation and Angulation

Module Overview

Moving the instrument working-end end over the tooth surface to produce an instrumentation stroke is a motor skill that is comprised of several small motor skills. Before you can move the working-end across the tooth surface, you need to learn how to position the working-end in relation to the tooth surface. The two skills used in positioning the working-end—adaptation and angulation—are introduced in this module. Other elements of the instrumentation stroke are covered in Modules 9 and 10.

Adaptation refers to the positioning of the first 1 or 2 millimeters of the lateral surface in contact with the tooth. Angulation refers to the relation between the face of a calculus removal instrument and the tooth surface to which it is applied. For successful instrumentation, correct adaptation and angulation of the working-end must be maintained throughout the instrumentation stroke.

Module Outline

Key Terms

Adaptation

Leading-third of working-end

Toe-third of working-end

Tip-third of working-end

Lower shank parallel

Shank "goes up and over the tooth"

Shank "goes down and around the tooth"

Angulation

Insertion

0- to 40-degree angle

45- to 90-degree angle

Closed angle

Learning Objectives

1. Identify the leading-, middle-, and heel-third of the working-end on a sickle scaler and curet.

2. Using a typodont and an anterior sickle scaler, describe and demonstrate correct adaptation of the working-end.

3. Using a typodont and a curet, describe and demonstrate insertion of the instrument working-end beneath the gingival margin.

4. Using a typodont, describe and demonstrate correct angulation for calculus removal.

5. Given a universal curet and a typodont, select the correct working-end for use on the distal surface of a mandibular posterior tooth.

Section 1
Adaptation

INTRODUCTION TO ADAPTATION

Adaptation is the positioning of the first 1 or 2 millimeters of the working-end's lateral surface in contact with the tooth.

1. Correct adaptation of the working-end to the tooth surface requires positioning the working-end so that only the *leading section of the working-end* is in contact with the tooth surface.
   a. Calculus removal instruments—for proper adaptation, only the toe-third or tip-third of the working-end is kept in contact with the tooth surface.
   b. Explorers—for proper adaptation, only one-third of the tip-side of the explorer is kept in contact with the tooth surface.
2. For successful instrumentation, adaptation of the leading-third of the working-end must be maintained throughout the instrumentation stroke. Two examples of working-end adaptation are shown below.

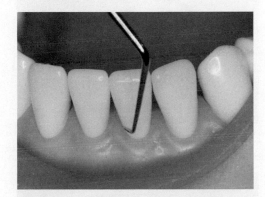

Adaptation of an Explorer. The first few millimeters of the side of the explorer working-end are adapted against the line angle of the incisor.

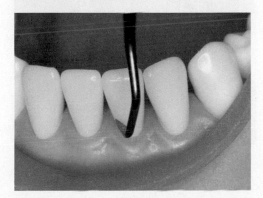

Adaptation of a Sickle Scaler. Adaptation of the tip-third of a sickle scaler to the line angle of the incisor.

THE LEADING-THIRD OF THE WORKING-END

A working-end has three imaginary sections: (1) the leading-third, (2) the middle-third, and (3) the heel-third. The leading-third is the portion of the working-end that is kept in contact with the tooth surface during instrumentation.

On curets, the leading-third is termed the toe-third of the working-end.

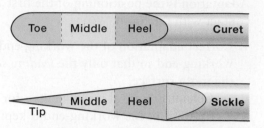

On sickle scalers, the leading-third is termed the tip-third of the working-end.

Correct Adaptation. The tip-third of this sickle scaler is correctly adapted to the tooth surface in this photograph.

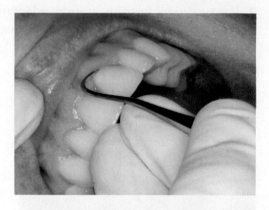

Incorrect Adaptation. Here, the middle-third of the working-end, rather than the tip-third, is incorrectly adapted to the tooth. Note how the instrument tip is sticking out and could cut the soft tissue (ouch!).

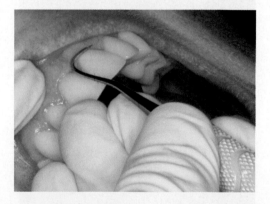

TECHNIQUE PRACTICE: ADAPTATION TO THE TOOTH CROWN

Directions:
1. Assemble the following equipment: anterior sickle scaler and dental typodont.
2. Treatment Area:
   RIGHT-Handed clinician: Mandibular anteriors, facial surfaces TOWARD your nondominant hand
   LEFT-Handed clinician: Mandibular anteriors, facial surfaces AWAY FROM your nondominant hand
3. Remember: "Me, My Patient, My Light, My Dominant Hand, My Nondominant Hand."

Right-Handed Clinicians   Left-Handed Clinicians

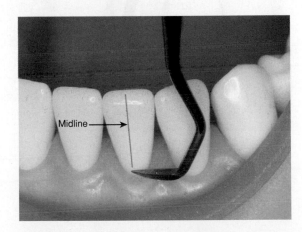

Practice Correct Adaptation on the Facial Surface.
1. Adapt the tip-third of a sickle scaler to the midline of the incisor.
2. Because you are working on the surfaces toward the tip of the instrument should be pointing toward your nondominant hand.
3. Note that the middle- and heel-thirds of the working-end are NOT in contact with the tooth surface.

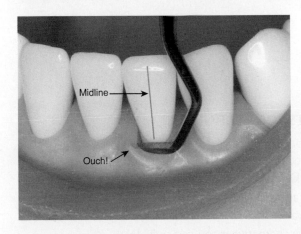

Experience the Results of Incorrect Adaptation at the Midline.
1. Adapt the middle-third of the working-end to the tooth.
2. Look carefully at the instrument, and note that now the tip-third of the working-end is not adapted to the tooth. In fact, it is sticking out.
3. What would happen if a curet were incorrectly adapted in this manner when working beneath the gingival margin?

Practice Correct Adaptation on the Line Angle.

1. Adapt the tip-third of a sickle scaler to the disto-facial line angle of the incisor.
2. Note that the middle- and heel-thirds of the working-end are not adapted to the tooth.

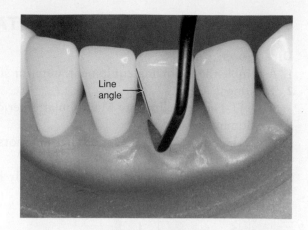

Experience the Results of Incorrect Adaptation at the Line Angle.

1. Adapt the middle-third of the working-end to the distofacial line angle.
2. This incorrect adaptation is a mistake commonly made by beginning clinicians when moving from the facial surface onto the distal surface.
3. Can you see why this is not the correct technique for adaptation?

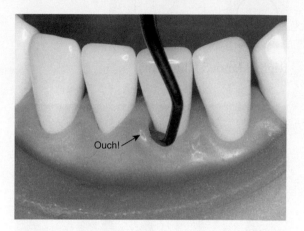

NOTE TO COURSE INSTRUCTOR: TYPODONTS FOR TECHNIQUE PRACTICE

One excellent source of periodontal typodonts for technique practice is Kilgore International, Inc. Telephone (800) 892-9999 or online at http://www.kilgoreinternational.com. The company has a dental hygiene typodont with flexible gingiva and synthetic calculus, as well as a variety of other periodontal typodonts with flexible gingiva.

If your school does not have typodonts, an inexpensive alternative is to use acrylic teeth with anatomically correct roots. The student holds the tooth with the nondominant hand and an instrument with the dominant hand. Of course, this method is not as realistic as using typodonts for technique practice.

Section 2
Selecting the Correct Working-End

INTRODUCTION: USE OF DOUBLE-ENDED INSTRUMENT ON POSTERIORS

Before using a double-ended instrument on a posterior tooth, the clinician must first determine which working-end to use. To select the correct working-end, the clinician observes the relation of the lower shank to the distal surface of the tooth. When the correct working-end is adapted to the distal surface, the lower shank will be parallel to the distal surface (Box 8-1).

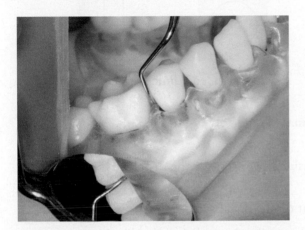

Correct Working-End. This photograph shows working-end 1 of the instrument adapted to the distal surface of the first premolar.

This is the correct working-end because the **lower shank is parallel** to the distal surface.

VISUAL CLUE: The *lower shank* is parallel to the proximal surface, and the *functional shank* "goes up and over the tooth".

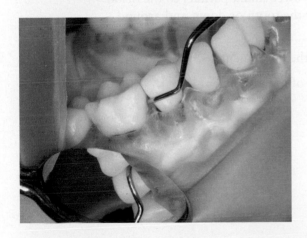

Incorrect Working-End. This photograph shows working-end 2 of the instrument adapted to the distal surface of the first premolar.

This is the incorrect working-end because the lower shank is not parallel to the proximal surface.

VISUAL CLUE: The *lower shank* is not parallel, and the *functional shank* is "down and around the tooth".

Box 8-1. Rule for Working-End Selection on Posterior Teeth

When the working-end is adapted to the distal surface, the correct working-end has the following relationship between the shank and the tooth:

- Lower shank is parallel to the distal surface
- Functional shank goes up and over the tooth

Think: Posterior = Parallel. Functional shank up and over!

TECHNIQUE PRACTICE: WORKING-END SELECTION, POSTERIOR TEETH

Directions

1. **Instrument:** Ask your instructor to help you pick an instrument for this technique practice. Use a universal curet, such as a Barnhart 1/2 or a Columbia 13/14. If you do not have a universal curet in your instrument kit, you can use a Langer 1/2 or a posterior sickle.

2. Position yourself for the quadrant shown in the icons below.

Right-Handed Clinicians   Left-Handed Clinicians

3. Remember: "Me, My Patient, My Light, My Dominant Hand, My Nondominant Hand."

4. Grasp the curet in your dominant hand and establish a finger rest for the distal surface of the first premolar.

5. Randomly place one working-end of the instrument on the distal surface.

6. Assess the visual clues for this working-end. Is the lower shank parallel to the distal surface? Does the functional shank go up and over the tooth or down and around the tooth?

7. Repeat the process with the other working-end of the instrument.

8. Based on the visual clues, the correct working-end of the instrument is
_____.

9. Ask your instructor to check your results.

Section 3
Angulation

INTRODUCTION TO ANGULATION

Angulation is the relation between the face of a calculus removal instrument and the tooth surface to which it is applied.

1. For insertion beneath the gingival margin, the *face-to-tooth surface angulation* should be an angle <u>between 0 and 40 degrees</u>.
2. For calculus removal, the *face-to-tooth surface angulation* should be an angle <u>between 45 and 90 degrees</u>.
3. For successful instrumentation, correct angulation of the working-end must be maintained throughout the instrumentation stroke.

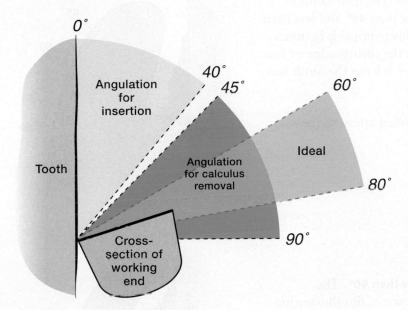

Angulation of the Working-End. The *face-to-tooth surface angulation* for insertion beneath the gingival margin is an angle between 0° and 40°.

The *face-to-tooth surface angulation* for calculus removal is an angle greater than 45° and less than 90°. An angulation between 60° and 80° is ideal for calculus removal.

ANGULATION FOR INSERTION BENEATH THE GINGIVAL MARGIN

Insertion is the action of moving the working-end beneath the gingival margin into the sulcus or pocket.

1. Care must be used during insertion when the gingival margin is closely adapted to the tooth. Curets are the primary calculus removal instruments for subgingival instrumentation.
2. The working-end is inserted at an angle between 0 and 40 degrees. This 0- to 40-degree angle is referred to as a **closed angle**.

Closed Angulation for Insertion. For insertion, position the instrument face as close to the tooth surface as possible. In this position, the curet is moved gently beneath the gingival margin and down the surface of the root to the base of the pocket.

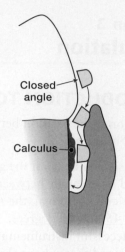

Closed angle

Calculus

ANGULATION FOR CALCULUS REMOVAL

Close-Up View of Correct Angulation. The *face-to-tooth surface angulation* should be greater than 45° and less than 90°. The ideal angulation for calculus removal is between 60°and 80°. This angulation allows the cutting edge to bite into the calculus deposit and fracture it from the tooth surface.

Note that the working-end is positioned apical to (below) the calculus deposit.

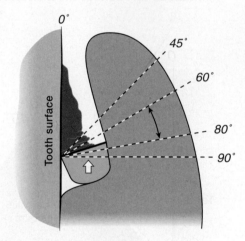

Incorrect Angulation—Angle Greater than 90°. The *face-to-tooth surface angulation* shown in this illustration is greater than 90°. The face is tilted away from the root surface. In this position, calculus removal will be difficult and tissue trauma is likely.

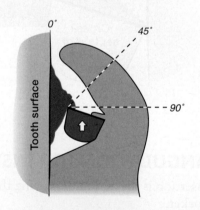

Incorrect Angulation—Angle Less than 45°. The *face-to-tooth surface angulation* shown here is less than 45°. The face is tilted too close to the root surface. In this position, the cutting edge cannot bite into the deposit; instead, it will slip over the calculus deposit.

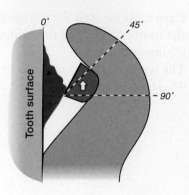

Section 4
Technique Practice

INSERTION ON A DISTAL SURFACE

Equipment: Periodontal typodont and a universal curet. *If the typodont has removable gingiva, remove it so that you can see the working-end of the instrument on the root.*

Right-Handed Clinicians   Left-Handed Clinicians

1. **Prepare:** *Me. My patient. My light. My dominant hand. My non-dominant hand.*
2. **Establish a Finger Rest.** Keep your fulcrum finger **out of the line of fire** by establishing a finger rest near but not directly over surface to be instrumented.

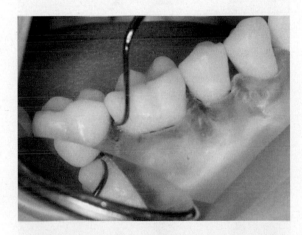

3. **Get Ready.**
   - Turn the toe of working-end toward the distal surface.
   - Place the working-end in the Get Ready Zone. *The Get Ready Zone is the middle-third of the crown.* In this case, the Get Ready Zone is at the distofacial line angle in the middle-third of the crown.

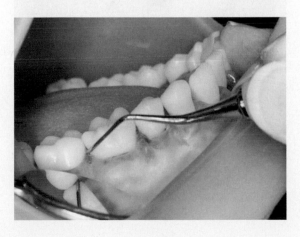

4. **Prepare for Insertion.**
   - Lower your hand and the instrument handle *until the face-to-tooth surface angulation is near to 0-degrees.*
   - *The face of the instrument should hug the distal surface.*

5. Insert.
  * Maintaining your hand position gently slide the working-end beneath the gingival margin and onto the distal surface of the root.
  * *Imagine the face of the working-end sliding along the distal surface, all the way to the base of the pocket*

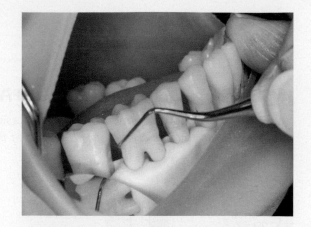

6. Establish Angulation. Establish an 80-degree instrument face-to-root surface angulation *by tilting the lower shank slightly toward the distal surface.*

Shank Tilt. The face of a universal curet is at a 90-degee angle to the lower shank. This means that the curet face and shank are tilted toward the tooth surface to achieve correct angulation.

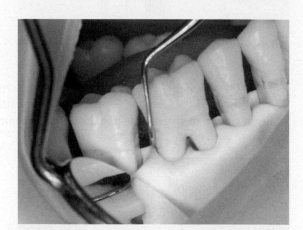

7. Lock on Toe-Third. Adapt the toe-third of the working-end to the distal surface of the root. *Imagine "locking the toe-third" against the tooth surface.*

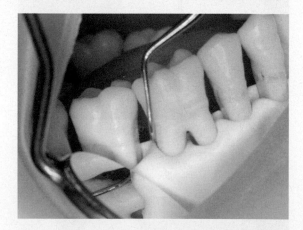

INSERTION ON THE FACIAL SURFACE

Equipment: Periodontal typodont and a universal curet. *If the typodont has removable gingiva, remove it so that you can see the working-end of the instrument on the root.*

Right-Handed Clinicians   Left-Handed Clinicians

1. **Prepare:** *Me. My patient. My light. My dominant hand. My non-dominant hand*
2. **Establish a Finger Rest.** Keep your fulcrum finger **out of the line of fire** by establishing a finger rest near but not directly over surface to be instrumented.

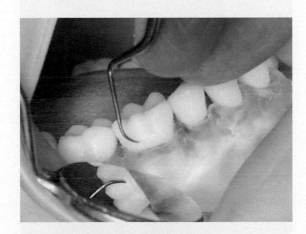

3. **Get Ready.**
   - Turn the working-end so that the toe of the curet is "pointing toward" the front of the mouth.
   - Place the working-end in the Get Ready Zone on the middle-third of the facial surface.

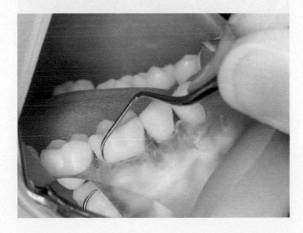

4. **Prepare for Insertion.**
   - Lower your hand and the instrument handle until the curet toe is pointing toward the gingival margin.
   - Insert at a 0-degree angulation with the lower shank close to the tooth.
   - *The face of the instrument should hug the facial surface.*

5. Insert.
- Maintaining your hand position gently slide the working-end beneath the gingival margin and onto the facial surface of the root.
- *Imagine the face sliding along the distal surface all the way to the base of the pocket*

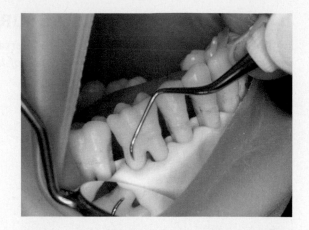

6. Establish Angulation. Establish an 80-degree instrument face-to-root surface angulation *by tilting the lower shank slightly toward the facial surface.*

Shank Tilt. The face of a universal curet is at a 90-degee angle to the lower shank. This means that the curet face and shank are tilted toward the tooth surface to achieve correct angulation.

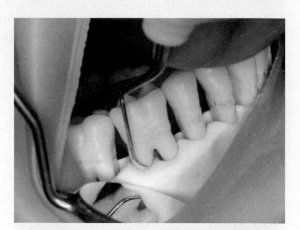

7. Lock on Toe-Third. Adapt the toe-third of the working-end to the facial surface of the root. *Imagine "locking the toe-third" against the tooth surface.*

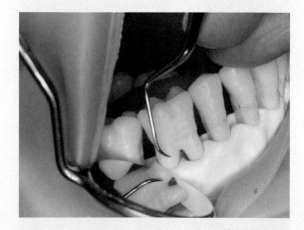

FLOW CHART: PREPARATION FOR INSTRUMENTATION

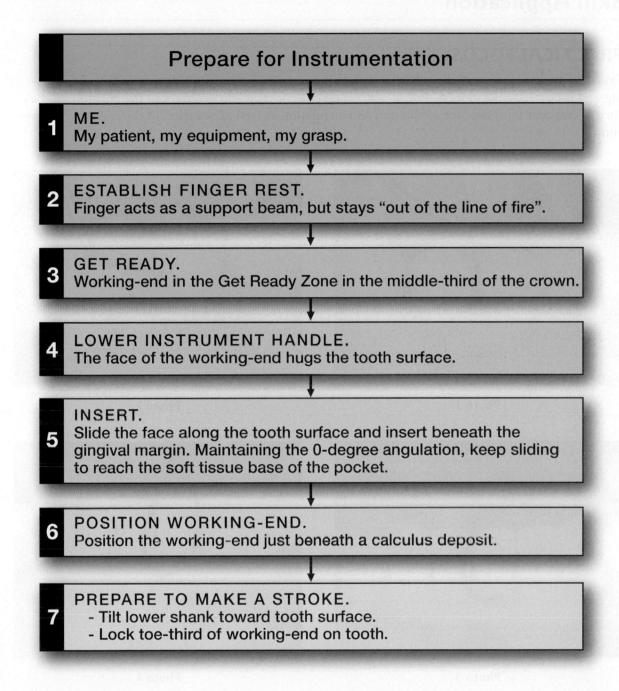

Prepare for Instrumentation

1 ME.
My patient, my equipment, my grasp.

2 ESTABLISH FINGER REST.
Finger acts as a support beam, but stays "out of the line of fire".

3 GET READY.
Working-end in the Get Ready Zone in the middle-third of the crown.

4 LOWER INSTRUMENT HANDLE.
The face of the working-end hugs the tooth surface.

5 INSERT.
Slide the face along the tooth surface and insert beneath the gingival margin. Maintaining the 0-degree angulation, keep sliding to reach the soft tissue base of the pocket.

6 POSITION WORKING-END.
Position the working-end just beneath a calculus deposit.

7 PREPARE TO MAKE A STROKE.
- Tilt lower shank toward tooth surface.
- Lock toe-third of working-end on tooth.

Section 5
Skill Application

PRACTICAL FOCUS

Evaluate the positioning of the working-end in photographs 1 through 4. Indicate (1) if the working-end is correctly positioned, and, if not, (2) describe what is incorrect about the positioning. Be sure to consider working-end adaptation and angulation as well as selection of the correct working-end.

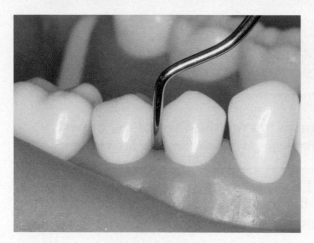

Photo 1

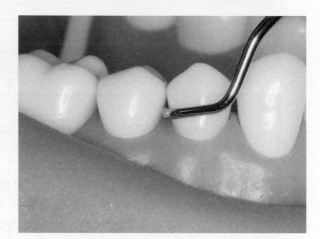

Photo 2

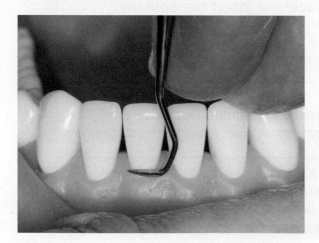

Photo 3

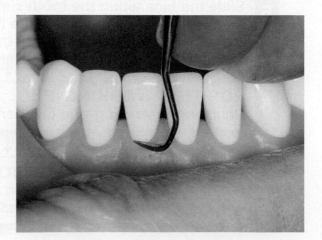

Photo 4

| SKILL EVALUATION MODULE 8 | ADAPTATION AND ANGULATION |

Student: _____

Evaluator: _____

Date: _____

DIRECTIONS FOR STUDENT: Use **Column S.** Evaluate your skill level as: **S** (satisfactory) or **U** (unsatisfactory).

DIRECTIONS FOR EVALUATOR: Use **Column E.** Indicate: **S** (satisfactory) or **U** (unsatisfactory). Each **S** equals 1 point, each **U** equals 0 points.

CRITERIA	S	E
Identifies the 1) tip-third or toe-third, 2) middle-third, and 3) heel-third of the cutting edge on a sickle scaler and a curet		
Using a typodont and an anterior sickle scaler, adapts the tip-third of the cutting edge to a canine and establishes correct face-to-tooth angulation		
Given a universal curet, selects the correct working-end for use on the distal surface of a mandibular premolar or molar		
Using a typodont and a curet, demonstrates a face-to-tooth angulation of 0– to 40-degrees (for insertion)		
Using a typodont and a curet, demonstrates a face-to-tooth angulation of less than 45-degrees (incorrect angulation)		
Using a typodont and a curet, demonstrates a face-to-tooth angulation of 90-degrees (incorrect angulation)		
Using a typodont and a curet, demonstrates a face-to-tooth angulation between 45- and 90 degrees (correct angulation for calculus removal)		
Demonstrates insertion and preparation for an instrumentation stroke in a step-by-step manner on a periodontal typodont with flexible "gingiva".		
OPTIONAL GRADE PERCENTAGE CALCULATION Total **S**'s in each E column.		

Sum of **S**'s _____ divided by Total Points Possible (**8**) equals the Percentage Grade _____%

| SKILL EVALUATION MODULE 8 | ADAPTATION AND ANGULATION |

Student: _____

EVALUATOR COMMENTS

_____

_____

_____

_____

_____

_____

_____

_____

_____

_____

_____

_____

_____

_____

_____

_____

_____

Box for sketches pertaining to written comments.

Activation, Pivot, and Handle Roll

Module Overview

Motion activation, the hand pivot, and the handle roll are three motor skills used to produce an instrumentation stroke. The first section of this module discusses how to move the instrument to produce a stroke. The second section explains how to pivot the hand and roll the instrument handle to maintain adaptation as the working-end moves around the tooth.

General recommendations for stroke production may not be suitable for everyone. If you experience any discomfort, consult a physician.

Module Outline

Key Terms

Motion activation   Pivoting
Wrist motion activation   Handle roll
Digital motion activation   Drive finger

Learning Objectives

1. Stabilize the hand and instrument to perform an instrumentation stroke by using an appropriate intraoral fulcrum and the ring finger as a "support beam" for the hand.

2. Define and demonstrate wrist motion activation.

3. Define and demonstrate digital motion activation.

4. Define and demonstrate the hand pivot and handle roll to maintain working-end adaptation to the tooth surface.

Section 1
Moving the Working-End

INTRODUCTION TO MOTION ACTIVATION

Motion activation is the act of moving the instrument to produce an instrumentation stroke on the tooth surface.

1. Two types of motion activation commonly used in periodontal instrumentation are wrist motion activation and digital motion activation.
2. As you move the instrument, your fulcrum finger supports the weight of your hand.
   a. When you initiate (begin) a stroke, press down with your fulcrum finger against the tooth; this action allows the fulcrum to function as a brake to allow you to stop the stroke.
   b. If you fly off the tooth at the end of a stroke, you did not stop the stroke by pressing down on your fulcrum.
3. It is important to remember that instrumentation strokes are tiny movements. You move the working-end only a few millimeters with each stroke.

On the following pages, you will practice using wrist motion activation and digital motion activation. In the Technique Practice, the movements you will make will be broad, large movements compared with the actual movements used to instrument a tooth.

WRIST MOTION ACTIVATION

Wrist motion activation is the act of rotating the hand and wrist as a unit to provide the power for an instrumentation stroke.

1. This movement is a rotating motion similar to the action of turning a doorknob.
2. Wrist motion activation is recommended for calculus removal with hand-activated instruments.
   a. This type of motion activation allows the clinician to use the power of the hand and wrist to move the instrument. Together, the hand and wrist are stronger than the fingers.
   b. You will experience less fatigue with wrist activation than would occur if you used your fingers to move the instrument for calculus removal.

A Technique Practice designed to help you experience wrist motion activation is found on the next page of this module.

TECHNIQUE PRACTICE: WRIST MOTION ACTIVATION

Technique Hint: Wrist motion activation is similar to the action of turning a doorknob.

1. Grasp a pencil or probe with a modified pen grasp in your *dominant hand*. The photographs show a right-handed clinician.

2. Place your ring finger on a countertop. Your thumb, middle, and index fingers should be in a curved position and relaxed. Your ring finger is straight and acts as a support beam for your hand.

3. Grasp a pencil in a modified pen grasp and establish a finger rest on a countertop. The pencil tip should be touching the countertop, and the long axis of the pencil should be perpendicular ($\perp$) to the countertop. Your wrist should be in neutral position so that the back of your hand and wrist are in straight alignment and your arm is parallel ($=$) to the countertop.

4. The photograph below shows the starting position, Position A, when viewed from behind.

5. Use wrist motion activation to move the pencil tip off of the counter, by rotating your hand and wrist away from your body into Position B shown below. Right-handed clinicians will rotate the hand and wrist to the right in a clockwise direction. Left-handed clinicians will rotate the hand and wrist to the left in a counter-clockwise direction. Your ring finger should remain motionless pressing down against the countertop.

6. Return the pencil to Position A by rotating your hand and wrist back toward your body.

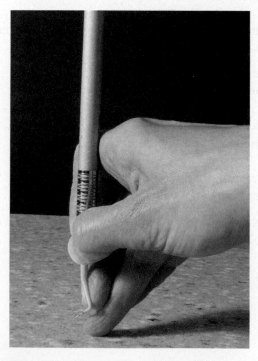

Position A. Starting position of your hand and wrist.

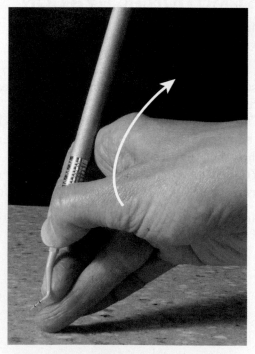

Position B. Finishing position of your hand and wrist.

DIGITAL MOTION ACTIVATION

Digital motion activation is moving the instrument by flexing the thumb, index, and middle fingers.

1. Digital motion activation is used whenever physical strength is not required during instrumentation.
2. It may be used with periodontal probes, explorers, and ultrasonic instruments. With ultrasonic instruments, the machine, not the clinician, provides the force necessary for calculus removal.
3. Digital motion activation also may be used to instrument areas where movement is very restricted, such as when instrumenting furcation areas.

TECHNIQUE PRACTICE: DIGITAL MOTION ACTIVATION

Technique Hint: Digital motion activation is made with pull-push motions of the thumb, index, and middle fingers.

1. Grasp a pencil or probe with a modified pen grasp in your *dominant hand*.
2. Assume the starting position, Position A. (The photographs show a right-handed clinician.)
3. Use digital motion activation to pull the pencil tip away from the countertop by pulling your thumb, index, and middle fingers toward the palm of your hand into Position B. Your ring finger should remain motionless pressing down against the countertop.
4. Return the pencil tip to Position A by pushing downward with your thumb, index, and middle fingers. Note that you have little strength when using this type of motion activation.

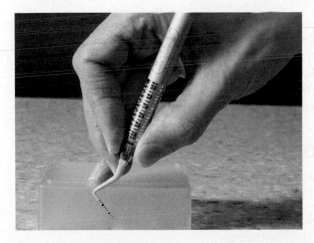

Position A. Starting position of the fingers.

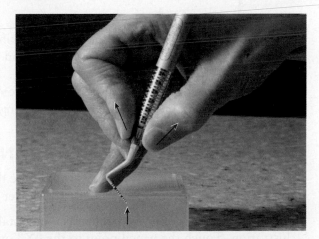

Position B. Finishing position of the fingers.

Section 2
Maintaining Adaptation

THE HAND PIVOT

Pivoting is a swinging motion of the hand and arm carried out by balancing on the fulcrum finger.

1. Pivoting the hand and arm assists the clinician in maintaining adaptation as the working-end moves around the tooth.
2. Neutral wrist position should be maintained during the pivot.
3. Pivoting is used principally when moving around line angles and onto proximal surfaces.

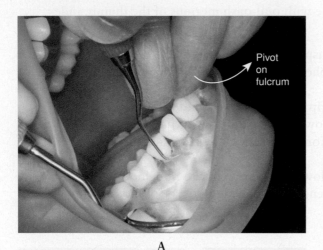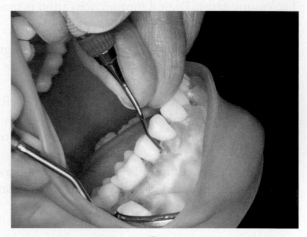

A   B

The Hand Pivot. As the clinician moves the working-end from the lingual surface and onto the proximal, he or she pivots on the fulcrum finger to aid in adaptation. **A,** Starting hand position as the clinician prepares to move on to the mesial surface. **B,** With a slight pivot of the clinician's hand, the working-end moves on to the mesial surface. Note that more of the side of the middle finger is visible in photograph B due to the slight repositioning of the hand.

TECHNIQUE PRACTICE: THE HAND PIVOT

Directions: *RIGHT-handed clinicians* should use the illustration at the *top* of the next page for practice. *LEFT-handed clinicians* should use the lower illustration on the next page for practice.

1. Grasp a pencil in a modified pen grasp and establish a fulcrum in the circle on the illustration. Touch the pencil point to the "**X**" on the illustration.
2. Begin with your hand and arm aligned with dotted line **A.**
3. Push down lightly and pivot on your fulcrum finger as you swing your hand and arm as a unit to align with dotted line **B.** Be sure to maintain neutral wrist position.

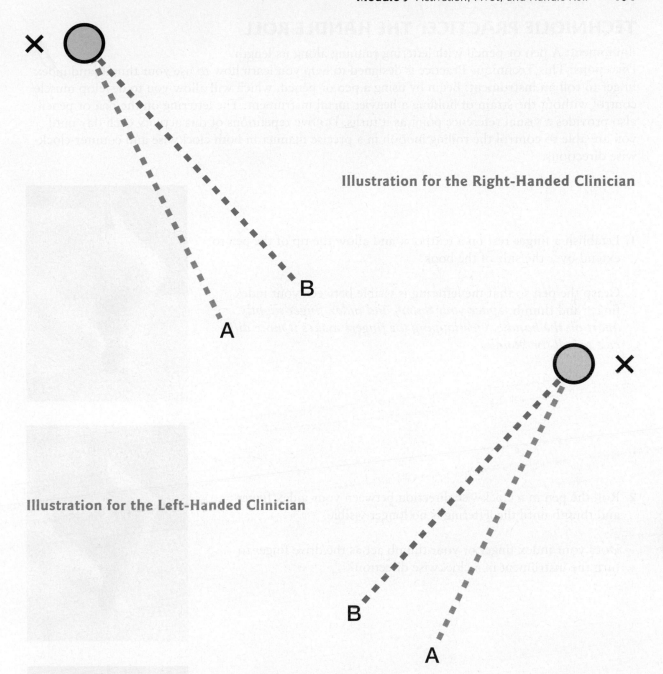

Illustration for the Right-Handed Clinician

Illustration for the Left-Handed Clinician

THE HANDLE ROLL

Handle Roll

The handle roll is the act of turning the instrument handle slightly between the thumb and index finger to readapt the working-end to the next segment of the tooth.

1. As the instrumentation strokes advance around the tooth surface, the working-end constantly is readjusted to maintain adaptation with the tooth surface. These readjustments are accomplished by rolling the instrument handle between strokes.
2. Either the index finger *or* the thumb acts as the **drive finger** to turn the instrument. The finger used to roll the handle determines the direction in which the working-end will turn.

TECHNIQUE PRACTICE: THE HANDLE ROLL

Equipment: A pen or pencil with lettering running along its length.

Directions: This Technique Practice is designed to help you learn how to use your thumb and index finger to roll an instrument. Begin by using a pen or pencil, which will allow you to develop muscle control without the strain of holding a heavier metal instrument. The lettering on the pen or pencil also provides a visual reference point as it turns. Do five repetitions of this activity each day until you are able to control the rolling motion in a precise manner in both clockwise and counter-clockwise directions.

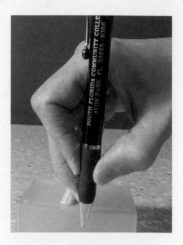

1. Establish a finger rest on a textbook and allow the tip of the pen to extend over the side of the book.

Grasp the pen so that the lettering is visible between your index finger and thumb. *Space your thumb and index finger slightly apart on the handle. Overlapping the fingers makes it more difficult to roll the handle.*

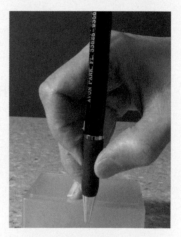

2. Roll the pen in a clockwise direction between your index finger and thumb until the lettering is no longer visible.

Does your index finger or your thumb act as the drive finger to turn the instrument in a clockwise direction?

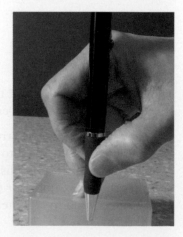

3. Finally, turn the pen in a counter-clockwise direction, back toward the starting position. Continue rolling until the handle has returned to the original starting position.

Does your index finger or your thumb act as the drive finger to turn the instrument in a counter-clockwise direction?

TECHNIQUE PRACTICE: MAINTAINING ADAPTATION

Equipment: an inexpensive pen, an anterior instrument, and a pad of paper

1. Draw a line around the pen about ½ inch (12 millimeters) from the top of the pen (see photographs below).
2. Sit in a comfortable seated position with the paper tablet on your lap. Hold the pen with your *nondominant* hand, and rest the pen point on the paper. The pen represents the tooth.

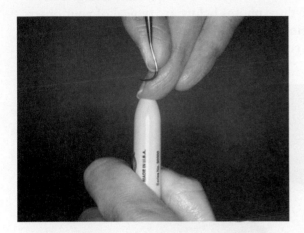

3. Grasp an anterior instrument and establish a finger rest on the edge of the pen top.

4. Adapt the leading-third of the cutting edge just above the line on the pen. (Imagine the line is the base of a periodontal pocket.) Look down at the pen top, and tilt the instrument face toward the pen until the face meets the pen's surface at a 70- to 80-degree angle.

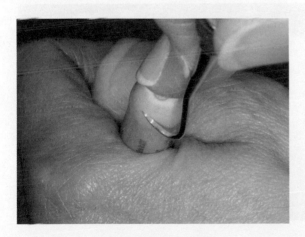

5. Use wrist motion to activate a short (3 mm) instrumentation stroke up the surface of the pen toward the pen top.

6. Make a series of strokes around the circumference of the pen, beginning each stroke near the line on the pen. Roll the instrument handle to keep the leading-third of the cutting edge adapted to the pen.

Section 3
Skill Application

PRACTICAL FOCUS

CASE 1. Your friend Marybeth has difficulty removing calculus on the mandibular teeth. In addition, she frequently lacerates the papillae when working on the mandibular anteriors. Marybeth simply does not know what she is doing wrong! She asks you to observe her in clinic and give her feedback about the problems she is encountering. The three photos below are typical of your observations as Marybeth worked on the mandibular anteriors, facial and lingual aspects. What problems, if any, did your observe? How might Marybeth correct these problems?

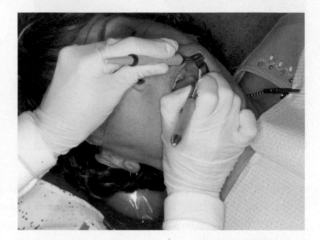

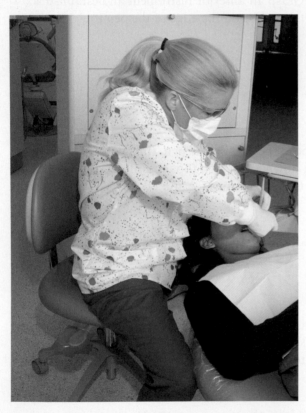

Case I

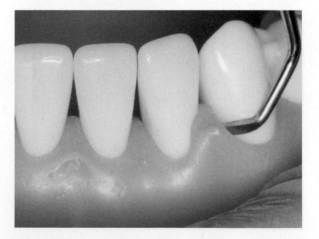

CASE 2. Your class assignment is to observe a classmate, Marie, as she practices determining the correct working-end of an explorer. The three photos on the next page are typical of your observations as Marie worked on the mandibular posterior sextant. (1) Evaluate each photograph. (2) If you find any problems, explain how each problem could be corrected.

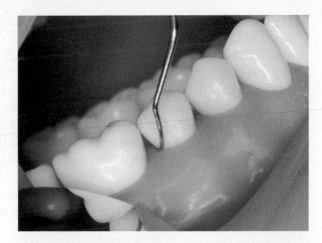

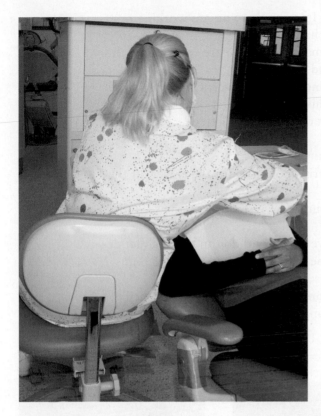

Case 2

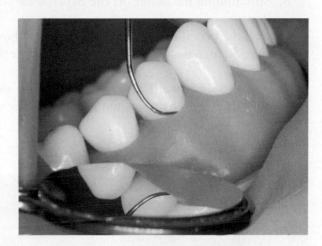

SKILL BUILDING: MAINTAINING ADAPTATION

This activity is designed to help you develop the ability the ability to roll an instrument between your index finger and thumb to maintain adaptation. This activity uses a pencil and an abstract line to provide practice in the handle roll.

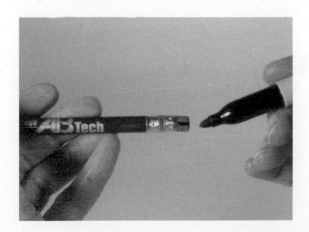

1. **Use a pen to draw a *vertical line* on the eraser.** The line should run vertically from the base of the eraser to the top of the eraser. In this activity, you will try to adapt the vertical mark to the abstract design on the next page.

2. **Hold the pencil in a modified pen grasp.** Assume that the vertical **mark** is the leading-third of the working-end.

3. Right-handed clinicians: Begin near the letter **R**. Imagine that you are working on the anterior surfaces toward your *nondominant* hand.

   Left-handed clinicians: Begin near the letter **L**. Imagine that you are working on the anterior surfaces toward your nondominant hand.

4. **Establish a fulcrum near the end of the abstract line.** Touch the vertical mark on the eraser to the first dot. If you are right-handed, this will be the first dot beside the letter **R**. If you are left-handed, this will be the first dot beside the letter **L**. The **mark** is now adapted to the first dot.

5. **Adapt to the second dot by following these steps:**
   a. Keep your finger rest on the book, and use wrist motion to lift the eraser off the paper.
   b. Still holding the eraser off the paper, slide your finger rest closer to the second dot.
   c. Roll the pencil until the **mark** is directly above the second dot on the abstract design. Return the eraser to the paper so that the mark is adapted to the second dot.

6. **Continue to slide your finger rest as you move along the design,** rolling the pencil to adapt the mark to each dot until you reach the opposite end of the line.

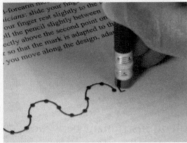 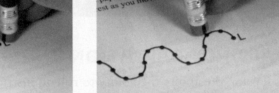 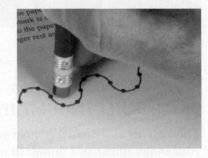

START   CONTINUE   FINISH

SKILL EVALUATION MODULE 9	ACTIVATION, PIVOT, AND HANDLE ROLL

Student: _____

Evaluator: _____

Date: _____

DIRECTIONS FOR STUDENT: Use **Column S.** Evaluate your skill level as: **S** (satisfactory) or **U** (unsatisfactory).

DIRECTIONS FOR EVALUATOR: Use **Column E.** Indicate: **S** (satisfactory) or **U** (unsatisfactory). Each **S** equals 1 point, each **U** equals 0 points.

CRITERIA	S	E
Wrist Motion:		
Uses a pencil to demonstrate wrist motion activation		
Uses modified pen grasp		
Uses ring finger as a support beam		
Maintains neutral wrist position throughout wrist activation		
Digital Motion:		
Uses a pencil to demonstrate digital motion activation		
Uses modified pen grasp		
Uses ring finger as a support beam		
Maintains neutral wrist position throughout digital activation		
Pivot:		
Uses a pencil and the illustration from the Hand Pivot Technique Practice to demonstrate pivoting		
Uses ring finger as a support beam during pivot		
Maintains neutral wrist position during pivot		
Handle Roll:		
Demonstrates rolling a pencil in clockwise and counter-clockwise directions		
Uses modified pen grasp		
Uses ring finger as a support beam		
Maintains neutral wrist position		
OPTIONAL GRADE PERCENTAGE CALCULATION Total **S**'s in each E column.		

Sum of **S**'s _____ divided by Total Points Possible (**12**) equals the Percentage Grade _____

SKILL EVALUATION MODULE 9   ACTIVATION, PIVOT, AND HANDLE ROLL

Student: _____

EVALUATOR COMMENTS

_____
_____
_____
_____
_____
_____
_____
_____
_____
_____
_____
_____
_____
_____
_____
_____
_____
_____

Box for sketches pertaining to written comments.

Instrumentation Strokes

Module Overview

Moving the working-end end over the tooth surface to produce an instrumentation stroke is a complex motor skill. The components of an instrumentation stroke are covered in Modules 8–10. Modules 8 and 9 introduced the concepts of adaptation, angulation, activation, the hand pivot, and handle roll. This module discusses the three types of instrumentation strokes, patterns and directions for making instrumentation strokes.

Module Outline

Key Terms

Assessment stroke

Calculus removal stroke

Root debridement stroke

Burnished deposit

Instrumentation zones

Vertical strokes

Oblique strokes

Horizontal strokes

Learning Objectives

1. Compare and contrast the different types of instrumentation strokes.

2. Differentiate the uses of three instrumentation strokes.

3. Demonstrate vertical, oblique, and horizontal strokes.

4. Demonstrate how to stabilize the hand and instrument to perform an instrumentation stroke by using an appropriate intraoral fulcrum and the ring finger as a "support beam" for the hand.

5. Demonstrate the elements of an assessment stroke in a step-by-step manner.

6. Demonstrate the elements of a calculus removal stroke in a step-by-step manner.

7. Demonstrate the elements of a root debridement stroke in a step-by-step manner.

8. Describe how a deposit of calculus is fractured from a tooth surface and differentiate that from burnishing.

Section 1
Introduction to Instrumentation Strokes

TYPES OF INSTRUMENTATION STROKES

1. **Assessment Stroke.** (Also known as an exploratory stroke)
   - An assessment stroke is used to evaluate the tooth surface. Assessment strokes are used with explorers to locate calculus deposits or other tooth surface irregularities hidden beneath the gingival margin.
   - No pressure is applied against the tooth surface during an assessment stroke. For an assessment stroke, keep the fingers relaxed in the grasp and make feather-light strokes across the tooth surface.

2. **Calculus Removal Stroke.** (Also known as a scaling stroke.)
   - A calculus stroke is used with sickle scalers, universal and area-specific curets to remove calculus deposits from the tooth.
   - A calculus removal is a very short, controlled, biting stroke made with moderate pressure against the tooth surface.
   - Hand activation is used to create a brief, short stroke to snap the deposit from the tooth.
   - A calculus removal stroke is only made in a direction away from the soft tissue base of the pocket.
   - After each calculus removal stroke is made, the clinician should pause, and then use a feather-light assessment stroke to lightly reposition the curet beneath a calculus deposit.
   - Calculus removal strokes are never used on tooth surfaces that are free of calculus deposits.
   - *Use of a curet in a healthy sulcus for the detection of calculus deposits may result in periodontal attachment loss.[1]*
     - *For this reason, dental hygiene students learning to use curets should not practice on student partners who have healthy shallow sulci.*
     - *Periodontal typodonts with flexible "gingiva" are recommended for students learning instrumentation. Periodontal typodonts allow students to practice insertion into periodontal pockets and instrumentation of root surfaces.*

3. **Root Debridement Stroke.** (Also known as a root planing stroke.)
   - The root debridement stroke is used to remove residual calculus deposits, bacterial plaque and byproducts from (1) root surfaces that are exposed in the mouth due to gingival recession or (2) root surfaces within deep periodontal pockets.
   - A root debridement stroke is a shaving stroke made with light pressure against the tooth surface. The root debridement stroke is slightly longer than a calculus removal stroke.
   - Conservation of cementum is a goal of instrumentation. Within deep periodontal pockets, a plastic "implant" curet or a slim-tipped ultrasonic instrument should be used for plaque removal when no calculus deposits are present.

REFERENCE SHEET: CHARACTERISTICS OF INSTRUMENTATION STROKES

TABLE 10-1.	Stroke Characteristics With Hand-Activated Instruments		
	Assessment Stroke	**Calculus Removal Stroke**	**Root Debridement Stroke**
Purpose	To assess tooth anatomy; detect calculus and other plaque-retentive factors	To lift calculus deposits off of the tooth surface	To remove residual calculus; disrupt bacterial plaque from root surfaces within deep periodontal pockets
Used with	Probes/explorers, curets	Sickle scalers, curets, files	Curets
Insertion	0° to 40°	0° to 40°	0° to 40°
Working angulation	50° to 70°	70° to 80°	60° to 70°
Lateral pressure	Contacts tooth surface, but no pressure	Moderate pressure	Light pressure
Character	Flowing, feather-light stroke of moderate length	Brief, tiny biting stroke to snap a calculus deposit from tooth	Lighter shaving stroke of moderate length
Direction	Vertical, oblique, and horizontal	Vertical, oblique, and horizontal	Vertical, oblique, and horizontal
Number	Many, to evaluate the entire root surface	Limited to areas where needed	Many, covering entire root surface

Section 2
Technique Practice: Assessment/Exploratory Stroke With an Explorer

Directions:

- *For this technique practice, you will be working on the* mandibular right first molar, facial aspect.
- *Use a* periodontal typodont with flexible "gingiva" *so that you can practice as if working in a deep periodontal pocket. Use an* explorer *such as an* 11/12-type explorer *for this technique practice.*

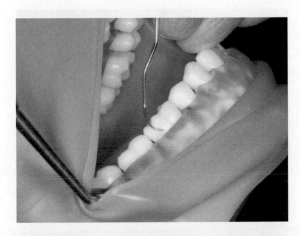

1. **Get Ready.** Place the working-end of the explorer in the Get Ready Zone in the middle-third of the crown.

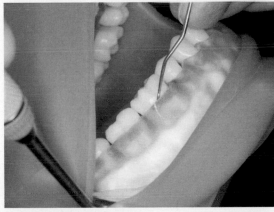

2. **Insert.** Slide the tip of the explorer beneath the gingival margin.
   - When working on a periodontal typodont, insert the tip of the explorer well into the "periodontal pocket".
   - *In a real mouth, the explorer is inserted until the back of the explorer tip touches the junctional epithelium at the base of the pocket.*

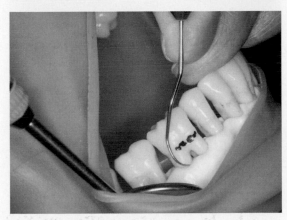

3. **Prepare for Stroke: Position the Working-End.** Place the *toe-third of the working-end (side of the tip—not the point)* against the tooth surface.

4. Make a Stroke.
- Make an instrumentation stroke, away from the soft tissue at the base of the pocket.
- *Assessment strokes are feather-light strokes.*
- Keep the fingers in your grasp very relaxed when making assessment strokes.
- A tight grasp will prevent you from feeling calculus deposits.

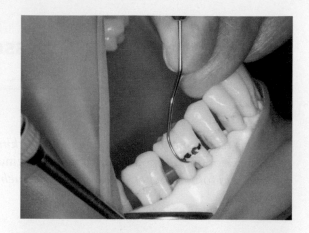

5. Stop the Stroke.
- End each stroke just beneath the gingival margin.
- At the gingival margin, do not remove the explorer tip from the pocket. Removing and reinserting with each stroke will traumatize the gingival tissue.

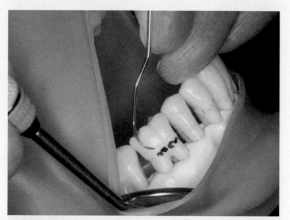

6. Make a Series of Strokes.
- Practice making a series of feather-light strokes across the facial surface.
- Remember to *keep your fingers very relaxed in the grasp.*
- Keep your touch *feather-light against the tooth surface.*

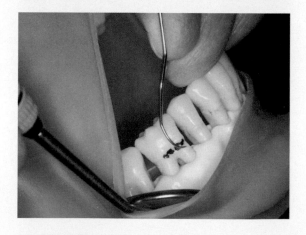

Section 3
Technique Practice: Calculus Removal Stroke With Universal Curet

Directions:

* For *this technique practice, you will be working on the* mandibular right first molar, facial aspect.
* Use *a* periodontal typodont with flexible "gingiva" *so that you can practice as if working in a deep periodontal pocket. Use a* universal curet *for this technique practice.*

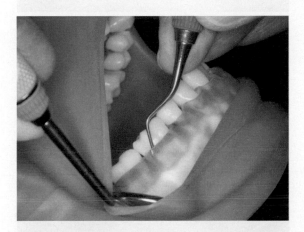

1. **Get Ready and Insert.**
   * Refer to *pages 179 and 180 if you need to review the steps in insertion.*
   * Insert at a 0-degree angulation with the lower shank close to the tooth surface.
   * Gently slide the working-end beneath the gingival margin and onto the facial surface of the root.
   * *Imagine the face sliding along the facial surface all the way to the base of the pocket.*

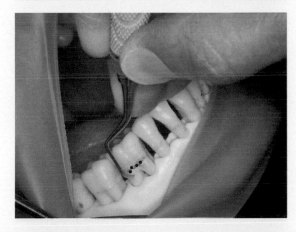

2. **Prepare for Stroke: Position Working-End Beneath Deposit.** Slide the tip of the curet beneath the gingival margin.
   * Slide the working-end up the root until it is positioned just beneath a calculus deposit.
   * If there are no calculus deposits on your typodont, imagine one.

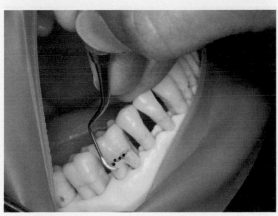

3. **Prepare for Stroke: Tilt the Lower Shank Toward Tooth Surface.**
   * Establish an 80-degree face-to-root surface angulation *by tilting the lower shank toward the facial surface.*
   * The face of a universal curet is at a 90-degee angle to the lower shank. This means that the curet face and shank are tilted toward the root surface to achieve correct angulation.

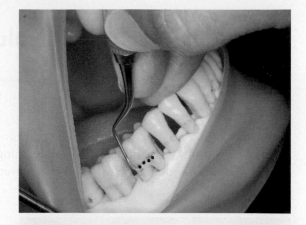

4. **Prepare for Stroke: Lock on Toe-Third.**
   "Lock" the toe-third of the working-end against the facial surface of the root.

5. **Make a Calculus Removal Stroke.**
   - Make an instrumentation stroke, away from the soft tissue at the base of the pocket.
   - Keep the toe-third locked against the facial surface.
   - *Use a tiny, biting stroke upward against the calculus deposit to snap the deposit off of the tooth.*

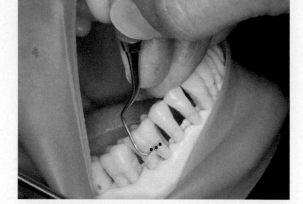

6. **Stop the Stroke.**
   - Each calculus removal stroke should be a short, precise stroke to lift the deposit from the tooth.
   - End each stroke with precision, by pressing down with your fulcrum finger against the occlusolingual surface of the tooth.
   - *Each stroke is distinct; make only one upward stroke and then pause.* **Do NOT make a series of back and forth strokes.**

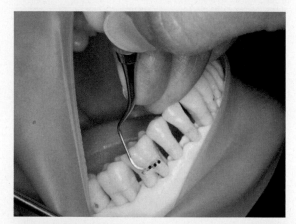

7. **Relax Between Strokes One and Two.**
   - Relax your fingers after a stroke.
   - *Make a single calculus removal stroke, stop the stroke, and immediately relax your fingers.*
   - Pause momentarily after each stroke to prevent strain to the muscles of your hand.
   - *Repeat Step 1.* At a 0-degree angulation, reposition in preparation for a second stroke.

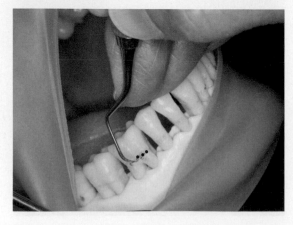

Section 4
Technique Practice: Calculus Removal Stroke With Area-Specific Curet

Directions:

- *For this technique practice, you will be working on the* mandibular right first molar, facial aspect.
- *Use a* periodontal typodont with flexible "gingiva" *so that you can practice as if working in a deep periodontal pocket. Use an* area-specific curet *such as a* Gracey curet *for this technique practice. Ask your instructor for assistance in selecting the correct working-end.*

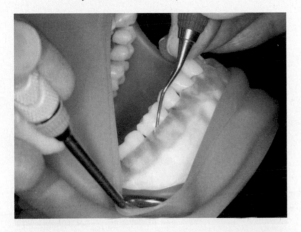

I. Insert.
- *Refer to pages 179 and 180 if you need to review the steps in insertion.*
- Insert at a 0-degree angulation with the lower shank close to the tooth surface.
- Gently slide the working-end beneath the gingival margin and onto the facial surface of the root.
- *Imagine the face sliding along the facial surface all the way to the base of the pocket.*

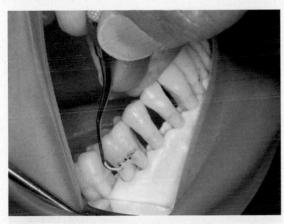

2. Position Working-End Beneath Deposit.
- Slide the working-end up the root until it is positioned just beneath a calculus deposit.
- If there are no calculus deposits on your typodont, imagine one.

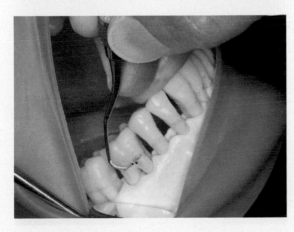

3. Make a Calculus Removal Stroke.
- Tilt shank toward the tooth surface.
- Lock the toe-third against the tooth surface.
- *Make a tiny, biting stroke upward against the calculus deposit.*
- *Repeat Step 1.* At a 0-degree angulation, reposition the working-end in preparation for a second stroke.

Section 5
Technique Practice: Root Debridement Stroke With Area-Specific Curet

Directions:

- *For this technique practice, you will be working on the* mandibular right first molar, facial aspect.
- *Use a* periodontal typodont with flexible "gingiva" *so that you can practice as if working in a deep periodontal pocket. Use an* area-specific curet *such as a* Gracey curet *for this technique practice.*

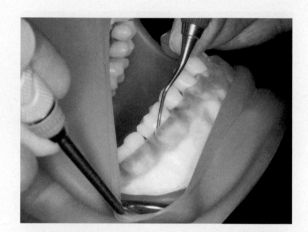

1. **Insert.**
   - Refer to *pages 179 and 180 if you need to review the steps in insertion.*
   - Insert at a 0-degree angulation with the lower shank close to the tooth surface.
   - Gently slide the working-end beneath the gingival margin and onto the facial surface of the root.
   - *Imagine the face sliding along the facial surface all the way to the base of the pocket.*

2. **Prepare for Stroke: Tilt Lower Shank Toward Root Surface.**
   - *A root debridement stroke is a shaving stroke.*
   - To accomplish a shaving stroke, the face should be approximately at a *60 degree angle to the tooth surface.*
   - To create this angulation, simply tilt the lower shank toward the root surface.

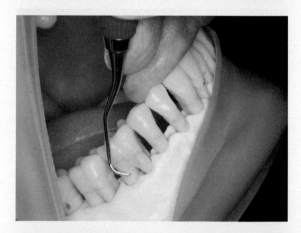

3. **Make a Root Debridement Stroke.**
   - Initiate *a light, shaving stroke away from the base of the pocket.*
   - A root debridement stroke is a *lighter* and *longer stroke* than a calculus removal stroke.
   - *Repeat Step 1.* At a 0-degree angulation, reposition the working-end in preparation for a second stroke.

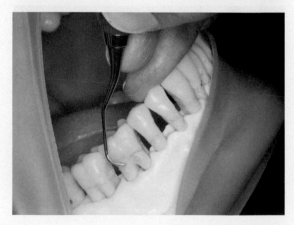

Section 6
Stroke Pattern

PATTERN FOR REMOVING LARGE SUPRAGINGIVAL DEPOSITS

Often a calculus deposit will be too large to be removed in one piece. Large calculus deposits *should be removed in sections* using a series of short, firm instrumentation strokes.

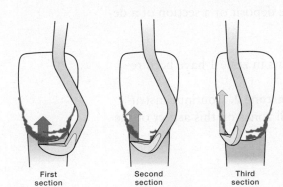

First section   Second section   Third section

Correct Technique: Remove Deposit in Sections.
- Large calculus deposits should be removed in sections.
- Use a series of calculus removal strokes to remove the deposit one section at a time.

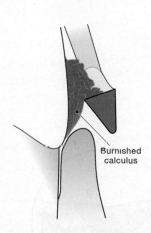

Burnished calculus

Incorrect Technique: Remove Outer Layer.
- The deposit *should not be removed in layers* since removing the outermost layer will leave the deposit with a smooth surface.
- A calculus deposit that has had the outermost layer removed is referred to as a **burnished deposit.**
- Burnished calculus is difficult to remove since the cutting edge tends to slip over the smooth surface of the deposit.

PATTERN FOR LOCATING AND REMOVING SUBGINGIVAL DEPOSITS

Locating and removing subgingival calculus deposits is a challenging task since the clinician is working beneath the gingival margin and cannot see the calculus deposits or root surface. For this reason, the clinician must adopt a very systematic pattern of instrumentation strokes. A haphazard stroke pattern will result in sections not being instrumented and unsuccessful treatment of the root surface.

Use Systematic Approach.
- It is helpful to think of the root surface as being divided into a series of long narrow instrumentation zones.
- Each instrumentation zone is only as wide as the toe-third of the instrument's cutting edge.

Use of Instrumentation Zones. The steps in employing instrumentation strokes in a series of narrow tracts is as follows:

1. **Begin in "instrumentation zone 1".**
   - Use an assessment stroke to locate the calculus deposit closest to the soft tissue base of the periodontal pocket.
   - Calculus deposits adjacent to the junctional epithelium are removed first; those near the gingival margin are removed last.
2. **Place the curet working-end beneath a deposit in zone 1.**
   - Use a tiny calculus removal stroke to snap the entire deposit or a section of a deposit from the root surface.
   - Reassess the area using a relaxed assessment stroke.
3. **Continue working in a coronal direction** until all deposits in zone 1 have been removed.
4. Once you have completed zone 1, **repeat the process in zone 2**. Continue instrumenting each narrow zone in a similar manner until all zones on this aspect of the tooth have been completed.

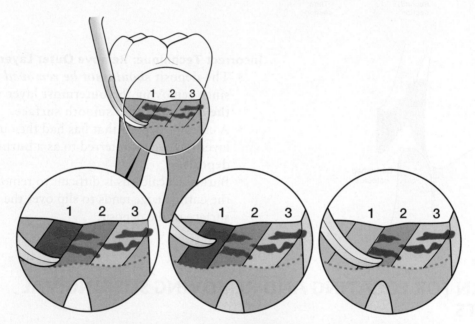

Instrumentation Zones for Subgingival Calculus Removal. The root surface is divided into a pattern of instrumentation zones or tracts for the systematic removal of calculus deposits located beneath the gingival tissues. First, all deposits are removed from zone 1, then zone 2, and so on, until all zones are completed.

Section 7
Stroke Direction

VERTICAL, OBLIQUE, AND HORIZONTAL STROKES

Instrumentation strokes are initiated in a coronal direction *away from the soft tissue base of the sulcus or periodontal pocket.*

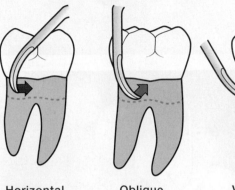

Horizontal direction

Oblique direction

Vertical direction

Stroke Directions. Three stroke directions can be used when assessing and instrumenting subgingival root surfaces within periodontal pockets:

- Vertical
- Oblique
- Horizontal

REFERENCE SHEET: STROKE DIRECTIONS ON ANTERIOR AND POSTERIOR TEETH

TABLE 10-2.	Stroke Directions on Anterior and Posterior Teeth	
Tooth Surface	**Primary**	**Secondary**
Mesial and distal surfaces	vertical	horizontal, oblique
Facial and lingual surfaces	oblique	vertical, horizontal
Line angles	horizontal	oblique, vertical
Facial or lingual root surfaces of anteriors	horizontal	vertical
Furcation crotch areas	horizontal	vertical
Narrow pockets	horizontal	vertical

Vertical Strokes.
- On *anterior teeth*, vertical strokes are used on the facial, lingual, and proximal surfaces.
- On *posterior teeth*, vertical strokes are used on the mesial and distal surfaces.

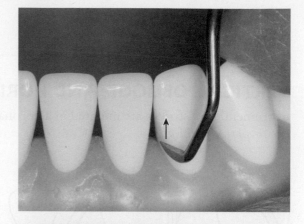

Oblique Strokes. Oblique strokes are used most commonly on the *facial and lingual surfaces* of anterior and posterior teeth.

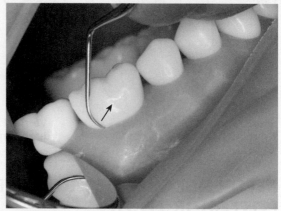

Horizontal Strokes. Horizontal strokes are used:
- At the line angles of posterior teeth
- In furcation areas
- In areas that are too narrow to allow vertical or oblique strokes

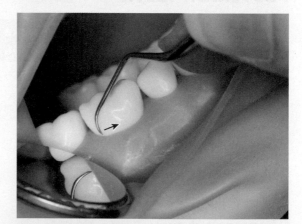

Horizontal Strokes on Anterior Teeth.
- The *facial and lingual surfaces* of anterior teeth are difficult to instrument because these teeth have a narrow mesial-distal width. Horizontal strokes are very effective in removing calculus from these narrow root surfaces.
- The working-end is used in a toe-down position. A short, controlled horizontal stroke is made on the tooth surface.

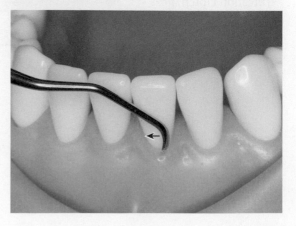

Section 8
Skill Application

PRACTICAL FOCUS

CASE 1. Your friend, Beatrix, is having difficulty removing calculus on the mandibular anteriors. She asks you to observe her and give her feedback about the problems she is encountering. What problems, if any, did you observe? How might Beatrix correct these problems?

Your Observations:

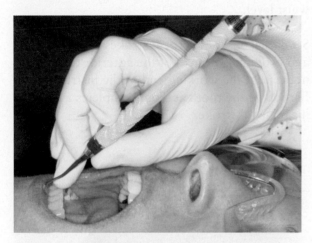

Photo 1. Beatrix's grasp and fulcrum for the anterior surfaces away.

Beatrix is a right-handed clinician.

Beatrix's position: she sits at 8-9:00 for anterior surfaces toward and at 12:00 for surfaces away. Her lower arms are at waist-level.

The patient's head is chin-down.

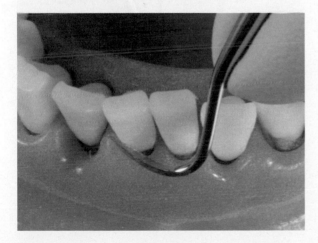

Photo 2. Beatrix's adaptation and angulation on facial surface.

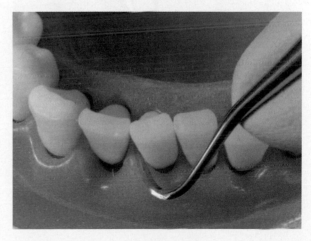

Photo 3. Beatrix's adaptation and angulation on mesial surface.

CASE 2. Your friend, Tom, is having difficulty removing calculus on the mandibular anterior teeth. He asks you to observe him and give him feedback about the problems he is encountering. What problems, if any, did you observe? How might Tom correct these problems?

Your Observations:

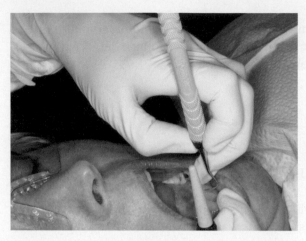

Photo 1. Tom's grasp and fulcrum for the surfaces away.

Tom is a *left-handed* clinician.

Tom's position: He sits at 4-3:00 for anterior surfaces toward and at 12:00 for surfaces away. Tom's forearms are parallel to the floor and at waist level.

Strokes: Tom uses vertical strokes on the facial and proximal surfaces of the anterior teeth. You notice that the working-end of the instrument flies off of the tooth as Tom completes a calculus removal stroke.

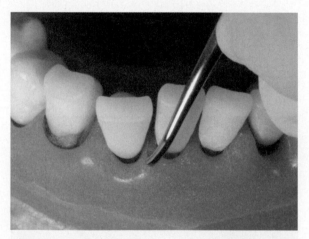

Photo 2. Tom's adaptation and angulation to the distal surface.

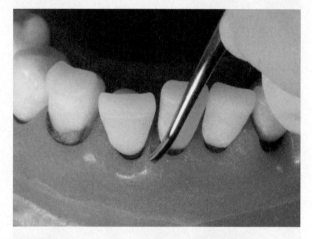

Photo 3. Tom's adaptation and angulation to the facial surface.

MODULE REFERENCE:

1. Dufour, L.A. and Bissell, H.S., *Periodontal attachment loss induced by mechanical subgingival instrumentation in shallow sulci.* The Journal of Dental Hygiene, 2002. **76**(3): p. 207-212.

SKILL EVALUATION MODULE 10	INSTRUMENTATION STROKES

Student: _____

Evaluator: _____

Date: _____

DIRECTIONS FOR STUDENT: Use **Column S.** Evaluate your skill level as: **S** (satisfactory) or **U** (unsatisfactory).

DIRECTIONS FOR EVALUATOR: Use **Column E.** Indicate: **S** (satisfactory) or **U** (unsatisfactory). Each **S** equals 1 point, each **U** equals 0 points.

CRITERIA	S	E
Assessment Stroke on Facial Surface of Mandibular First Molar		
Places explorer working-end in the Get Ready Zone in the middle-third of the crown.		
Inserts explorer working-end beneath gingiva.		
Places toe-third of working end (side of tip) against tooth surface.		
Using a relaxed grasp, initiates a feather-light stroke away from the junctional epithelium.		
Stops each stroke just beneath the gingival margin.		
Calculus Removal Stroke With Universal Curet on Facial Surface of Mandibular First Molar		
Places the working-end of a universal curet in the Get Ready Zone.		
Inserts the working-end beneath the gingival margin to the soft tissue base of the pocket.		
Positions the working-end beneath a calculus deposit.		
Establishes 80-degree angulation: Tilts lower shank toward tooth surface.		
Locks the toe-third of the cutting edge against the root surface.		
Makes a tiny, biting stroke to snap deposit off the tooth surface.		
Precisely stops the stroke and pauses to relax grasp.		
Root Debridement Stroke With Area-Specific Curet		
Places the working-end of the area-specific curet in the Get Ready Zone.		
Establishes 60-degree angulation.		
Makes a light shaving stroke away from the base of the pocket.		
OPTIONAL GRADE PERCENTAGE CALCULATION Total **S**'s in the E column.		

Sum of **S**'s _____ divided by Total Points Possible (**15**) equals the Percentage Grade _____

SKILL EVALUATION MODULE 10   INSTRUMENTATION STROKES

Student: _____

EVALUATOR COMMENTS

_____
_____
_____
_____
_____
_____
_____
_____
_____
_____
_____
_____
_____
_____
_____
_____
_____
_____
_____
_____

Box for sketches pertaining to written comments.

Calibrated Periodontal Probes and Basic Probing Technique

Module Overview

This module presents the (1) design characteristics of calibrated periodontal probes and (2) step-by-step instructions for use of a calibrated periodontal probe.

Module Outline

Key Terms

Calibrated periodontal probe
Gingiva
Free gingiva
Gingival margin
Gingival sulcus
Sulci

Junctional epithelium
Attached gingiva
Mucogingival junction
Alveolar mucosa
Interdental gingiva
Col

Periodontal pocket
Probing
Probe tip
Walking stroke
Probing depth
Periodontal chart

Learning Objectives

1. Identify the design characteristics of a calibrated periodontal probe.

2. Identify the millimeter markings on several calibrated periodontal probes including some probe designs that are not in your instrument kit.

3. Describe the rationale and technique for periodontal probing.

4. Discuss the characteristics of effective probing technique in terms of adaptation and angulation of the tip, amount of pressure needed, instrumentation stroke, and number and location of probe readings for each tooth.

5. Using calibrated periodontal probe, demonstrate correct adaptation on facial, lingual, and proximal surfaces and beneath the contact area of two adjacent teeth.

6. Activate a calibrated periodontal probe using a walking stroke and correct probing technique.

7. Determine the probing depth accurately to within 1 mm of the instructor's reading.

8. Define the term junctional epithelium.

9. Differentiate between a normal sulcus and a periodontal pocket, and describe the position of the probe in each.

NOTE TO COURSE INSTRUCTORS: Refer to Module 21, Advanced Probing Techniques, for content on advanced assessments with periodontal probes: (1) gingival recession, (2) tooth mobility, (3) oral deviations, (4) width of attached gingiva, (5) clinical attachment level, (6) furcation involvement, and (7) the Periodontal Screening and Recording (PSR) System assessment.

Section 1
Calibrated Periodontal Probes

GENERAL DESIGN CHARACTERISTICS

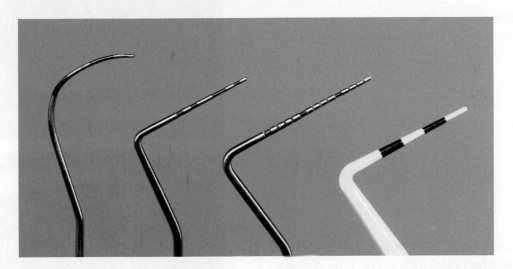

The calibrated periodontal probe is a periodontal instrument that is marked in millimeter increments and used to evaluate the health of the periodontal tissues.

1. **Design of Calibrated Probes.** Calibrated probes have blunt, rod-shaped working-ends that may be circular or rectangular in cross section.
2. **Function of Periodontal Probes.**
   a. Findings from an examination with a calibrated probe are an important part of a comprehensive periodontal assessment to determine the health of the periodontal tissues.
   b. The calibrated periodontal probe is used to measure sulcus and pocket depths, to measure clinical attachment levels, to determine the width of attached gingiva, to assess for the presence of bleeding and/or purulent exudate (pus), and to measure the size of oral lesions.

MILLIMETER MARKINGS

Calibrated probes are marked in millimeter increments and are used like miniature rulers for making intraoral measurements.

1. **Millimeter Markings.**
   a. The working-end of the probe is marked at millimeter intervals. Indentations or grooves, colored indentations, or colored bands may be used to indicate the millimeter markings on the working-end.
   b. Each millimeter may be indicated on the probe or only certain millimeter increments may be marked (Table 11-1).
   c. If you are uncertain how a probe is calibrated, you can use a millimeter ruler to determine the millimeter markings.
2. **Color Coding.** Color-coded probes are marked in bands (often black in color) with each band being several millimeters in width.

EXAMPLES OF PROBE MARKINGS

Markings at Each Millimeter. The UNC 15 probe has millimeter markings at 1, 2, 3, 4, 5, 6, 7, 8, 9, 10, 11, 12, 13, 14, and 15 millimeters.

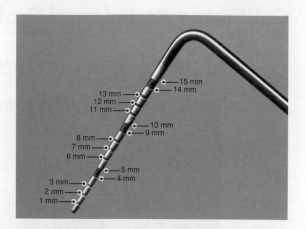

Markings at Certain Millimeters. This probe has millimeter (mm) markings at 1-2-3-5-7-8-9-10.

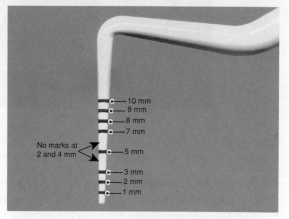

Color-Coded Probe. This probe has black bands; each band is 3 millimeters in length. The millimeter markings on this particular probe are at 3-6-9-12 mm.

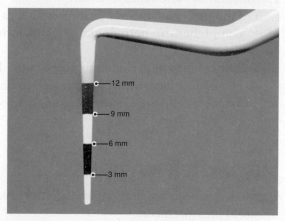

COMPUTER-ASSISTED PROBES

Computer-Assisted Probe. The Florida Probe is an example of a computer-assisted probe. The probe handpiece automatically standardizes the probing force at 15 grams. (Photograph courtesy of Florida Probe Corporation.)

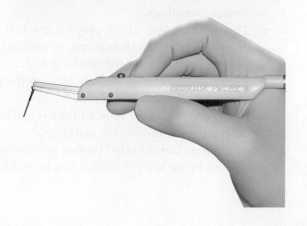

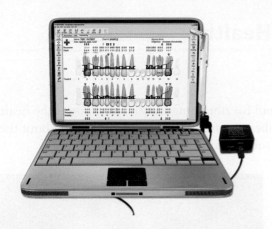

Data Entry with Computer-Assisted Probe. The computer-assisted probe is connected to a computer. Probing depths are entered via the computer keyboard on the computerized anatomical dental chart. The software program stores information on recession, pocket depth, furcation involvement, and mobility. (Photograph courtesy of Florida Probe Corporation.)

TABLE 11-1. Examples of Millimeter Markings

Probe Design	Marking Pattern	Millimeter Increments
UNC15	All mm from 1 to 15 marked	1–15
Glickman 26G	No mark at 6 mm	1-2-3-5-7-8-9-10
Goldman Fox	No mark at 6 mm	1-2-3-5-7-8-9-10
Merritt	No mark at 6 mm	1-2-3-5-7-8-9-10
Williams	No mark at 6 mm	1-2-3-5-7-8-9-10
Maryland Moffitt	No mark at 6 mm; ball-end	1-2-3-5-7-8-9-10
Michigan "O"	Marks at 3, 6, and 8 mm	3-6-8
PSR Screening	Colored band from 3.5 to 5.5 Marks at 8.5 and 11.5 mm; ball-end	3.5-5.5-8.5-11.5
CP-18	Colored bands from 3 to 5 and 8 to 10 mm	3-5-8-10
CP-11	Colored bands from 3 to 6 and 8 to 11 mm	3-6-8-11
CP-12	Colored bands from 3 to 6 and 9 to12 mm	3-6-9-12

Section 2
Use of Probe to Assess Tissue Health

FUNCTION OF CALIBRATED PROBE

The periodontal probe is the most important clinical tool for obtaining information about the health status of the periodontium. Calibrated periodontal probes are used to gather information about the health of the gingival tissues and bone loss and to measure the size of intraoral lesions.

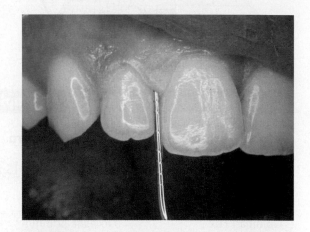

Probe in a Healthy Sulcus. This photograph shows a periodontal probe inserted into a healthy gingival sulcus, the space between the free gingiva and the tooth. In health, the depth of the sulcus is from 1 to 3 millimeters (mm).

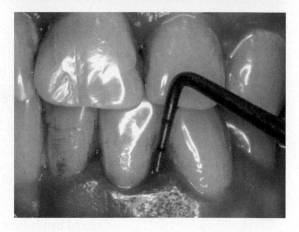

Probe in a Periodontal Pocket. This photograph shows a periodontal probe inserted into a periodontal pocket. A periodontal pocket is a sulcus that has deepened because of disease. The depth of a periodontal pocket is greater than 3 mm. The depth of the periodontal pocket shown here is 6 mm.

REVIEW OF PERIODONTAL ANATOMY IN HEALTH

The gingiva is the tissue that covers the cervical portions of the teeth and the alveolar processes of the jaws.

1. **The Free Gingiva.**
   a. The free gingiva is the unattached portion of the gingiva that surrounds the tooth in the region of the cemento-enamel junction. It is also known as the unattached gingiva or the marginal gingiva.
   b. The free gingiva surrounds the tooth in a turtleneck or cufflike manner.
   c. The tissue of the free gingiva fits closely around the tooth but is not directly attached to it. This tissue, because it is unattached, may be stretched away from the tooth surface with a periodontal probe.
   d. The free gingiva also forms the soft tissue wall of the gingival sulcus.
   e. The free gingiva meets the tooth in a thin, rounded edge called the gingival margin.

2. **The Gingival Sulcus.**
   a. The gingival sulcus is the *space* between the free gingiva and the tooth surface.
   b. The sulcus is a V-shaped, shallow space around the tooth. The plural form of sulcus is sulci.
   c. The base of the sulcus is formed by the junctional epithelium—a specialized type of epithelium that attaches to the tooth surface. The junctional epithelium forms the base of a gingival sulcus or periodontal pocket.

3. **The Attached Gingiva.**
   a. The attached gingiva is the part of the gingiva that is tightly connected to the cementum on the cervical-third of the root and to the periosteum (connective tissue cover) of the alveolar bone.
   b. The attached gingiva lies between the free gingiva and the alveolar mucosa.
   c. In health, the attached gingiva is pale or coral pink. In dark-skinned individuals, it may be pigmented. The pigmented areas of the attached gingiva may range from light brown to black.
   d. The attached gingiva ends at the mucogingival junction where the gingiva meets the alveolar mucosa. The alveolar mucosa can be distinguished easily from the attached gingiva by its dark red color and smooth, shiny surface.

4. **The Interdental Gingiva.**
   a. The interdental gingiva is the portion of the gingiva that fills the area between two adjacent teeth apical to (beneath) the contact area.
   b. The col is a valleylike depression in the portion of the interdental gingiva that lies directly apical to the contact area of two adjacent teeth. The col is not present if the adjacent teeth are not in contact or if the gingiva has receded.

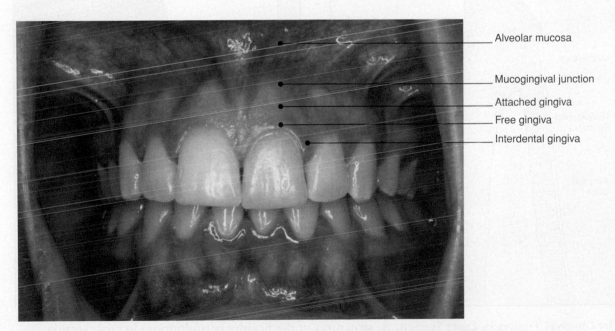

Healthy Gingival Tissues. (Used with permission from Nield-Gehrig, J.S. and Willmann, D., Foundations of Periodontics for the Dental Hygienist, Edition 2, 2007. Philadelphia: Lippincott Williams & Wilkins: p. 3.)

PROBING HEALTHY VERSUS DISEASED TISSUE

1. **Clinically Normal Sulcus.**
    a. In health, the tooth is surrounded by a sulcus. The junctional epithelium (JE) forms the base of the sulcus by attaching to the enamel of the crown near the cemento-enamel junction (CEJ).
    b. The depth of a clinically normal gingival sulcus is from 1 to 3 mm, as measured by a periodontal probe.

2. **Periodontal Pocket.**
    a. A periodontal pocket is a gingival sulcus that has been deepened by disease. In a periodontal pocket, the JE forms the base of the pocket by attaching to the root surface somewhere apical to the CEJ. A periodontal pocket results from destruction of alveolar bone and the periodontal ligament fibers that surround the tooth.
    b. The depth of a periodontal pocket, as measured by a periodontal probe, is greater than 3 mm. It is common to have pockets measuring 5 to 6 mm in depth.

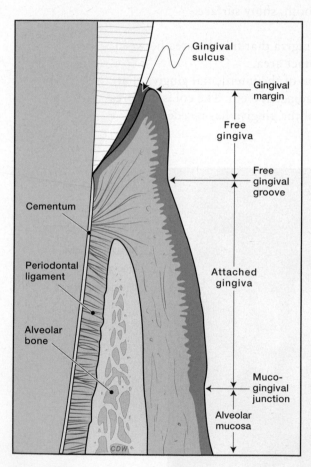 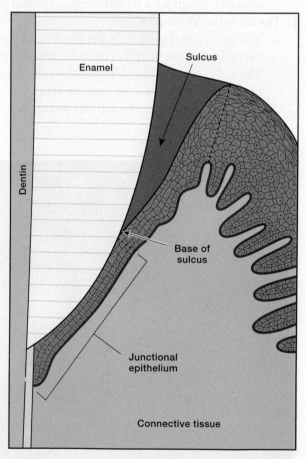

The Gingival Tissues in Cross Section. **A,** structures of the healthy periodontium in cross section. **B,** The sulcus is a V-shaped, shallow space around the tooth. The base of the sulcus is formed by the junctional epithelium. (Used with permission from Nield-Gehrig, J.S. and Willmann, D., Foundations of Periodontics for the Dental Hygienist, Edition 2, 2007. Philadelphia: Lippincott Williams & Wilkins: p. 35.)

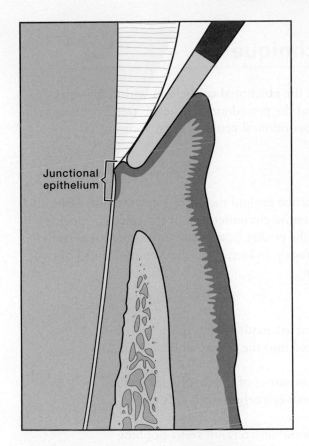

Position of Probe in a Healthy Sulcus. In health, the probe tip touches the junctional epithelium located above the cemento-enamel junction. A healthy sulcus is 1 to 3 mm deep, as measured with a periodontal probe.

(Used with permission from Nield-Gehrig, J.S. and Willmann, D., Foundations of Periodontics for the Dental Hygienist, Edition 2, 2007. Philadelphia: Lippincott Williams & Wilkins: p. 35.)

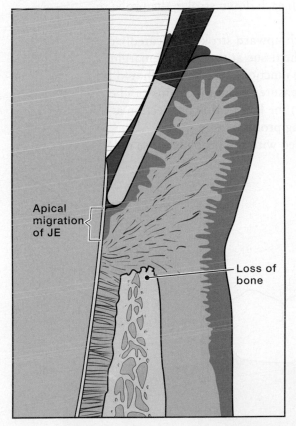

Position of Probe in a Periodontal Pocket. In a periodontal pocket, the probe tip touches the junctional epithelium (JE) located on the root somewhere below the cemento-enamel junction. The depth of a periodontal pocket, as measured by a periodontal probe, will be greater than 3 mm.

(Used with permission from Nield-Gehrig, J.S. and Willmann, D., Foundations of Periodontics for the Dental Hygienist, Edition 2, 2007. Philadelphia: Lippincott Williams & Wilkins: p. 36.)

Section 3
Basic Concepts of Probing Technique

Probing is the act of walking the tip of a probe along the junctional epithelium within the sulcus or pocket for the purpose of assessing the health status of the periodontal tissues. Careful probing technique is essential if the information obtained with a periodontal probe is to be accurate.

THE WALKING STROKE

The walking stroke is the movement of a calibrated probe around the perimeter of the base of a sulcus or pocket. Walking strokes are used to cover the entire circumference of the sulcus or pocket base. It is essential to evaluate the entire "length" of the pocket base because the junctional epithelium is not necessarily at a uniform level around the tooth. In fact, differences in the depths of two neighboring areas along the pocket base are common.

Production of the Walking Stroke

1. Walking strokes are a series of bobbing strokes that are made within the sulcus or pocket. The stroke begins when the probe is inserted into the sulcus while *keeping the probe tip against the tooth surface.*
2. The probe is inserted until the tip encounters the resistance of the junctional epithelium that forms the base of the sulcus. The junctional epithelium feels soft and resilient when touched by the probe.
3. Create the walking stroke by moving the probe up and down (↕) in short bobbing strokes and forward in 1-mm increments (↔). With each down stroke, the probe returns to touch the junctional epithelium.
4. The probe is not removed from the sulcus with each upward stroke. Repeatedly removing and reinserting the probe can traumatize the tissue at the gingival margin.
5. The pressure exerted with the probe tip against the junctional epithelium should be between 10 and 20 grams. A sensitive scale that measures weight in grams can be used to standardize your probing pressure. Refer to the Practical Focus section at the end of this module for instructions in calibrating probing force.
6. Either wrist or digital (finger) activation may be used with the probe because only light pressure is used when probing.

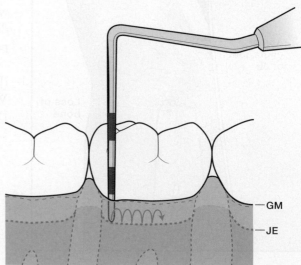

The Walking Stroke. The walking stroke is a series of bobbing strokes along the junctional epithelium (JE). Each up-and-down stroke should be approximately 1 to 2 mm in length (↕). The strokes must be very close together, about 1 mm apart (↔).

ADAPTATION

The side of the probe tip should be kept in contact with the tooth surface. The **probe tip** is defined as 1 to 2 mm of the side of the probe.

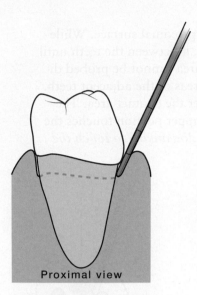

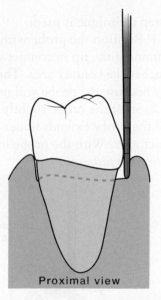

Correct Adaptation. The probe tip is kept in contact with the tooth surface.

Incorrect Adaptation. The probe tip should not be held away from the tooth.

PARALLELISM

The probe is positioned as *parallel as possible to the tooth surface*. The probe must be parallel in the mesiodistal dimension and faciolingual dimension.

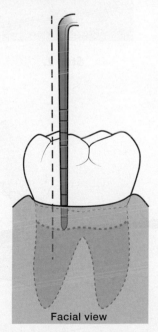

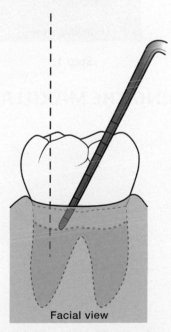

Probe Parallel to Long Axis. This probe is correctly positioned parallel to the long axis of the tooth.

Probe Not Parallel to Long Axis. This probe is incorrectly positioned in relation to the long axis of the tooth.

INTERPROXIMAL TECHNIQUE

When two adjacent teeth are in contact, a special technique is used to probe the area directly beneath the contact area.

A two-step technique is used:

1. **Step 1:** Position the probe with the tip in contact with the proximal surface. While maintaining the tip in contact with the tooth surface, walk it between the teeth until it touches the contact area. The area beneath the contact area cannot be probed directly because the probe will not fit between the contact areas of the adjacent teeth.

2. **Step 2:** Slant the probe slightly so that the tip reaches under the contact area. The tip of the probe extends under the contact area while the upper portion touches the contact area. With the probe in this position, *gently press downward to touch the junctional epithelium.*

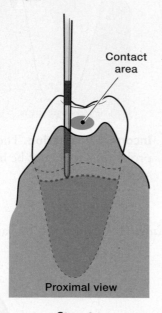

Step 1.

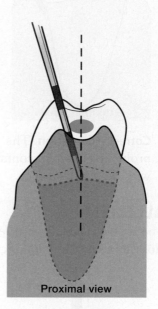

Step 2.

PROBING THE MAXILLARY MOLARS

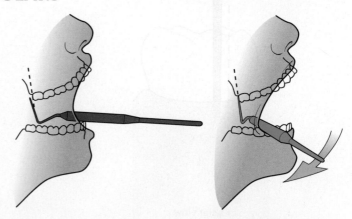

Technique for the Maxillary Molars. Often it is difficult to probe the distal surfaces of the maxillary molars because the mandible is in the way. This problem can be overcome by repositioning the instrument handle to the side of the patient's face.

Section 4
Probing Depth Measurements

PROBING DEPTHS

A probing depth is a measurement of the depth of a sulcus or periodontal pocket. It is determined by measuring the distance from the gingival margin to the base of the sulcus or pocket with a calibrated periodontal probe (Box 11-1).

Box 11-1. Probing Depths

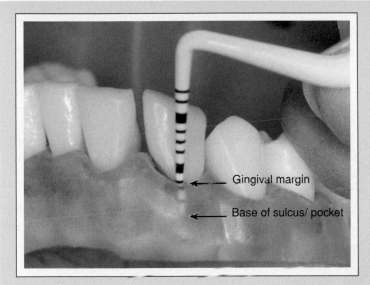

Gingival margin

Base of sulcus/ pocket

A **probing depth** is the distance in millimeters from the *gingival margin* to the base of the sulcus or periodontal pocket as measured with a calibrated probe.

CHARTING PROBING DEPTHS

Probing depth measurements are recorded on a periodontal chart and become a permanent part of the patient chart.

1. **Six Sites Per Tooth.** Probing depth measurements are recorded for 6 specific sites on each tooth: (1) distofacial, (2) facial, (3) mesiofacial, (4) distolingual, (5) lingual, and (6) mesiolingual (Box 11-2).
2. **One Reading Per Site.** Only one reading per site is recorded. If the probing depths vary within a site, the deepest reading obtained in that site is recorded. For example, if the probing depths in the facial site were to range from 2 to 6 mm, only the 6 mm reading would be entered on the chart for that site.
3. **Full Millimeter Measurements.** Probing depths are recorded to the nearest full millimeter. Round measurements to the next higher whole number; for example, a reading of 3.5 mm is recorded as 4 mm, and a 5.5 mm reading is recorded as 6 mm.

Box 11-2. Measurements for Six Sites Are Recorded Per Tooth

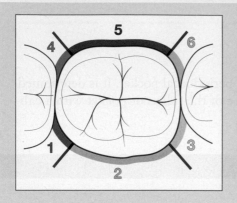

Probing depth measurements are recorded for 6 specific sites on each tooth:

1—distofacial line angle to the midline of distal surface

2—facial surface

3—mesiofacial line angle to the midline of mesial surface

4—distolingual line angle to the midline of distal surface

5—lingual surface

6—mesiolingual line angle to the midline of mesial surface

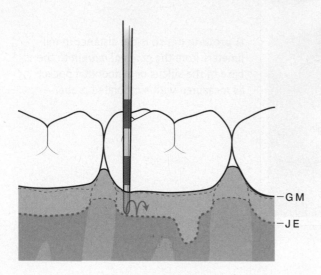

Stroke Technique. It is common for the depth of the pocket base to vary considerably from one spot to the next.

What would happen if only one or two probing strokes were made on the facial surface of the tooth illustrated here?

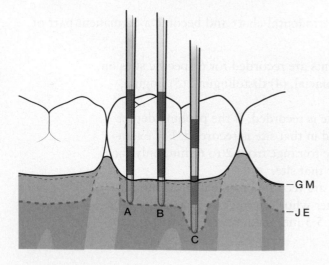

Record the Deepest Reading Per Site. In the illustration shown here, the depth of the pocket base varies considerably at points **A**, **B**, and **C** in the facial site. Because only a single reading can be recorded for the facial site, the deepest reading at point **C** is recorded.

PERIODONTAL CHART

Probing depth measurements are recorded on a periodontal chart. Most periodontal charts include rows of boxes that are used to record the probing depths on the facial and lingual aspects of the teeth.

On the sample chart shown below, the probing depths on the maxillary right first molar are as follows:

Facial Aspect of Tooth 3

Site 1—distofacial line angle to midline of distal surface—the deepest reading is 5 mm.
Site 2—facial surface—the deepest reading is 3 mm.
Site 3—mesiofacial line angle to midline of mesial surface—the deepest reading is 4 mm.

Lingual Aspect of Tooth 3

Site 4—distolingual line angle to midline of the distal surface—the deepest reading is 8 mm.
Site 5—lingual surface—the deepest reading is 6 mm.
Site 6—mesiolingual line angle to midline of the mesial surface—the deepest reading is 7 mm.

Sample Periodontal Chart for the Maxillary Right Posterior Teeth

POSITIONING AND SEQUENCE FOR PROBING

The technique used for probing is different from that used with other periodontal instruments. For example, it is not necessary to use different clock positions when probing the anterior surfaces toward and away from your nondominant hand. The diagrams on this page show (1) the recommended clinician clock positions and (2) a suggested sequence for probing the maxilla and mandible. This sequence is a logical one to follow as you probe the dentition and record the probing measurements on a periodontal chart. You may want to photocopy this diagram to use for reference as you practice probing the dentition.

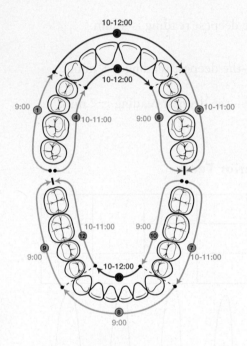

Right-Handed Clinicians

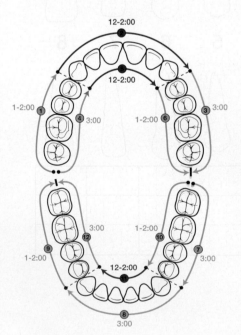

Left-Handed Clinicians

Section 5
Technique Practice: Posterior Teeth

Directions:
1. For this technique practice, you will be working on the *mandibular right first molar, facial aspect.*
2. Remember: "Me, My Patient, My Light, My Dominant Hand, My Nondominant Hand, My Finger Rest, My Adaptation."

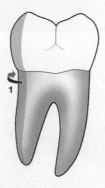

3. **Insert at the Distofacial Line Angle.** Insert the probe into the sulcus near the distofacial line angle of the *first molar.* Keep the side of the tip in contact with the tooth surface as you gently slide the probe to the sulcus base. (Illustration shows the facial view.)

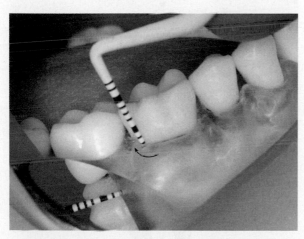

4. **Begin to Probe Site 1.** Your probe is now positioned to evaluate Site 1 of this tooth—the distofacial line angle to the midline of the distal surface.

    Keeping the tip in contact with the tooth, initiate a series of short, bobbing strokes *toward the distal surface.* Use a walking stroke, keeping your strokes close together.

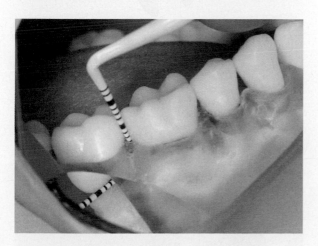

5. **Walk the Probe Onto the Proximal Surface.** Walk the probe across the distal surface until it touches the contact area.

6. **Assess Beneath the Contact Area.** Tilt the probe so that the tip reaches beneath the contact area (the upper portion of the probe touches the contact area).

   Gently press downward to touch the junctional epithelium.

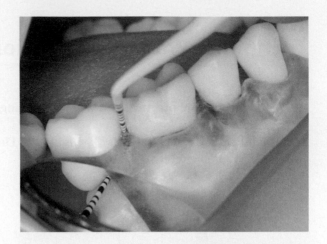

7. **Technique Check: Distal View.** *In this photo, the adjacent tooth has been removed* to provide a view of the correct probe position for assessing the tissue beneath the contact area from the facial aspect. Tilt your probe in a similar manner.

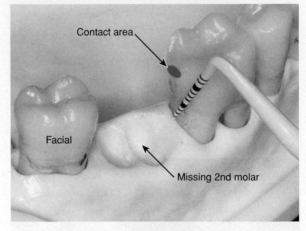

8. **Reinsert at the Distofacial Line Angle.** Remove the probe from the sulcus and reinsert it at the distofacial line angle. You are now in position to probe the facial surface.

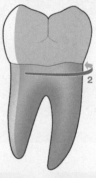

9. **Probe Site 2.** Make a series of tiny walking strokes across Site 2—the facial surface—moving in a forward direction toward the mesial surface.

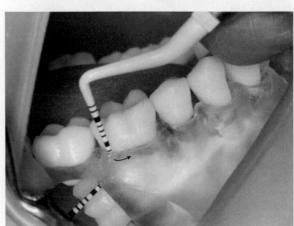

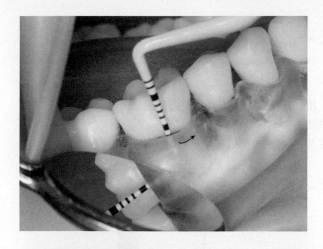

10. Probe Site 3. Walk the probe across the mesial surface until it touches the contact area.

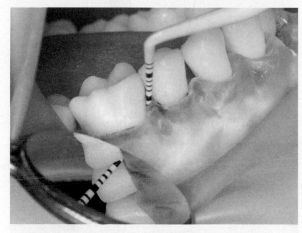

11. Assess Beneath the Contact Area. Tilt the probe and extend the tip beneath the contact area. Press down gently to touch the junctional epithelium.

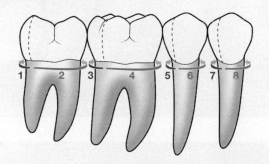

12. Probing Sequence for Sextant. This illustration shows the sequence for probing the entire mandibular right posterior sextant. This sequence allows you to probe the sextant in the most efficient manner.

Practice probing the facial and lingual aspects of the four posterior sextants using the sequence shown in the illustration above.

Section 6
Technique Practice: Anterior Teeth

Directions:

1. When probing an anterior sextant, begin on the distofacial or distolingual line angle of the canine farthest from your nondominant hand.

2. For this technique practice, you will be working on the *mandibular left canine, facial aspect.*

3. **Insert at the Distofacial Line Angle.** Begin by inserting the probe at the distofacial line angle of the left canine. You are now in position to assess the distal surface of the canine.

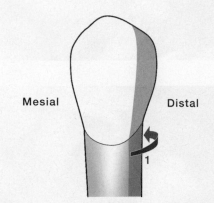

4. **Walk Toward the Distal Surface.** Walk the probe across the distal surface until it touches the contact area.

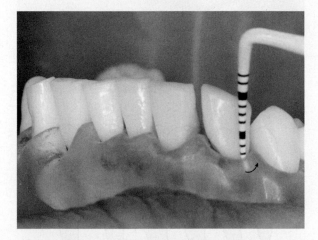

5. **Assess Beneath the Contact Area.** Tilt the probe and extend the tip beneath the contact area. Press down gently to touch the junctional epithelium.

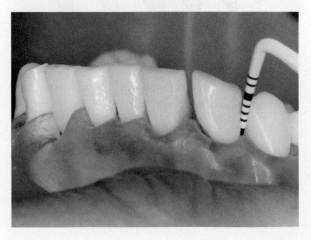

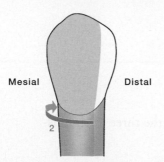

Mesial   Distal

6. **Reinsert at the Distofacial Line Angle.**
   Remove the probe from the sulcus and reinsert it at the distofacial line angle. You arc
   now in position to probe the facial surface of
   the canine.

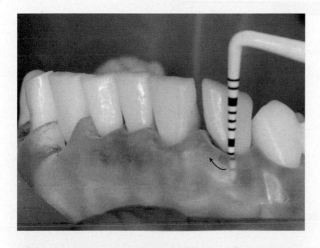

7. **Assess the Facial Surface.** Make a series of
   walking strokes across the facial surface.

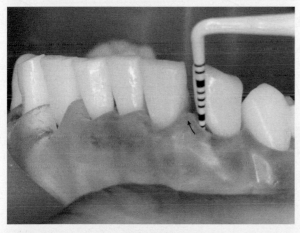

8. **Walk Toward the Mesial Surface.** Walk across
   the mesial surface until the probe touches the
   contact area.

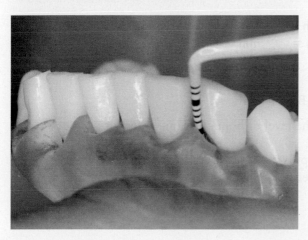

9. **Assess Beneath the Contact Area.** On adjacent *anterior teeth*, only a slight tilt is needed
   to probe the col area. Gently probe the col
   area.

Section 7
Skill Application

PRACTICAL FOCUS

1. **Probing Depths.** Measure and record the probing depths for the three teeth illustrated below.

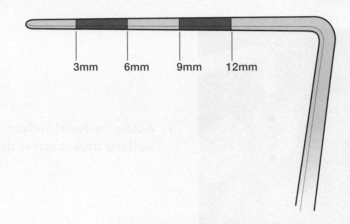

Probe Millimeter Markings

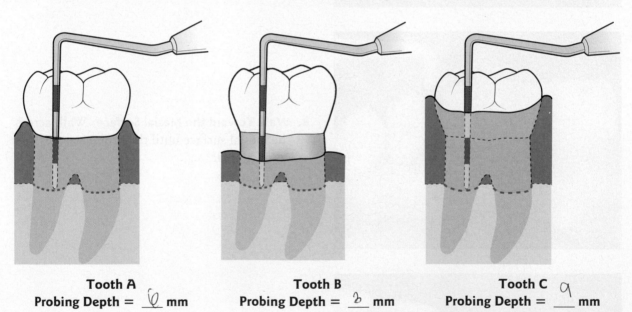

| **Tooth A** | **Tooth B** | **Tooth C** |
| Probing Depth = _6_ mm | Probing Depth = _3_ mm | Probing Depth = _9_ mm |

Assess the Probing Depths. Look closely at teeth **A, B,** and **C** above.

1. Compare the bone level on these three teeth. Is the level of bone the same or different for these teeth?
2. Compare the probing depths. Do the probing depths provide you with an accurate picture of the amount of bone lost from around each of the teeth?

2. **Calibrate Probing Pressure.** Obtain a scale calibrated in grams from a scientific supply company. Grasp a calibrated probe in a modified pen grasp. Apply pressure against the scale platform with the tip of the probe. Calibrate your pressure to between 10 and 20 grams.

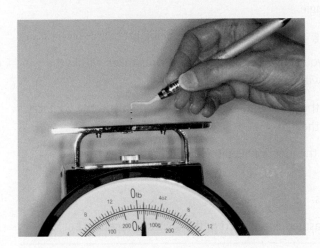

Scientific Scale Used to Measure Probing Force.

REFERENCE SHEET: FOR PROBING TECHNIQUE

TABLE 11-2. Probing Technique

1. Insert probe at the distofacial or distolingual line angle.

2. Position the probe as parallel as possible to the long axis of the tooth surface being probed.

3. Adapt the tip of the probe to the tooth surface as you activate short up-and-down strokes within the sulcus or pocket. Touch the junctional epithelium with each down stroke.

4. Assess the area beneath the contact area by tilting the probe and extending the tip beneath the contact area. Press down gently to touch the junctional epithelium.

5. Walk the probe around the entire circumference of the junctional epithelium using strokes that are about 1 mm apart.

6. Use light stroke pressure, between 10 and 20 grams.

7. Record 6 measurements per tooth (the deepest measurement in each of the 6 sites is recorded).

NOTE TO COURSE INSTRUCTORS: Refer to Module 21—Advanced Probing Techniques—for content on advanced assessments with periodontal probes: (1) gingival recession, (2) tooth mobility, (3) oral deviations, (4) width of attached gingiva, (5) clinical attachment level, (6) furcation involvement, and (7) the Periodontal Screening and Recording (PSR) System assessment.

SKILL EVALUATION MODULE 11	BASIC PROBING TECHNIQUE

Student: _____

Evaluator: _____

Date: _____

Anterior Area 1 = _____

Anterior Area 2 = _____

Posterior Area 3 = _____

Posterior Area 4 = _____

DIRECTIONS FOR STUDENT: Use **Column S.** Evaluate your skill level as: **S** (satisfactory) or **U** (unsatisfactory).

DIRECTIONS FOR EVALUATOR: Use **Column E.** Indicate: **S** (satisfactory) or **U** (unsatisfactory). Each **S** equals 1 point, each **U** equals 0 points.

	Area 1		Area 2		Area 3		Area 4	
CRITERIA:	S	E	S	E	S	E	S	E
Position:								
Positioned correctly on clinician stool								
Positioned correctly with relation to patient, equipment, and treatment area								
Establishes correct patient head position								
Dental Mirror:								
Uses correct grasp and establishes secure rest with mirror								
Uses the mirror correctly for retraction and/or indirect vision								
Modified Pen Grasp with Dominant Hand:								
Thumb and index finger pads positioned opposite one another on handle; fingers not touching or overlapped								
Pad of middle finger rests lightly on shank; touches the ring finger								
Handle rests between the 2nd knuckle of the index finger and the "V" of hand								
Grasp is relaxed (no blanching of fingers)								
Intraoral Fulcrum:								
Ring finger is straight and supports weight of hand								
Fulcrums on same arch, near tooth being instrumented								
Probing Technique:								
Positions probe parallel to the tooth surface								
Keeps tip in contact with the tooth surface								
Uses small walking strokes within the sulcus								
Tilts probe and extends tip beneath contact area to assess interproximal area								
Covers entire circumference of sulcus with walking strokes								
OPTIONAL GRADE PERCENTAGE CALCULATION Total **S**'s in each E column.								

Sum of **S**'s _____ divided by Total Points Possible (**64**) equals the Percentage Grade _____

SKILL EVALUATION MODULE 11   BASIC PROBING TECHNIQUE

Student: _____

EVALUATOR COMMENTS

_____
_____
_____
_____
_____
_____
_____
_____
_____
_____
_____
_____
_____
_____
_____
_____
_____
_____

Box for sketches pertaining to written comments.

Explorers

Module Overview

This module presents the design characteristics of explorers and step-by-step instructions for their use in the detection of root surface irregularities and calculus deposits.

Module Outline

Practical Focus
Reference Sheet: Explorers
Skill Evaluation Module 12: Explorers

Key Terms

Explorer	Tactile sensitivity	Spicule of calculus
Assessment instruments	Calculus	Calculus ledge
Explorer tip	Plaque retentive	Calculus ring
Supragingival instrumentation	Supragingival calculus deposits	Thin veneer of calculus
Subgingival instrumentation	Subgingival calculus deposits	Fingerlike calculus formation
Assessment stroke	Residual calculus deposits	Carious lesion

Learning Objectives

1. Identify the design characteristics of explorers.

2. Given a variety of explorer designs, identify the explorer tip.

3. Identify and describe the advantages and limitations of various explorer designs.

4. Describe how the clinician can use visual clues to select the correct working-end of a double-ended explorer.

5. Demonstrate correct adaptation and use of assessment strokes with an explorer.

6. Demonstrate calculus detection with an explorer and compressed air.

Section 1
Explorers

GENERAL DESIGN CHARACTERISTICS

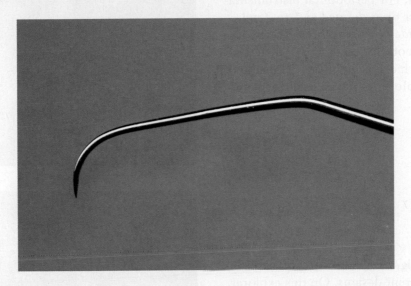

An explorer is an assessment instrument with a flexible wirelike working-end. Assessment instruments—such as periodontal probes and explorers—are used to determine the health of the periodontal tissues, tooth anatomy, and texture of tooth surfaces. The explorer's flexible working-end quivers as it is moved over tooth surface irregularities such as dental calculus (tartar). Dental calculus deposits frequently are located subgingivally below the gingival margin, where they cannot be detected visually. Because these subgingival calculus deposits cannot be seen, the clinician must rely on his or her sense of touch to find and remove these hidden deposits. The explorer with its highly flexible working-end is the instrument of choice for detection of subgingival calculus deposits.

1. **Design of Explorers.**
   a. Explorers are made of flexible metal that conducts vibrations from the working-end to the clinician's fingers on the instrument shank and handle.
   b. Explorers are circular in cross section and may have unpaired (dissimilar) or paired working-ends.
   c. The working-end is 1 to 2 mm in length and is referred to as the explorer tip.
   d. The actual point of the explorer is not used to detect dental calculus; rather, the side of the explorer tip is applied to the tooth surface.

2. **Function of Explorers.**
   a. Explorers are used to detect, by tactile means, the texture and character of tooth surfaces before, during, and after periodontal debridement to assess the progress and completeness of instrumentation.
   b. Explorers are used to examine tooth surfaces for calculus, decalcified and carious lesions, dental anomalies, and anatomic features such as grooves, curvatures, or root furcations.

EXPLORER TIP AND LOWER SHANK

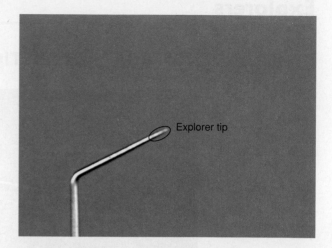

The Explorer Tip. For periodontal instrumentation, the explorer tip is defined as 1 to 2 millimeters of the *side* of the explorer. The tip is adapted to the tooth for detection of dental calculus or root surface irregularities. **The actual *point* of the explorer is never used for detection of calculus.**

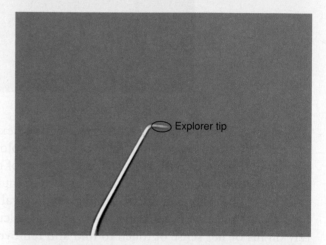

Explorer Tip Design. Explorers are available in a variety of different designs. On this explorer, the tip is bent at a 90-degree angle to the lower shank. Such an explorer design is ideal for subgingival instrumentation.

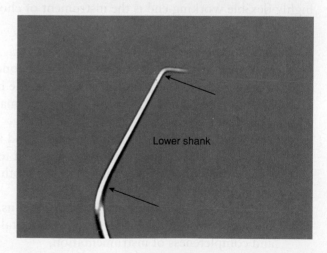

Lower Shank. The lower shank is the section of the shank nearest to the explorer tip.
The lower shank provides an important visual clue for the clinician when positioning the instrument. In posterior sextants, the lower shank should be parallel to the tooth surface being instrumented.

EXPLORER DESIGN TYPES

Explorers are available in a variety of design types. All design types are not well suited to subgingival use; therefore, the clinician should be knowledgeable about the recommended use of each design type.

1. **Supragingival instrumentation**—use of an instrument coronal to (above) the gingival margin, for example, use of an explorer to examine the occlusal surface for decay.
2. **Subgingival instrumentation**—use of an instrument apical to (below) the gingival margin, for example, use of an explorer to detect calculus deposits hidden beneath the gingival margin.

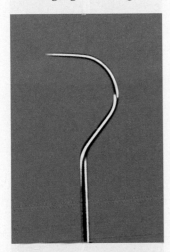

Shepherd Hook Explorer—gets its name because it resembles the long stick with a curved end that was used by ancient shepherds to catch sheep.

1. Use
   a. *Supragingival* examinations for dental caries (decay) and irregular margins of restorations.
   b. NOT recommended for subgingival use because the point could injure the soft tissue at the base of the sulcus or pocket.
2. Examples: 23 and 54 explorers.

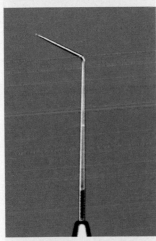

Straight Explorer.

1. Use
   a. Examinations for *supragingival* dental caries and irregular margins of restorations.
   b. NOT recommended for subgingival use because the point could injure the soft tissue at the base of the sulcus or pocket.
2. Examples: 6, 6A, 6L, and 6XL explorers.

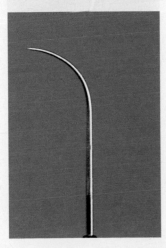

Curved Explorer.

1. Use
   a. Calculus detection in normal sulci or shallow pockets.
   b. Care must be taken not to injure the soft tissue base of the sulcus or pocket if the working-end is used subgingivally.
2. Examples: 3 and 3A.

Pigtail and Cowhorn Explorers—get their names because they resemble a pig's tail or a bull's horn.

1. Use
   a. Calculus detection in normal sulci or shallow pockets extending no deeper than the cervical-third of the root.
   b. The curved lower shank causes considerable stretching of the tissue away from the root surface.
2. Examples: 3ML, 3CH, and 2A.

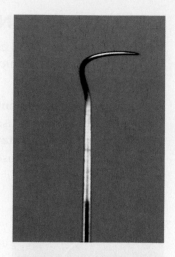

Orban-type Explorer.

1. Design Characteristics
   a. The tip is bent at a 90-degree angle to the lower shank; this feature allows the *back of the tip* (instead of the point) to be directed against the soft tissue at the base of the sulcus or pocket.
   b. The straight lower shank allows insertion in narrow pockets with only slight stretching of the tissue away from the root surface.
2. Use: Assessment of anterior root surfaces and the facial and lingual surfaces of posterior teeth. Difficult to adapt to the line angles and proximal surfaces of the posterior teeth.
3. Examples: 17, 20F, and TU17.

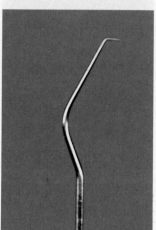

11/12-type Explorer—an explorer with several advantageous design characteristics

1. Design Characteristics
   a. Like the Orban-type explorers, the tip is at a 90-degree angle to the lower shank.
   b. The long complex shank design makes it equally useful when working on anterior and posterior teeth with normal sulci or deep periodontal pockets.
2. Use: Assessment of root surfaces on anterior and posterior teeth.
3. Examples: ODU 11/12 and 11/12AF.

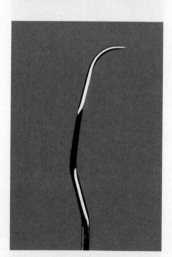

THE ASSESSMENT STROKE

An assessment stroke, also called an exploratory stroke, is used to detect calculus deposits or other tooth surface irregularities. Assessment strokes require a high degree of precision. The proper use of an explorer requires light, controlled strokes.

1. During subgingival instrumentation, the clinician relies on his or her sense of touch to locate calculus deposits hidden beneath the gingival margin.
2. Tactile sensitivity is the ability to detect tooth irregularities by feeling vibrations transferred from the explorer tip to the handle. For example, the explorer tip quivers slightly as it travels over rough calculus deposits on the tooth surface. These vibrations are transmitted from the tip, through the shank, and into the handle. The clinician feels the vibrations with his or her fingertips resting on the handle and instrument shank.
3. The fine working-end and flexible shank of an explorer are used to enhance tactile information to the clinician's fingers. The superior tactile conduction of an explorer makes it the instrument of choice for (1) *initially locating subgingival calculus deposits* and (2) *re-evaluating tooth surfaces* following calculus removal.
4. *During calculus removal,* the curet is used for calculus detection. When all deposits detectable with a curet have been removed, a definitive evaluation of the root surface should be made using an explorer. Because the explorer provides superior tactile information, it is common to detect some remaining calculus deposits with an explorer that could not be detected with a curet.

TABLE 12-1.	Assessment Stroke With an Explorer
Grasp	Relaxed grasp; middle finger rests lightly on shank
Adaptation	1 to 2 mm of the side of the tip is adapted
Lateral Pressure	Light pressure with working-end against tooth
Activation	Wrist activation is usually recommended; however, digital activation is acceptable with an explorer because physical strength is not required for assessment strokes
Stroke Characteristics	Fluid, sweeping strokes
Stroke Number	Many overlapping strokes are used to cover every square millimeter of the root surface
Common Errors	AVOID a tight, tense "death grip" on handle
	AVOID applying pressure with the middle finger against the instrument shank because this reduces tactile information to the finger

SUBGINGIVAL ASSESSMENT WITH AN EXPLORER

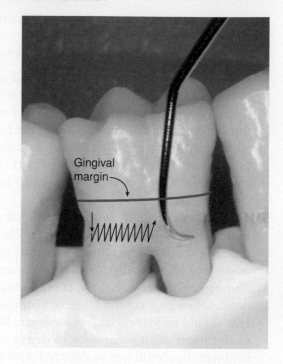

Subgingival Exploring. Subgingival assessment strokes should be short in length and involve many overlapping strokes covering every square millimeter of the root surface.

Steps for Subgingival Exploration

1. Adapt the explorer tip to the tooth surface above the gingival margin. Gently slide the tip under the gingival margin.

2. Keep the tip constantly in contact with the root surface. Gently slide the explorer in an apical direction until the back of the tip touches the soft tissue base of the sulcus or pocket. The attached tissue will have a soft, elastic feel.

3. Move the tip forward slightly, and use a vertical or oblique stroke to move the explorer up the surface of the root. Keep the tip in contact with the root surface as you pull the tip up toward the gingival margin. Concentrate as the tip moves over the tooth surface; be alert for quivers of the tip that indicate a calculus deposit.

4. Don't remove the explorer tip from the sulcus or pocket as you make an upward stroke. Removing and reinserting the tip repeatedly can traumatize the tissue at the gingival margin. Bring the explorer tip to a point just beneath the gingival margin and move the tip forward slightly.

5. Maintaining the tip in contact with the tooth surface, return the tip to the base of the sulcus or pocket. As you move the tip, remain alert for tactile information transmitted through the instrument shank.

6. Keep your assessment strokes short, approximately 2 to 3 mm in length. If you are working within a normal sulcus, your strokes will extend from the base of the sulcus to a point just beneath the gingival margin. When working within a periodontal pocket, you will need to explore the root in horizontal sections. First, explore the section next to the base of the pocket. Then, move the tip up and explore the midsection on the root. Finally, assess the section near the gingival margin. The depth of the pocket determines how many sections—3 mm in height—are needed to cover the entire root surface.

7. On the distal and mesial proximal surfaces, lead with the point of the tip. Do not "back" into the proximal surface. Your strokes should reach under the contact area so that half of the proximal surface is explored from the facial aspect and half from the lingual aspect of the tooth.

Section 2
Technique Practice: Anterior Teeth

INSTRUMENT SELECTION

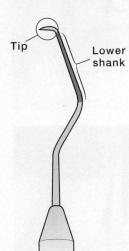

Tip

Lower shank

Instrument selection for anterior teeth. An Orban-type explorer, such as a TU17, is an excellent choice for subgingival assessment of the anterior teeth.

STEP-BY-STEP TECHNIQUE ON CENTRAL INCISOR

1. Equipment: an explorer.
2. Position yourself for the sextant shown in the icons below.

Right-Handed Clinicians

Left-Handed Clinicians

3. Remember: "Me, My Patient, My Light, My Dominant Hand, My Nondominant Hand, My Finger Rest, My Adaptation."

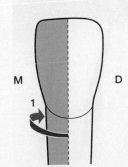

M   D

1

4. **Tooth.** As an introduction to exploring anterior teeth, first practice on the *mandibular left central incisor, facial aspect.*

   Right-handed clinicians—*surface toward.*
   Left-handed clinicians—*surface away.*

5. **Place the Tip in the Get Ready Zone.**
   - Place the tip in the Get Ready Zone near the midline of the facial surface.
   - The point of the explorer should face in the direction of the mesial surface.

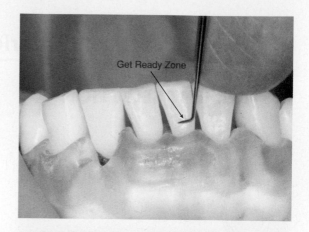

6. **Insert.** Insert the working-end beneath the gingival margin.

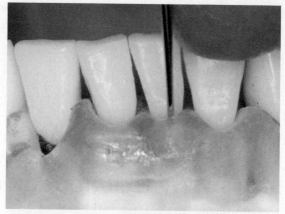

7. **Roll the Instrument Handle.** As you approach the mesiofacial line angle, roll the instrument handle to maintain adaptation.

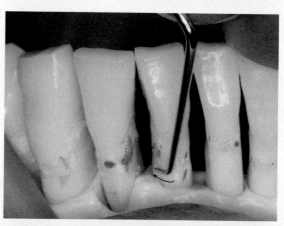

8. **Explore the Mesial Surface.** Continue making strokes under the contact area until you have explored at least halfway across the mesial proximal surface. (The other half of the mesial surface is reached from the lingual aspect of the tooth.)

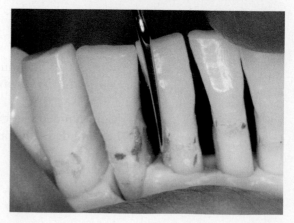

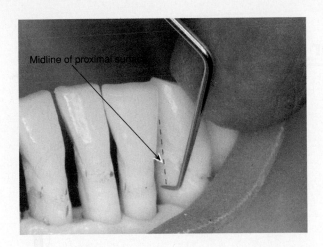

Midline of proximal surface

9. **Technique Check.** This photograph shows a dental typodont with the gingiva removed. Note the position of the explorer tip on the mesial of this canine tooth. Correct technique demands that the explorer reach at least the halfway point of the proximal surface under the contact area.

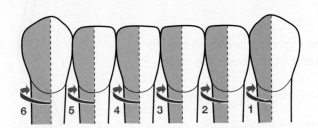

10. **Sequence 1.** Next, use the sequence shown in this illustration to explore the colored tooth surfaces of the facial aspect. Begin with the left canine and end with the right canine.

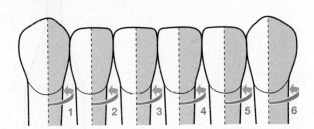

11. **Sequence 2.** Change your clock position and complete the remaining facial surfaces, beginning with the right canine and ending with the left canine.

Section 3
Technique Practice: Posterior Teeth

INSTRUMENT SELECTION

Tip

Lower
shank

Explorer Selection on Posterior Teeth. An 11/12-type explorer, such as an ODU 11/12, is an excellent choice for subgingival assessment of the posterior teeth.

The ODU 11/12 is a double-ended instrument with mirror image working-ends.

CHOOSING THE CORRECT WORKING-END

Before using a double-ended explorer, the clinician must first determine which working-end to use.

1. To select the correct working-end, observe the relationship of the lower shank to the distal surface of the tooth.
2. Pick a tooth that is easily seen, such as the first premolar tooth. Randomly select one of the explorer working-ends and adapt the tip to the distal surface of the first premolar.
   a. Correct working-end—the lower shank is parallel to the distal surface of the premolar.
   b. Incorrect working-end—the lower shank extends across the facial surface of the premolar.
3. Using the mandibular right posterior sextant as an example, one working-end of the explorer adapts to the facial aspect and the other working-end adapts to the lingual aspect of the sextant.

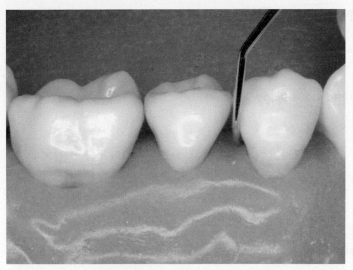

Correct Working-End

VISUAL CLUE—CORRECT:
The *lower shank* is parallel to the proximal surface and the *functional shank* goes "up and over the tooth."

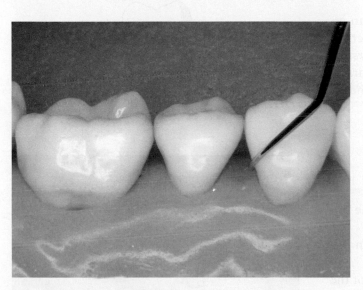

Incorrect Working-End

VISUAL CLUE—INCORRECT:
The *lower shank* is not parallel and the *functional shank* is "down and around the tooth."

Box 12-1. Rule for Working-End Selection on Posterior Teeth

When the working-end is adapted to the distal surface, the correct working-end has the following relationship between the shank and the tooth:

- Lower shank is parallel to the distal surface
- Functional shank goes up and over the tooth

Think: **Posterior = Parallel. Functional shank up and over!**

STEP-BY-STEP TECHNIQUE ON MANDIBULAR FIRST MOLAR

Directions:
- Equipment: an explorer.
- Position yourself for the sextant shown in the icons below.

Right-Handed Clinicians

Left-Handed Clinicians

- Remember: "Me, My patient, My light, My dominant hand, My non-dominant hand, My finger rest, My adaptation".

1. **Begin With Mandibular First Molar.** As an introduction to exploring the posterior teeth, first practice on the *mandibular right first molar*. The distal surface is completed first, beginning at the distofacial line angle and working onto the distal surface.

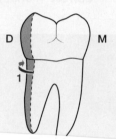

2. **Position the Tip Near the Distofacial Line Angle in the Get Ready Zone.**
   - Place the tip in the Get Ready Zone in the middle-third of the crown.
   - The tip should aim toward the back of the mouth because this is the direction in which you are working.

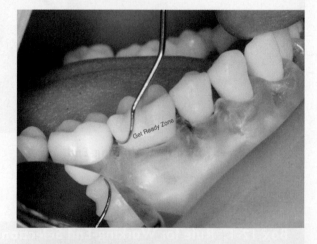

3. **Insert.**
   - Lower the instrument handle and adapt the "face" of the explorer tip to the tooth surface.
   - Slide the tip beneath the gingival margin.

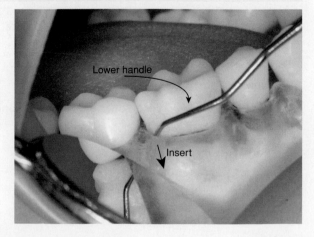

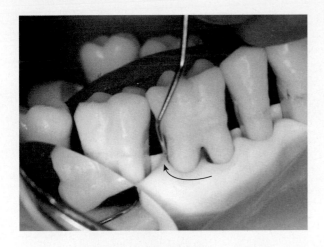

4. **Roll the Instrument Handle.** Roll the instrument handle slightly to adapt to the distal surface. Explore at least halfway across the distal surface from the facial aspect. Keep the tip adapted to the tooth surface at all times.

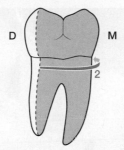

5. **Explore the Facial Surface.** You are now ready to explore the facial and mesial surfaces of the tooth, beginning at the distofacial line angle.

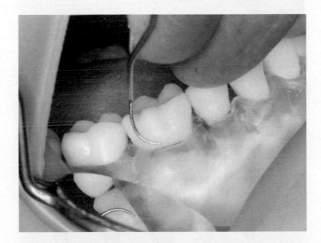

6. **Reposition the Tip for Facial Surface.**
   * While maintaining your fulcrum, remove the tip from the sulcus and turn it so that it aims toward the front of the mouth.
   * Place the tip in the Get Ready Zone.
   * Reinsert the tip and reposition it just to the left of the distofacial line angle.

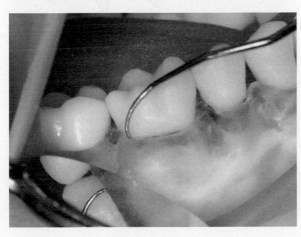

7. **Insert.**
   * Lower the instrument handle and place the "face" of the explorer against the facial surface in preparation for insertion.
   * Reinsert the tip and reposition it just to the left of the distofacial line angle.

8. **Roll the Handle.** As you approach the mesio-facial line angle, roll the handle slightly to maintain adaptation.

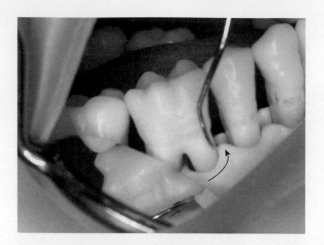

9. **Continue Strokes.** Explore at least halfway across the mesial surface from the facial aspect. (The other half will be explored from the lingual aspect.)

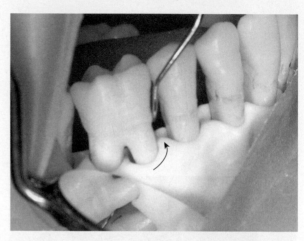

10. **Sequence for Sextant.** Next, use the sequence shown in this illustration to explore the facial aspect of the entire sextant, beginning with the posterior-most molar.

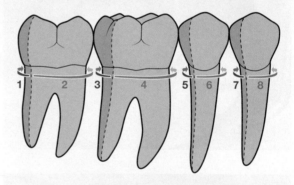

NOTE TO COURSE INSTRUCTOR: Exploration of root surfaces is covered in Module 22.

Section 4
Technique Alerts

USE OF HORIZONTAL STROKES FOR CALCULUS DETECTION

New clinicians often fail to detect calculus deposits that are located (1) near the distofacial or distolingual line angle of posterior teeth and (2) at the midline of the facial or lingual surfaces of anterior teeth. Undetected calculus deposits may result from not overlapping the assessment strokes sufficiently at line angles and midlines of teeth. Horizontal strokes are extremely useful for calculus detection in these areas.

　　Horizontal strokes were discussed in Module 10, Instrumentation Strokes. Refer to this module if you need to review basic information about horizontal instrumentation strokes.

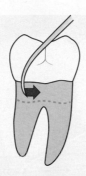

Horizontal Strokes. Horizontal strokes are made in a perpendicular direction to the long axis of the tooth.

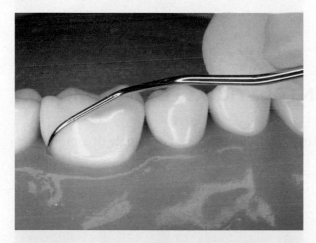

Handle Position. For a horizontal stroke, the instrument handle is lowered until the explorer working-end is oriented with the explorer point toward—but not touching—the base of the sulcus or pocket.

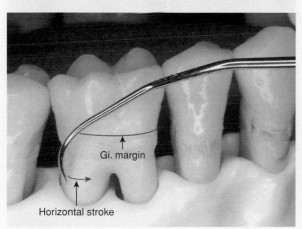

Gi. margin

Horizontal stroke

Working-End Position. This photograph was taken on a typodont with the gingiva removed so that the explorer working-end is visible. The tip is positioned at the line angle, and a short horizontal stroke is made around the line angle.

Reassume Oblique Strokes. After completing several horizontal strokes, the explorer is repositioned at the line angle. Oblique strokes are made across the facial surface in the usual manner.

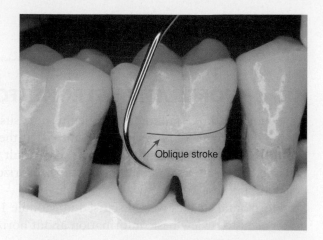

Oblique stroke

Horizontal Strokes on Anterior Teeth. Horizontal strokes are useful for detection of calculus deposits located at the midline of facial or lingual surfaces on anterior teeth.

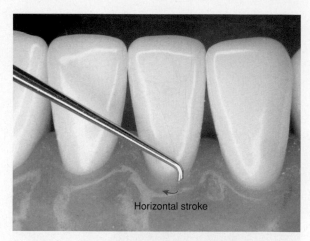

Horizontal stroke

TECHNIQUE PRACTICE 1: HORIZONTAL STROKES ON MOLAR TOOTH

Follow the directions below to practice horizontal strokes at the distofacial line angle of a molar tooth.

1. **Explore the Distal Surface.** Begin at the distofacial line angle on the mandibular first molar and work across the distal surface in the usual manner.

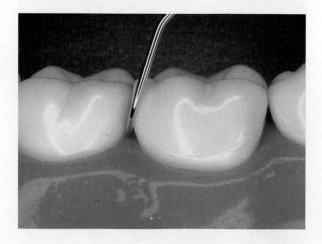

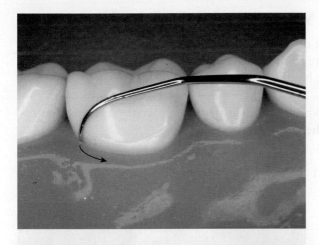

2. **Reposition for Horizontal Strokes.** Reinsert the explorer slightly distal to the distofacial line angle. Lower the instrument handle until the explorer's point is toward—but not touching—the base of the pocket. Make several short, controlled horizontal strokes around the line angle.

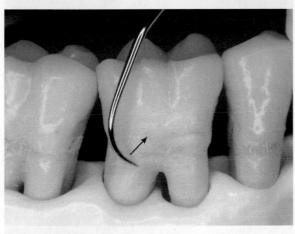

3. **Reposition for Oblique Strokes.** Reposition the working-end, and begin making oblique strokes across the facial surface.

TECHNIQUE PRACTICE 2: HORIZONTAL STROKES ON CENTRAL INCISOR

Follow the directions below to practice making horizontal strokes at the midline of the facial surface of a central incisor.

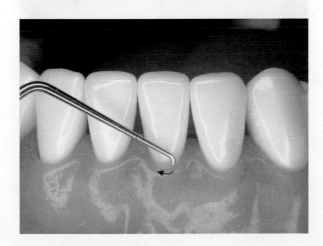

1. **Position for Horizontal Strokes.** Insert the explorer tip just distal to the midline.

   Lower the handle until the explorer's point is toward—but not touching—the base of the pocket. Make several short, controlled horizontal strokes across the midline.

TECHNIQUE PRACTICE: NEUTRAL WRIST POSITION

The most common positioning error when working on the maxillary posterior treatment areas is failing to maintain a neutral wrist position. A failure to maintain neutral wrist position occurs when the clinician bends the wrist rather than adjusts the handle position in the grasp.

Directions: This technique practice allows you to experience the difference in wrist positions that results from using two different handle positions in the grasp.

1. Equipment: an ODU 11/12-type explorer
2. Tooth: maxillary left first premolar, facial aspect

RIGHT-HANDED CLINICIANS

Incorrect Handle Position

1. Rest the instrument handle against your 2nd knuckle.
2. Place the explorer tip on the distal surface of the first premolar. Note that with the handle in this position, you must bend your wrist to position the lower shank parallel to the distal surface of the tooth.

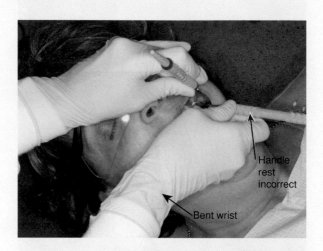

Correct Handle Position

1. Rest the handle somewhere between the 3rd knuckle and the "V" of your hand.
2. Place the tip of the explorer on the distal surface of the first premolar. Note that with the handle in this position you can maintain neutral wrist position and place the lower shank parallel to the distal surface of the tooth.

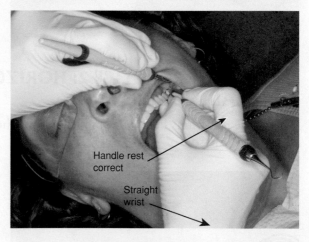

LEFT-HANDED CLINICIANS

Directions: This technique practice allows you to experience the difference in wrist positions that result from using two different handle positions in the grasp.

1. Equipment: an ODU 11/12-type explorer
2. Tooth: maxillary right first premolar, facial aspect

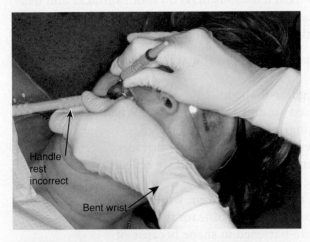

Handle
rest
incorrect

Bent wrist

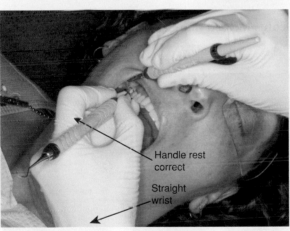

Handle rest
correct

Straight
wrist

Incorrect Handle Position

1. Rest the instrument handle against your 2nd knuckle.
2. Place the explorer tip on the distal surface of the first premolar. Note that with the handle in this position, you must bend your wrist to position the lower shank parallel to the distal surface of the tooth.

Correct Handle Position

1. Rest the handle somewhere between the 3rd knuckle and the "V" of your hand.
2. Place the tip of the explorer on the distal surface of the first premolar. Note that with the handle in this position you can maintain neutral wrist position and place the lower shank parallel to the distal surface of the tooth.

Section 5
Detection of Dental Calculus and Caries

TYPES AND CHARACTERISTICS OF CALCULUS DEPOSITS

Calculus is calcified bacterial plaque that forms as a hard tenacious mass on tooth surfaces and dental prostheses. It is commonly known as tartar. Calculus deposits are plaque retentive, meaning that the outer surface of a calculus deposit is covered with a layer of dental plaque biofilm.

1. Supragingival calculus deposits are located coronal to the gingival margin (above the gingival margin).
   a. Supragingival deposits often are large and irregular-shaped.
   b. These deposits can be detected using compressed air and a dental mirror. When dried with a stream of compressed air, supragingival calculus has a rough, chalky appearance, which contrasts visually with the smooth enamel surfaces. Wet supragingival calculus is difficult to detect because the wet surface reflects light and blends in with the shiny tooth enamel.
2. Subgingival calculus deposits are hidden beneath the gingival margin within the gingival sulcus or periodontal pocket. (Think "*sub*marines travel beneath the surface of the water.") Subgingival calculus deposits often are flattened in shape because of the pressure of the pocket wall against the tooth.
3. Residual calculus deposits are tiny remnants of calculus located on the surface of a tooth root.

Detection of Supragingival Calculus Deposits. Examine the tooth surfaces visually while applying a continuous stream of air with the air syringe.

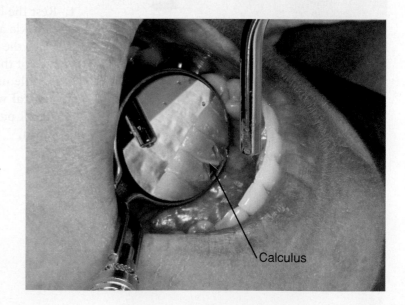

Calculus

TABLE 12-2. Characteristics of Dental Calculus

	Supragingival Deposits	Subgingival Deposits
Location	Above the gingival margin; detected visually	Beneath the gingival margin; detected by tactile means
Color	White, beige; may be discolored from food, beverages, or tobacco	Brown, black
Occurrence	Lingual aspect of mandibular anteriors, facial surfaces of maxillary molars, crowded or poorly aligned teeth	May be localized in certain areas or generalized throughout the mouth; heaviest on mesial and distal surfaces

THE NATURE OF CALCULUS FORMATION

When attempting to imagine the nature of subgingival deposits, remember that the deposits are built up layer by layer slowly over time. It may be helpful to imagine that you have taken a bucket of wet cement into your classroom! Once there, everyone takes turns throwing handfuls of cement against a plywood wall. Some individuals fling large globs of cement; some throw small handfuls. One aims at a new spot on the wall each time, another tries to hit the same area over and over. Now, imagine how the wall will appear when the cement has hardened. The cement mounds will be irregular and randomly spread over the wall. If you can imagine this absurd wall in your mind's eye, you have a fairly accurate concept of what subgingival calculus deposits look like on the root surface. To develop your ability to form a mental picture of the deposits that you detect, it is helpful to diagram what you are feeling and get feedback on your performance. For an activity designed to develop your ability to visualize calculus, refer to "Diagramming Calculus Deposits" in the Practical Focus section of this module.

Spicules   Ledge   Ring

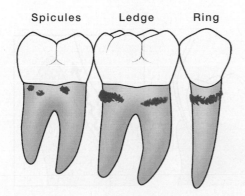

Common Calculus Formations. Three common types of calculus formations are (1) spicules, (2) calculus ledges, and (3) calculus rings.

Box 12-2. Common Calculus Formations

Spicule (or nodule)—an isolated, minute particle or speck of calculus. Commonly found under contact areas, at line angles, and at the midline line of a tooth.

Ledge—a long ridge of calculus running parallel to the gingival margin. Common on all tooth surfaces.

Ring—a ridge of calculus running parallel to the gingival margin that encircles the tooth.

Thin veneer—a thin, smooth coating of calculus on a portion of the root surface.

Fingerlike formation—a long, narrow deposit running parallel or oblique to the long axis of the root.

INTERPRETATION OF SUBGINGIVAL CONDITIONS

The ability to recognize what you are feeling beneath the gingival margin is a skill that takes time and concentration to develop. The following descriptions should aid you in interpreting what you feel. (From Trott, J.R.: The cross-subgingival calculus explorer. Dental Digest 67:481–483, 1961.)

Normal Conditions. Your fingers do not feel any interruptions in the path of the explorer as it moves from the junctional epithelium to the gingival margin.

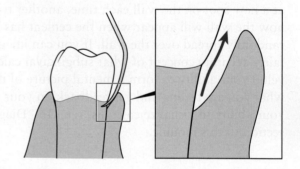

Spicules of Subgingival Calculus. The explorer tip transmits a gritty sensation to the clinician's fingers as it passes over fine, granular deposits. This can be compared with the sensation experienced when inline skating over a few pieces of gravel scattered on one area of a paved surface.

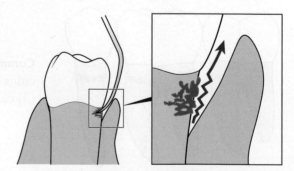

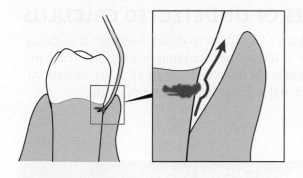

Ledge of Subgingival Calculus. As the explorer tip moves along the tooth surface, it moves out and around the raised bump and returns to the tooth surface. This is similar to the sensation of skating over speed bumps in a parking lot or over a cobblestone surface.

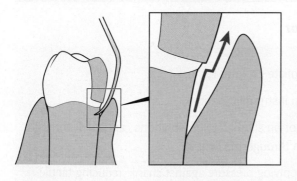

Restoration With Overhanging Margin. The explorer's path is blocked by the overhang and must move away from the tooth surface and over the restoration. This is similar to encountering the edge of a section of pavement that is higher than the surrounding pavement. Your skates must move up and over the higher section of pavement.

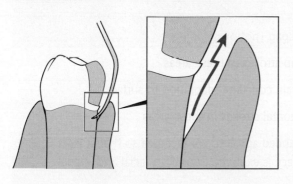

Restoration With Deficient Margin. The explorer passes over the surface of the tooth and then dips in to trace the surface of the restoration. This is similar to encountering the edge of a section of pavement that is lower than the surrounding pavement. Your skates must move down onto this section of pavement.

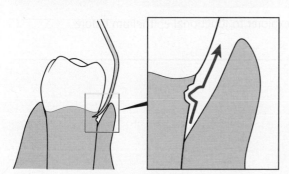

Carious Lesion (Decay). The explorer dips in and then comes out again as it travels along the tooth surface. This would be like skating into a pothole, across the pothole, and then back onto the pavement.

REFERENCE SHEET: COMMON CAUSES OF UNDETECTED CALCULUS

Errors in exploring technique are the most common cause of a failure to detect subgingival calculus deposits. As this reference sheet shows, a small change in technique often makes a big difference in the ability to detect calculus deposits. Calculus detection is the most difficult of all skills for new clinicians to develop. Attention to instrumentation basics will aid you in acquiring this skill.

TABLE 12-3.	Causes of Undetected Calculus Deposits
Location	**Technique Error**
No particular pattern of undetected deposits	• Use of inappropriate explorer for task • "Death-grip" on instrument handle • Middle finger not on shank (fewer vibrations can be felt through the handle than through the shank) • Middle finger applying pressure against shank, reducing tactile information • Strokes too far apart (not overlapping)
Undetected deposits at midlines of anteriors, or line angles of posteriors	• Failure to overlap strokes in these areas • Failure to maintain constant adaptation to surface • Not using horizontal strokes in these areas
Undetected deposits on mesial or distal surfaces	• Strokes not extended apical to contact area so that at least one-half of surface is explored from both facial and lingual aspects
Undetected deposits at base of sulcus or pocket	• Failure to insert explorer to junctional epithelium before initiating stroke

DENTAL CARIES

A carious lesion is a decayed area on the tooth crown or root. Enamel caries often can be detected visually by changes in the appearance of the enamel. An enamel lesion may appear chalky-white, gray, brown, or black in color. If explored, the walls of the lesion feel soft, tacky, or leathery in consistency. Root caries are common in older adults and periodontal patients. Subgingivally, root surface caries is detected as a rough, concave area on the surface of the root.

Technique for Caries Detection

1. An obvious carious lesion that can be detected visually *should not be explored.*
2. It is not a good idea to use the same explorer for both calculus and caries detection. The tip of an 11/12-type or a pigtail explorer can be damaged if used for caries detection. Once damaged, the burred working-end will not provide accurate tactile information to the clinician's fingers for detection of calculus. A straight or shepherd hook explorer is a good choice for caries detection.
3. The general technique for caries detection is to apply pressure with the point of the explorer against the region of suspected caries. Light pressure should be exerted with the explorer tip against the tooth surface. Firm pressure should not be used to force the explorer tip to penetrate the tooth surface.
   a. *Pit and Fissure Caries:* Direct the point straight into the pit or fissure using light pressure. Trace the entire length of a fissure with the explorer while applying light pressure downward into the developmental depression. If decay is present, the tip will "catch" in the surface of the enamel.
   b. *Smooth Surface Caries:* Move the tip of the explorer over the enamel surface; be alert for roughness, discontinuity, or change in hardness of the tooth surface. Visually check for discoloration of enamel surfaces.
   c. *Root Surface Caries:* While assessing the root surface, you will feel the explorer dip in and then come out again as it proceeds along the surface of the root. The depressed area of caries may feel rough or leathery.
   d. *Recurrent Decay:* Trace the margin of the restoration with the explorer. Be careful to check for overhanging margins on restorations that extend over the incisal or occlusal surface of a tooth.

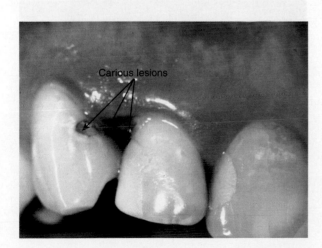

Dental Decay. Smooth surface caries on the canine and lateral incisor.

Section 6
Skill Application

PRACTICAL FOCUS

1. **Case 1.** Your classmate Ian is practicing using an ODU 11/12 type of double-ended explorer. Ian asks you to observe him and give him suggestions for improvement. The two photographs below are typical of Ian's grasp, finger rests, and adaptation as he works on the mandibular and maxillary teeth. What problems, if any, did you observe? How might Ian correct these problems?

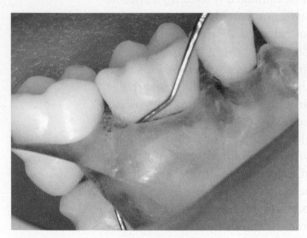

Case 1

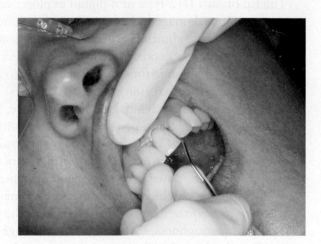

Case 1

2. **Case 2.** You are using a UNC 14 probe similar to the one shown at the top of page 220. Based on the information obtained by probing, which explorer design(s) discussed in this module would be recommended for calculus detection on the patient shown in Case 2A? On the patient shown in Case 2B?

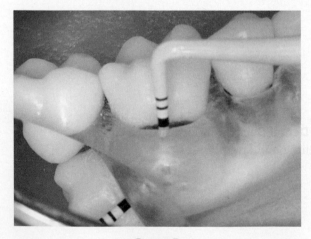

Case 2A

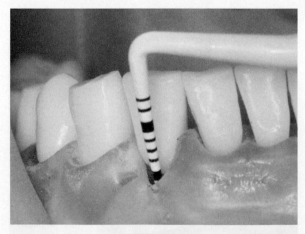

Case 2A

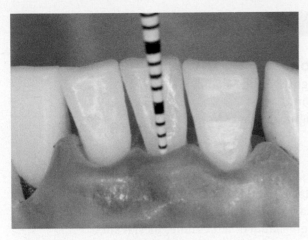

Case 2B

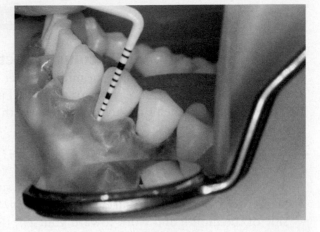

Case 2B

3. **Diagramming Calculus Deposits.** This activity will help you to develop tactile detection skills and the ability to form a mental picture of the deposits you detect.

Directions:

1) Begin by creating some objects that will represent tooth roots with calculus deposits. If possible, locate some discarded pieces of old copper or PVC tubing. The maintenance department at your college or university might be able to supply some. Use synthetic calculus to create "ledges and spicules of calculus" on the surface of the copper tubes. The "calculus deposits" should have a random pattern and each copper tube should have a unique pattern of deposits. Allow the calculus to dry overnight. Obtain a small *opaque* trash bag.

2) Put an explorer, a copper tube, and both your hands inside the trash bag. Use your mirror hand to hold the copper tube. Grasp the explorer in your other hand, and establish a finger rest on the side of the copper tube. Initiate assessment strokes along the surface of the tube. As you form a mental picture of the calculus deposits, diagram them on a piece of paper on which you have drawn a rectangle representing the copper tube. Indicate the location and relative size of the calculus deposits on the tube.

3) Finally, remove the copper tube from the bag. Compare the actual calculus deposits with your drawing. How did you do? Repeat this activity with different copper tubes to improve your detection and visualization skills.

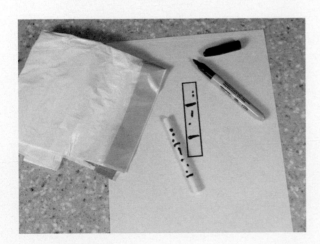

Check Your Diagram. Compare the actual deposits on the copper tube with your diagram.

TABLE 12-4. Explorers

General Technique for Calculus Detection

1. Use a relaxed grasp, resting your middle finger lightly on the shank.
2. Use the side of the explorer tip, not the actual point.
3. Cover every millimeter of the root surface with light, flowing strokes.

Anterior Teeth

1. Position: For surfaces toward, sit at 8–9:00 if you are a right-handed clinician or at 4–3:00 if you are a left-handed clinician. For surfaces away, sit at 12:00.
2. Sequence: Begin with the surfaces toward you. Start on the canine on the opposite side of the mouth and work toward yourself. (Right-handed: left canine, mesial surface; left-handed: right canine, mesial surface.)

Posterior Teeth

1. Position: For aspects toward, sit at 9:00 (or 3:00). For aspects away, sit at 10–11:00 (or 2–1:00).
2. Selection of working-end: Lower shank is parallel to tooth surface ("posterior parallel").
3. Sequence: Begin with the posterior-most tooth in the sextant. On each tooth, do the distal surface first, followed by facial and mesial (or lingual and mesial) surfaces.

NOTE TO COURSE INSTRUCTORS: See Module 22, Instruments for Advanced Root Debridement, for content on the exploration of root surfaces.

SKILL EVALUATION MODULE 12 | **EXPLORERS**

Student: _____

Evaluator: _____

Date: _____

Anterior Area 1 = _____
Anterior Area 2 = _____
Posterior Area 3 = _____
Posterior Area 4 = _____

DIRECTIONS FOR STUDENT: Use **Column S.** Evaluate your skill level as: **S** (satisfactory) or **U** (unsatisfactory).

DIRECTIONS FOR EVALUATOR: Use **Column E.** Indicate: **S** (satisfactory) or **U** (unsatisfactory). Each **S** equals 1 point, each **U** equals 0 points.

CRITERIA:	Area 1		Area 2		Area 3		Area 4	
	S	E	S	E	S	E	S	E
Position:								
Positioned correctly on clinician stool								
Positioned correctly with relation to patient, equipment, and treatment area								
Establishes correct patient head position								
Dental Mirror:								
Uses correct grasp and establishes secure rest with mirror								
Uses the mirror correctly for retraction and/or indirect vision								
Modified Pen Grasp with Dominant Hand:								
Thumb and index finger pads positioned opposite one another on handle; fingers not touching or overlapped								
Pad of middle finger rests lightly on shank; touches the ring finger								
Handle rests between the 2nd knuckle of the index finger and the "V" of hand								
Grasp is very relaxed (no blanching of fingers)								
Intraoral Fulcrum:								
Ring finger is straight and supports weight of hand								
Fulcrums on same arch, near tooth being instrumented								
Exploring Technique:								
Selects appropriate explorer for the task and the correct working-end if using a double-ended explorer								
Maintains correct adaptation of tip; rolls handle when needed for adaptation								
Uses light, overlapping strokes of an appropriate length								
Uses correct sequence in sextant								
Uses overlapping strokes (1) at midline of anterior teeth, (2) under the contact area, (3) at line angles of posterior teeth								
OPTIONAL GRADE PERCENTAGE CALCULATION Total **S**'s in each E column.								

Sum of **S**'s _____ divided by Total Points Possible (**64**) equals the Percentage Grade _____

SKILL EVALUATION MODULE 12   EXPLORERS

Student: _____

EVALUATOR COMMENTS

_____
_____
_____
_____
_____
_____
_____
_____
_____
_____
_____
_____
_____
_____
_____
_____
_____

Box for sketches pertaining to written comments.

Concepts in Periodontal Debridement

Module Overview

This module discusses (1) the role of periodontal instrumentation in the prevention and treatment of gingivitis and periodontitis, (2) changes in instrumentation terminology prompted by recent research findings, (3) healing after instrumentation, and (4) dental hypersensitivity.

Module Outline

Key Terms

Periodontal disease
Gingivitis
Periodontitis
Periodontally involved tooth
Plaque biofilm
Plaque-retentive factors

Dental calculus
Evidence-based care
Scaling
Root planing
Periodontal debridement
Long junctional epithelium

Exposed dentin
Dentinal hypersensitivity
Dentinal tubules
Odontoblastic process

Learning Objectives

1. Define the terms periodontal disease, gingivitis, and periodontitis.

2. Differentiate the terms gingivitis and periodontitis.

3. Describe the condition of the periodontal tissues surrounding a periodontally involved tooth.

4. Define plaque biofilm.

5. Discuss the roles of plaque biofilms and dental calculus in periodontal disease.

6. Discuss evidence-based care and how it benefits the patient.

7. Discuss instrumentation terminology and how terminology has evolved to reflect recent research findings.

8. Define periodontal debridement and explain how it differs from scaling and root planing.

9. List the goals of periodontal debridement.

10. Describe healing after periodontal debridement.

11. Define dental hypersensitivity and discuss patient education about hypersensitivity.

Section 1
Disease Prevention

THE ROLE OF DENTAL CALCULUS IN PERIODONTAL DISEASE

Periodontal disease is a bacterial infection of the periodontium. The two categories of periodontal disease are gingivitis and periodontitis.

1. Gingivitis is a bacterial infection that is confined to the gingiva. It results in damage to the gingival tissues that is reversible.
2. Periodontitis is a bacterial infection of all parts of the periodontium including the gingiva, periodontal ligament, bone, and cementum. It results in irreversible destruction to the periodontal tissues.
3. A periodontally involved tooth is a tooth that is experiencing destruction of the gingival tissues, periodontal ligament, bone, and cementum. A periodontally involved tooth exhibits bone loss in combination with pocket formation and/or gingival recession.
4. Research investigations have shown that the primary cause of most periodontal diseases is plaque biofilms.
   a. Plaque biofilm is a well-organized community of bacteria that adheres tenaciously to tooth surfaces, restorations, and prosthetic appliances.
   b. Plaque-retentive factors are conditions that foster the establishment and growth of plaque biofilms, such as calculus deposits and overhanging restorations.
5. Removal of calculus deposits from tooth surfaces is a critical step in the prevention and treatment of periodontal disease.
   a. Dental calculus is mineralized bacterial plaque, covered on its external surface with a living layer of plaque biofilm.
   b. Because the surface of a calculus deposit is irregular and is always covered with disease-causing bacteria, dental calculus plays a significant role in causing periodontal disease.
   c. It is difficult to prevent or control periodontal diseases if calculus deposits are present, and so it is important that these deposits be removed from the teeth.

EVIDENCE-BASED CARE

Dental healthcare providers have an obligation to provide evidence-based care. Evidence-based care is clinical care that is based on the best available scientific evidence. Every day the clinician makes decisions regarding patient care recommendations.

1. Evidence-based decision making emphasizes the use of scientific knowledge as the foundation for clinical decision making.
2. The ultimate purpose of using the evidence-based decision-making process is to provide better treatment to patients.
3. As with all treatment procedures, evidence-based decision making should be the basis for instrumentation of the teeth for the removal of calculus and plaque biofilms.
4. Recent scientific knowledge has resulted in changes in the way that calculus deposits and plaque biofilms are removed from the teeth during instrumentation.

Section 2
Periodontal Debridement

INSTRUMENTATION TERMINOLOGY

The body of scientific knowledge in dentistry is growing rapidly. As recently as 15 years ago, basic scientific knowledge about the nature and treatment of periodontal diseases was quite limited. Increased scientific knowledge about periodontal disease has inspired changes in the terminology associated with calculus and plaque removal instrumentation. The careful reader will note that different instrumentation terminology appears in books and journals written several years ago compared with recent publications. Periodontal debridement is a newer term used in the dental hygiene literature to replace the terms scaling and root planing.

1. Traditional Instrumentation Terminology.

   a. Traditionally, the terms scaling and root planing were used to describe nonsurgical periodontal instrumentation procedures. Scaling is the instrumentation of the crown and/or root surfaces to remove plaque, calculus, and stains.

   b. Root planing is instrumentation of periodontally involved teeth to remove cementum that is rough or contaminated with harmful bacterial products. Root planning was performed on the roots of all periodontally involved teeth (teeth with bone loss combined with periodontal pockets and/or tissue recession).

      1) As traditionally defined, root planing involved the intentional removal of cementum from the roots of periodontally involved teeth until the root surfaces were a glassy smooth texture.

      2) Until recently, it was thought that bacterial products were firmly held in the cementum of periodontally involved teeth and that the only way to remove these bacterial products was to remove the cementum from the root surfaces.

      3) *It is now clear that cementum removal is not necessary on most root surfaces.* Rather than root planing to remove most or all of the cementum, it is now known that the bacterial products can be removed from the root surfaces by using modern ultrasonic instruments or very light instrumentation strokes with hand-activated instruments.

2. Emerging Instrumentation Terminology.

   1. Periodontal debridement is a newer term used to replace the terms scaling and root planing. Periodontal debridement is the removal of bacterial plaque biofilms and calculus deposits from crown and/or root surfaces and from within the pocket space.

      a. Periodontal debridement includes instrumentation of root surfaces for the removal of plaque and calculus, but it does not include the deliberate, aggressive removal of cementum.

      b. Conservation of cementum is a goal of periodontal debridement. In health, an important function of cementum is to attach the periodontal ligament fibers to the root surface. During the healing process after disease, cementum is thought to contribute to repair of the periodontal tissues.

      c. The extent of instrumentation should be limited to that needed to obtain a favorable tissue response. Root surfaces should be instrumented only to a level that results in tissue healing.

      d. The differences between scaling/ root planing and periodontal debridement are summarized in Table 13-1.

TABLE 13-1.	Comparison of Scaling/Root Planing and Periodontal Debridement	
	Scaling and Root Planing	**Periodontal Debridement**
Focus	Removal of calculus from all tooth surfaces and the removal of cementum from root surfaces	Removal of the bacterial plaque biofilms and calculus from tooth surfaces and within the pocket space
Instrumentation of Root Surfaces	Aggressive instrumentation removes significant amounts of cementum	Conservation of cementum is a goal; bacterial products are removed easily with ultrasonic instruments or light instrumentation strokes
Method	Hand-activated instrumentation	A combination of hand-activated and ultrasonic instrumentation preferred

RATIONALE FOR PERIODONTAL DEBRIDEMENT

The goals of periodontal debridement are to maintain or reestablish periodontal health by:

1. Arresting the progress of periodontal disease by removing bacterial plaque biofilms and plaque retentive calculus deposits.
2. Creating an environment that assists in maintaining tissue health or permits the gingival tissue to heal, therefore eliminating inflammation.
3. Increasing the effectiveness of patient self-care by eliminating areas of plaque retention that are difficult or impossible for a patient to clean.

HEALING AFTER INSTRUMENTATION

1. The tissue damage of gingivitis can be reversed with periodontal debridement, good patient self-care, and the removal of local factors (such as a faulty dental restoration).
2. After the instrumentation of a periodontally involved tooth, some healing of the periodontal tissues will occur. For a periodontally involved tooth, the primary pattern of healing after instrumentation is through the formation of a long junctional epithelium.
   a. *No* new formation of bone, cementum, or periodontal ligament during the healing process occurs after periodontal debridement of a periodontally involved tooth.
   b. Periodontal debridement can result in reduced probing depths caused by the formation of a long junctional epithelium combined with the gingival recession that often occurs following periodontal instrumentation.

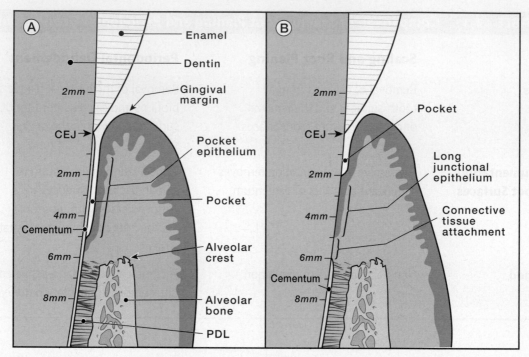

Healing after nonsurgical periodontal debridement. A. Periodontal pocket of 6 mm before periodontal debridement. **B.** After periodontal debridement, the pocket depth is 2 mm owing to healing by formation of a long junctional epithelium and a reduction in tissue swelling. (Used with permission from Nield-Gehrig, J.S. and Willmann, D., Foundations of Periodontics for the Dental Hygienist Edition 2, 2007, Philadelphia: Lippincott Williams & Wilkins: p. 258, Figure 17-1.)

Section 3
Dentinal Hypersensitivity

Exposed dentin is dentin that has been exposed to the oral cavity because of an absence of the enamel or cementum that normally covers it. Dentin may be exposed on a tiny or extensive area of the tooth. Usually, dentin is exposed as a result of loss of cementum on an area of the root surface.

1. Common causes of exposed dentin include toothbrush abrasion and root planing.
2. Dentinal hypersensitivity is a short, sharp painful reaction that occurs when an area of exposed dentin is subjected to a mechanical, thermal, or chemical stimulus.
   a. An individual may experience dentinal hypersensitivity when brushing a certain tooth (mechanical stimulus) or when eating sweet, sour, or acidic foods (chemical stimuli).
   b. Drinking hot coffee while eating ice cream or breathing in cold air while walking outside on a cold day might produce a similar painful reaction (thermal stimuli).
3. Hypersensitivity is associated with exposed dentin; however, not all exposed dentin is hypersensitive.
4. The pain of hypersensitivity is sporadic. A patient may experience sensitivity for a period of time and then other periods of time during which sensitivity is not a problem.
5. Instrumentation of root surfaces also can result in dentinal hypersensitivity. The possibility of creating dentinal hypersensitivity underscores that conservation of cementum should be a goal of nonsurgical instrumentation.

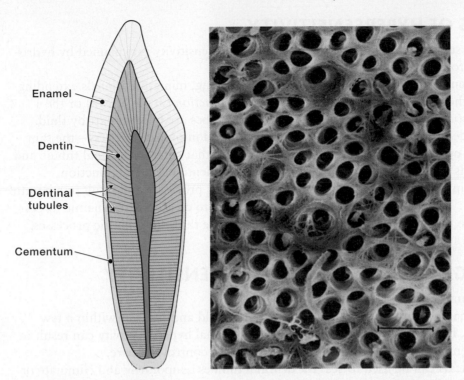

Dentinal Tubules. A. Diagram of dentin showing the numerous *dentinal tubules* that penetrate the dentin. **B.** A scanning electron micrograph of the dentinal tubules of a human tooth. (Used with permission from Melfi, R.C., Permar's Oral Embryology and Microscopic Anatomy, ed. 10. 2000, Philadelphia: Lippincott Williams & Wilkins: page 120, Figure 5-8.)

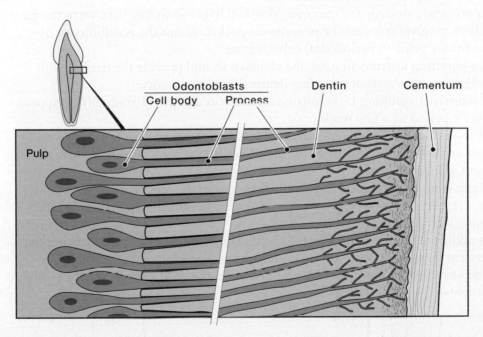

Odontoblastic Processes. An odontoblastic process is a thin tail of cytoplasm from a cell in the pulp that enters a dentinal tubule and extends from the pulp to the dentinoenamel or dentinocemental junction. (Used with permission from Nield-Gehrig, J.S. and Willmann, D., Foundations of Periodontics for the Dental Hygienist Edition 2, 2007, Philadelphia: Lippincott Williams & Wilkins: p. 259, Figure 17-2.)

ORIGINS OF HYPERSENSITIVITY

1. Evidence suggests that the origin of dentinal hypersensitivity is explained by hydrodynamic forces within the dentinal tubules.
   a. The dentinal tubules penetrate the dentin like long, miniature tunnels extending from the pulp chamber to the *dentinoenamel junction* (in the crown) or the *dentinocemental* junction (in the root). These tubes are filled in part by fluid.
   b. Each dentinal tubule is partially filled with an odontoblastic process—the thin tail of cytoplasm from a cell in the tooth pulp—that enters a dentinal tubule and extends from the pulp to the dentinoenamel or dentinocemental junction.
2. Changes in temperature stimulate the odontoblastic processes and result in a painful sensation. The changes in temperature are believed to create hydrodynamic forces within the fluid-filled dentinal tubules that stimulate the odontoblastic processes.

STRATEGIES FOR TREATING HYPERSENSITIVITY

1. Professional Care.
   a. Fortunately, most dentinal hypersensitivity is mild and resolves within a few weeks. In its more severe forms, however, dentinal hypersensitivity can result in a patient's inability to perform thorough plaque control self-care.
   b. Chemicals can be used to seal the dentinal tubules temporarily and eliminate or minimize the dentinal sensitivity.
      a. Fluorides can be used to precipitate fluoride-rich crystals on the tooth surface.
      b. Calcium hydroxide can be burnished into the root surface.
      c. Cavity varnishes can be used to cover the tooth surface temporarily.
2. Educating Patients About Hypersensitivity.
   a. An appropriate strategy for managing dentinal hypersensitivity is to warn the patient with gingival recession or periodontal pockets about the possibility of hypersensitivity prior to periodontal debridement.
   b. Before initiating instrumentation, the clinician should provide the patient with the following information regarding dentinal hypersensitivity:
      1) If sensitivity resulting from instrumentation occurs, it will gradually disappear over a period of a few weeks.
      2) Thorough daily plaque removal is *the most important factor* in the prevention and control of sensitivity. Without meticulous plaque control, no treatment will be successful.
      3) There is no treatment that will immediately stop the sensitivity. If sensitivity occurs, there are several agents that can be professionally applied to reduce sensitivity.
      4) In addition, there are toothpastes specifically formulated for desensitizing the teeth at home. Those pastes containing potassium nitrate or strontium chloride as the active ingredient have been demonstrated to provide relief in some patients.

Section 4
Practical Focus

Situation 1. You are a recent graduate of a dental hygiene program and have just started working in a new dental office. You learn that the other dental hygienist in the practice, Samantha, believes that aggressive root planing should be completed on all periodontally involved teeth. Samantha states she has been practicing for 20 years and that removal of cementum is what she learned in school. You feel a little intimidated because you just graduated 5 months ago; nevertheless, you mention to her that you were taught that vigorous root planing should not be performed as a routine procedure on all teeth with periodontal pockets. For a while, you accept that you and she have a difference of opinion about cementum removal, but you and Samantha see the same patients and it is not unusual for a patient to question you about your instrumentation. For example, Mr. Riveras asked: "Why don't you use a lot of pressure against my teeth and scrape, scrape, scrape over each tooth like Samantha always does? Are you getting my teeth clean?" Questions such as this make you feel that you should discuss periodontal debridement with Samantha. How would approach this issue with Samantha?

Situation 2. Mr. Rothenburger is a regular patient in the dental office. You saw him for periodontal debridement yesterday, and today he returned to the office complaining of a sensation "like a tiny electric shock" every time he brushes his maxillary right first molar. He also experiences "a sharp tingle" when he consumes cold water. (a) What do you think is causing the sensations that Mr. Rothenburger is experiencing? (b) How would you explain the problem to Mr. Rothenburger? (c) Is there any treatment that you can provide to temporarily alleviate this problem? (d) What self-care instructions should you give Mr. Rothenburger with regard to dentinal sensitivity?

Situation 3. Mrs. Starnes has bone loss and periodontal pockets throughout her mouth. She has agreed to a treatment plan consisting of patient education and periodontal debridement. Mrs. Starnes asks you if the bone support around her teeth will improve after you have finished "cleaning her teeth." How would you reply to Mrs. Starnes' question?

NOTE TO COURSE INSTRUCTORS: There is a separate module devoted to each design classification. Modules 14 to 17 cover sickle scalers, universal curets, area-specific curets, and periodontal files. Modules 21 to 23 cover advanced probing techniques and advanced root instrumentation.

Each of these modules provides step-by-step instructions for instrument use and does not rely on the content from any previous instrument module. *This module structure means that the instrument modules can be covered in any order that you prefer.* In addition, it is not necessary to include all modules. For example, if sickle scalers are not part of your school's instrument kit, this module does not need to be included in the course.

Sickle Scalers

Module Overview

This module presents the design characteristics of anterior and posterior sickle scalers and step-by-step instructions for using sickle scalers to remove medium-sized or heavy calculus deposits from the anterior and posterior teeth. *Module 13, Concepts in Periodontal Debridement, should be completed before beginning this module.*

NOTE TO COURSE INSTRUCTORS: There is a separate module devoted to each design classification (sickle scalers, universal curets, area-specific curets, periodontal files) and modules covering advanced probing techniques and advanced root instrumentation. Each module provides step-by-step instructions for instrument use and does not rely on content from any previous instrument module. *This module structure means that the instrument modules can be covered in any order that you prefer.* In addition, it is not necessary to include all modules. For example, if sickle scalers are not part of your school's instrument kit, this module does not need to be included in the course.

Module Outline

Key Terms

Sickle scaler   Face at 90 degrees to the lower shank
Anterior sickle scaler   Outer cutting edge
Posterior sickle scaler   Inner cutting edge

Learning Objectives

1. Identify the design characteristics of sickle scalers.

2. List the uses of sickle scalers.

3. Explain why the lower shank of a sickle scaler should be tilted slightly toward the tooth surface being instrumented to obtain correct angulation.

4. Using a sickle scaler, demonstrate correct adaptation and use of calculus removal strokes on the anterior teeth.

5. Describe how the clinician can use visual clues to select the correct working-end of a posterior sickle scaler.

6. Using a sickle scaler, demonstrate correct adaptation and use of calculus removal strokes on the posterior teeth.

Section 1
Sickle Scalers

GENERAL DESIGN CHARACTERISTICS

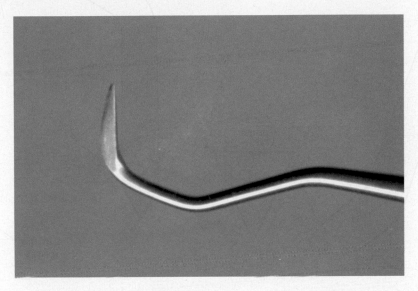

A sickle scaler is a periodontal instrument used to remove calculus deposits from the crowns of the teeth. Sickle scalers are confined to *supra*gingival use and should NOT be used on root surfaces.

1. Sickle scalers are available in either anterior or posterior designs.
   a. Anterior sickle scalers are limited to use on anterior treatment sextants.
      1) Often they are single-ended instruments because only one working-end is needed to instrument the crowns of the anterior teeth.
      2) It is common, however, to combine two different anterior sickles on a double-ended instrument.
   b. Posterior sickle scalers are designed for use on posterior sextants, but they also may be used on anterior teeth.
      1) Usually, two posterior sickles are paired on a double-ended instrument (the working-ends are mirror images of one another).
      2) For example, the Jacquette 34 is paired with the Jacquette 35 (the working-end of the Jacquette 34 is a mirror image of the working-end of the Jacquette 35).
2. The working-end of a sickle scaler has several unique design characteristics:
   a. A pointed back; some newer sickle scaler designs have working-ends with rounded backs
   b. A pointed tip
   c. Triangular in cross section
   d. Two cutting edges per working-end
   e. The face perpendicular to the lower shank
3. Some examples of sickle scaler instruments are:
   a. Anterior sickle scalers—OD-1, Jacquette-30, Jacquette-33, Whiteside-2, USC-128, Towner-U15, Goldman-H6, and Goldman-H7
   b. Posterior sickle scalers—Jacquette 34/35, Jacquette 14/15; Jacquette 31/32; Ball 2/3; Mecca 11/12; and the Catatonia 107/108

WORKING-END DESIGN

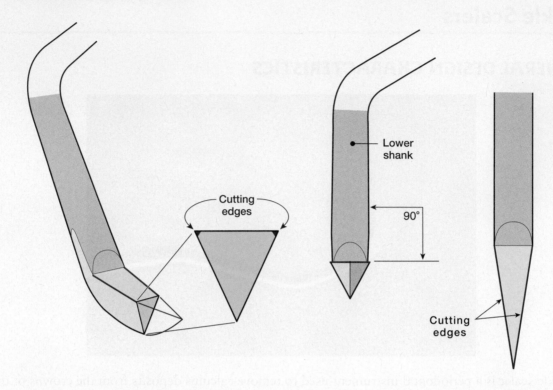

REFERENCE SHEET: SICKLE SCALER

TABLE 14-1. Sickle Scaler	
Cross Section	Triangular cross section; this design limits use to above the gingival margin because the pointed tip and back could cause tissue trauma
Working-End	Pointed back and tip Two cutting edges per working-end
Face	Face is perpendicular to the lower shank so that cutting edges are level with one another; *level cutting edges mean that the lower shank must be tilted slightly toward the tooth surface to establish correct angulation*
Application	Anterior teeth—only one single-ended instrument is needed Posterior teeth—one double-ended instrument is needed
Primary Functions	Removal of medium- to large-sized supragingival calculus deposits Excellent for calculus removal on the (1) proximal surfaces of anterior crowns and (2) enamel surfaces apical to the contact areas of posterior teeth NOT recommended for use on root surfaces

Section 2
Calculus Removal Concepts

CHARACTERISTICS OF THE CALCULUS REMOVAL STROKE

Before beginning the step-by-step technique practice with sickle scalers, review the (1) characteristics of the calculus removal stroke and (2) steps for calculus removal. These concepts are the same for use of a sickle scaler, universal curet, and area-specific curet.

TABLE 14-2. The Calculus Removal Stroke	
Stabilization	Apply pressure with the index finger and thumb inward against the instrument handle and press the tip of the fulcrum finger against a tooth surface
Adaptation	Tip-third (sickles) or toe-third (curets) of cutting edge is adapted
Angulation	70 to 80 degrees; for sickle scalers and universal curets, the lower shank must be tilted slightly toward the tooth surface to achieve correct angulation
Lateral Pressure for Calculus Removal	Moderate to firm pressure against the tooth surface is maintained throughout the pull stroke that is used for calculus removal. (Note: Lateral pressure is NOT used with the placement stroke when positioning the working-end beneath a calculus deposit)
Characteristics	Powerful controlled strokes, short in length
Stroke Direction	Vertical strokes are most commonly used on anterior teeth and on the mesial and distal surfaces of posterior teeth. Oblique strokes are most commonly used on the facial and lingual surfaces of posterior teeth. Horizontal strokes are used at the line angles of posterior teeth and the midlines of the facial or lingual surfaces of anterior teeth
Stroke Number	Strokes should be limited to areas where calculus is present; use the minimum number of strokes needed to remove calculus deposits

FLOW CHART: STEPS FOR CALCULUS REMOVAL

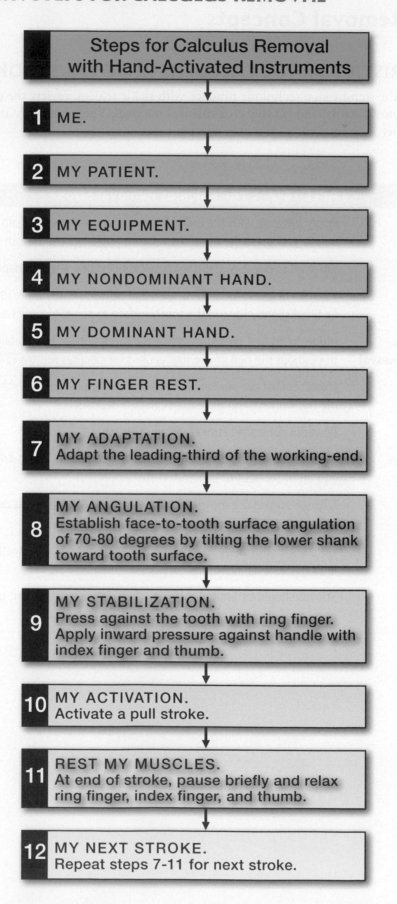

Steps for Calculus Removal with Hand-Activated Instruments

1 ME.

2 MY PATIENT.

3 MY EQUIPMENT.

4 MY NONDOMINANT HAND.

5 MY DOMINANT HAND.

6 MY FINGER REST.

7 MY ADAPTATION.
Adapt the leading-third of the working-end.

8 MY ANGULATION.
Establish face-to-tooth surface angulation of 70-80 degrees by tilting the lower shank toward tooth surface.

9 MY STABILIZATION.
Press against the tooth with ring finger. Apply inward pressure against handle with index finger and thumb.

10 MY ACTIVATION.
Activate a pull stroke.

11 REST MY MUSCLES.
At end of stroke, pause briefly and relax ring finger, index finger, and thumb.

12 MY NEXT STROKE.
Repeat steps 7-11 for next stroke.

Section 3
Technique Practice: Anterior Teeth

ESTABLISHING 70- TO 80-DEGREE ANGULATION

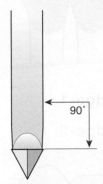

Working-end design. In establishing correct angulation, it is important to remember that on a sickle scaler *the face of the working-end is at a 90° angle to the lower shank.*

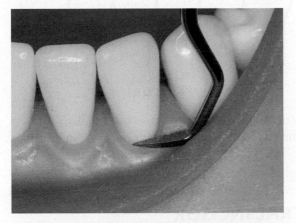

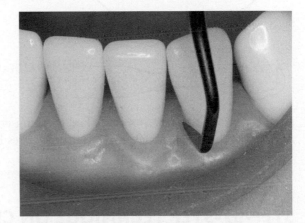

Incorrect angulation. Because the lower shank is at a 90-degree angle to face, positioning the lower shank parallel to the tooth surface results in an angulation of 90 degrees.

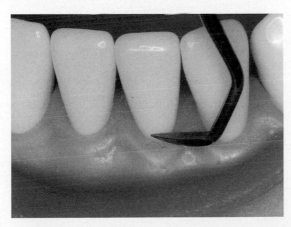

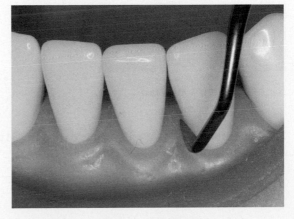

Correct angulation. Correct angulation is achieved by tilting the lower shank slightly toward the tooth surface to be instrumented. In this position, the face-to-tooth surface angulation is between 70 and 80 degrees.

APPLICATION OF THE CUTTING EDGES

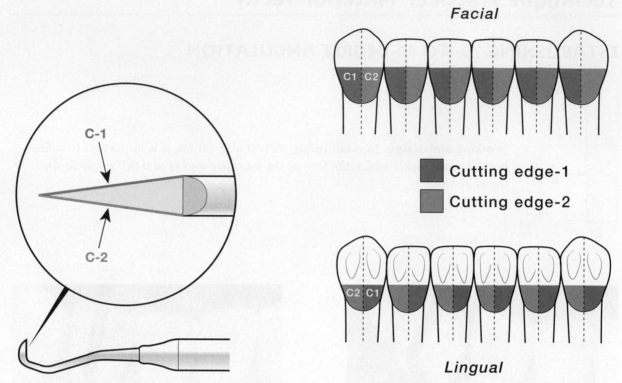

Facial

C-1

C-2

C1 C2

Cutting edge-1

Cutting edge-2

C2 C1

Lingual

Application to Anterior Surfaces. The working-end of an anterior sickle has two cutting edges (C-1 and C-2). The illustration on the right indicates how the two cutting edges are applied to the tooth surfaces of the anterior teeth.

STEP-BY-STEP TECHNIQUE ON CENTRAL INCISOR

1. Equipment: an anterior sickle scaler.
2. Position yourself for the sextant shown in the icons below.

   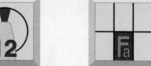

Right-Handed Clinicians

Left-Handed Clinicians

3. Remember: "Me, My Patient, My Light, My Dominant Hand, My Nondominant Hand, My Finger Rest, My Adaptation."

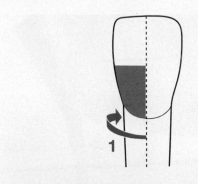

4. Tooth. As an introduction to using a sickle scaler on the anterior teeth, first practice on the *mandibular left central incisor, facial aspect.*

Right-handed clinicians—*surface toward.*
Left-handed clinicians—*surface away.*

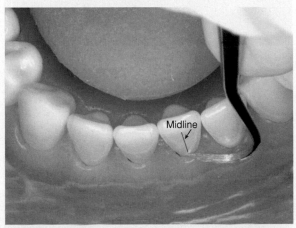

5. Position Working-End Near the Midline of Left Central Incisor. Establish a 70- to 80-degree instrument face-to-tooth surface angulation. The tip should be aimed toward the mesial surface of the tooth.

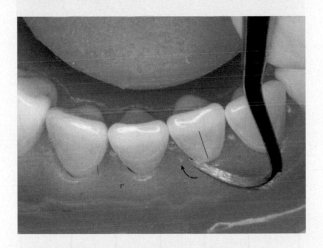

6. Continue Across the Facial Surface. Use overlapping strokes as you work across the facial surface in the direction of the mesial surface.

Roll the instrument handle slightly between strokes to maintain adaptation.

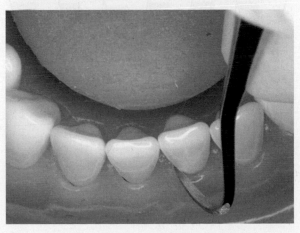

7. Roll the Instrument Handle. As you approach the mesiofacial line angle, roll the instrument handle to maintain adaptation of the tip-third of the working-end.

8. **Instrument the Mesial Surface.** Continue making strokes as you work your way along the mesial surface. Check to make sure that you have maintained an angulation of 70 to 80 degrees.

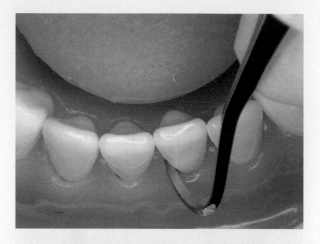

9. **Instrument Under the Contact Area.** Continue strokes until you work at least halfway across the mesial surface. (The other half of the mesial surface will be instrumented from the lingual aspect of the tooth.)

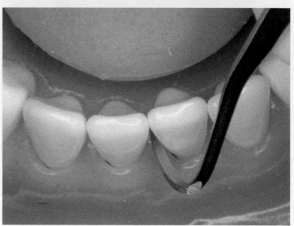

10. **Sequence.** Next, use the sequence shown in this illustration to instrument the colored tooth surfaces of the facial aspect. Begin with the left canine and end with the right canine.

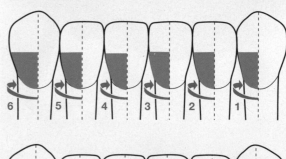

11. **Sequence.** Change your clock position and complete the remaining facial surfaces, beginning with the right canine and ending with the left canine.

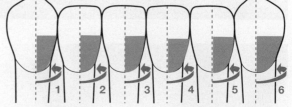

Section 4
Technique Practice: Posterior Teeth

CHOOSING THE CORRECT WORKING-END

Method 1: The Lower Shank as a Visual Clue

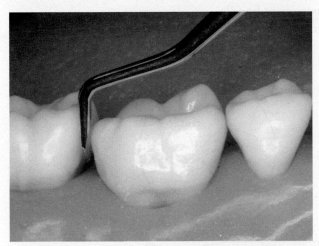

Correct Working-End

VISUAL CLUE—CORRECT: The *lower shank* is parallel to the proximal surface, and the *functional shank* goes "up and over the tooth."

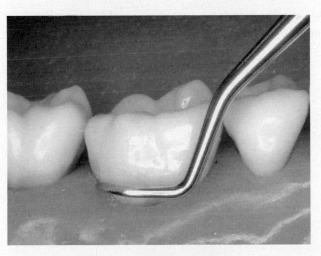

Incorrect Working-End

VISUAL CLUE—INCORRECT: The *lower shank* is not parallel, and the *functional shank* is "down and around the tooth."

Box 14-1. The Lower Shank as a Visual Clue

When the working-end is adapted to the distal surface, the correct working-end has the following relationship between the shank and the tooth:

- Lower shank is parallel to the distal surface
- Functional shank goes up and over the tooth

Think: Posterior = Parallel. Functional shank up and over!

Method 2: The Inner and Outer Cutting Edges as a Visual Clue

There is a second method that you can use to choose the correct working-end of a posterior sickle scaler. For this method, the cutting edges provide the visual clue. It is not important whether you use Method 1 or Method 2 to select the working-end. Use the method that is easiest for you.

Method 2: Each of the working-ends has two cutting edges, an inner and an outer cutting edge:

1. The outer cutting edges are *farther* from the instrument handle.
2. The inner cutting edges are *closer* to the instrument handle.

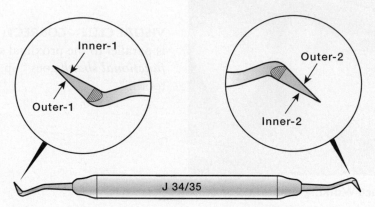

The Cutting Edges as a Visual Clue. Each of the two working-ends of a posterior sickle scaler has two cutting edges, an inner and an outer cutting edge.

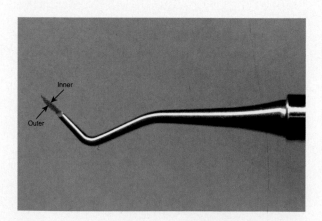

Inner and Outer Cutting Edges. To identify the cutting edges, hold the instrument so that you are looking at the face of the working-end.

Box 14-2. The Inner and Outer Cutting Edges as Visual Clues

The inner cutting edges are used to instrument the distal surfaces.

The outer cutting edges are used to instrument the facial (lingual) and mesial surfaces.

ESTABLISHING 70- TO 80-DEGREE ANGULATION

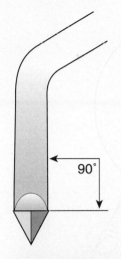

Working-End Design. In establishing correct angulation, it is important to remember that on a sickle scaler *the face of the working-end is at a 90° angle to the lower shank.*

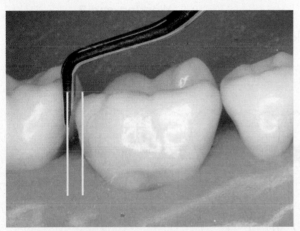

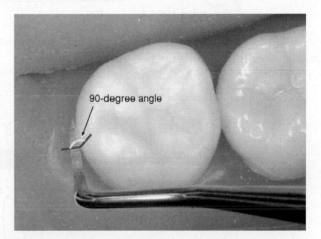

Incorrect angulation. Because the lower shank is at a 90-degree angle to the face, positioning the lower shank parallel to the tooth surface results in an angulation of 90 degrees.

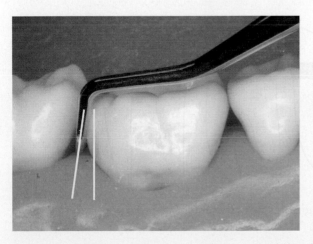

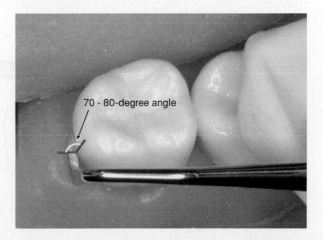

Correct angulation. Correct angulation is achieved by tilting the lower shank slightly toward the tooth surface to be instrumented. In this position the face-to-tooth surface angulation is between 70 and 80 degrees.

APPLICATION OF THE CUTTING EDGES

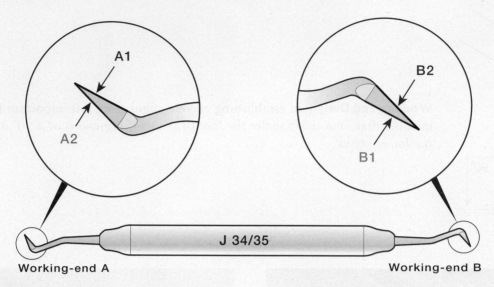

Cutting Edges. A posterior sickle scaler has two working-ends. Working-end **A** has two cutting edges and Working-end **B** has two cutting edges.

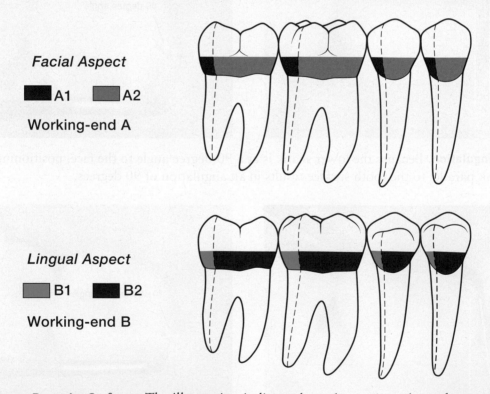

Application to Posterior Surfaces. The illustration indicates how the cutting edges of a posterior sickle scaler are applied to the tooth surfaces.

STEP-BY-STEP TECHNIQUE ON MANDIBULAR FIRST MOLAR

1. Equipment: a posterior sickle scaler.
2. Position yourself for the sextant shown in the icons below.

Right-Handed Clinicians

Left-Handed Clinicians

3. Remember: "Me, My Patient, My Light, My Dominant Hand, My Nondominant Hand, My Finger Rest, My Adaptation."

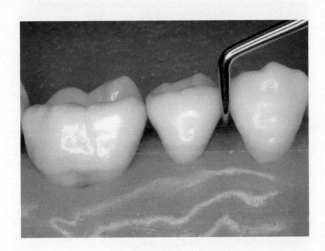

4. **Select the Correct Working-End.** When using the lower shank as a visual clue, use a tooth that is easily seen, such as the distal surface of the first premolar, to select the correct working-end.

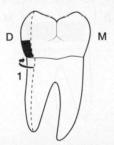

5. **Begin With the Mandibular First Molar.** As an introduction to the posterior sickle, first practice on the *mandibular right first molar*. The distal surface is completed first, beginning at the distofacial line angle and working onto the distal surface.

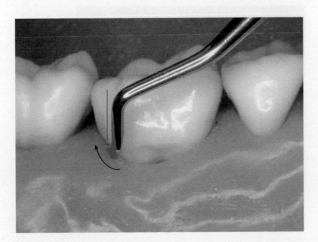

6. **Position the Working-End Near the Distofacial Line Angle.** Establish a face-to-tooth surface angulation of between 70 and 80 degrees. The tip should aim toward the back of the mouth because this is the direction in which you are working.

7. **Check Your Angulation to the Distal Surface.** Remember that the sickle's face is at a 90-degree angle to the lower shank. Tilt the lower shank toward the distal surface until the face-to-tooth surface angulation is between 70 and 80 degrees.

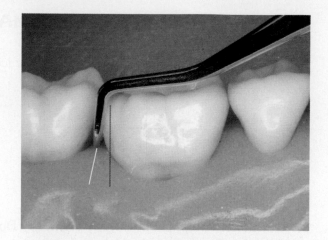

8. **Technique Check.** This photograph shows an "aerial view" looking down at the occlusal surface. The sickle's face should be at a 70- to 80-degree angulation to the distal surface. To obtain this angulation, the lower shank will be tilted toward the distal surface.

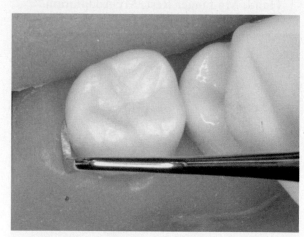

9. **Instrumentation of the Facial Surface.** You are now ready to instrument the facial and mesial surfaces of the tooth, beginning at the distofacial line angle.

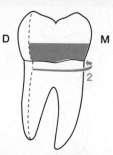

10. **Reposition the Working-End at the Line Angle.** While maintaining your fulcrum, lift the working-end away from the tooth and turn it so that it aims toward the front of the mouth. Reposition the working-end at the distofacial line angle.

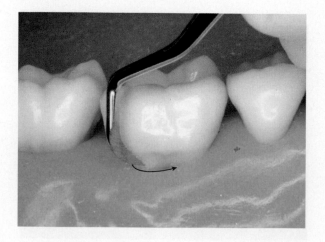

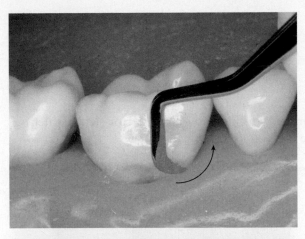

11. **Work Across Facial Surface.** Continue working across the facial surface. Remember to maintain adaptation at all times.

As you approach the mesiofacial line angle, roll the handle slightly to maintain adaptation.

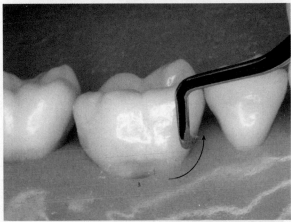

12. **Instrument the Mesial Surface.** Tilt the lower shank slightly toward the mesial surface to maintain correct angulation. Check your shank position to ensure that you have maintained a 70- to 80-degree face-to-tooth surface angulation.

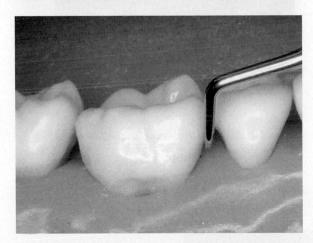

13. **Continue Strokes.** Work at least halfway across the mesial surface from the facial aspect. (The other half will be instrumented from the lingual aspect.)

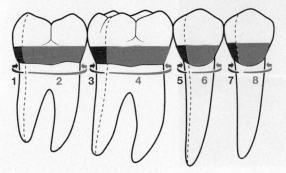

14. **Sequence for Sextant.** Next, use the sequence shown in this illustration to instrument the facial aspect of the entire sextant, beginning with the posterior-most molar. This sequence allows you to instrument the sextant in an efficient manner.

Section 5
Skill Application

PRACTICAL FOCUS

Task 1: Use visual clues to determine whether the correct working-end of a posterior sickle scaler is being used in photographs 1 and 2. What visual clue did you use?

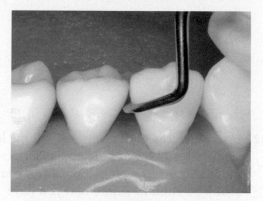

Photo 1

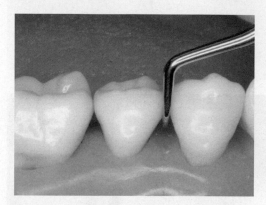

Photo 2

Task 2: What is the tooth-to-face angulation of the sickle scaler shown in photographs 3 and 4?

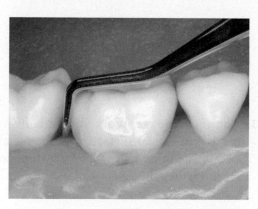

Photo 3

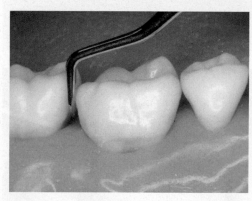

Photo 4

Task 3: Identify the inner and outer cutting edges in photograph 5. Should cutting edge A or B be used on the distal surfaces of the posterior teeth?

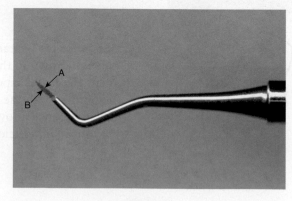

Photo 5

SUMMARY SHEET: SICKLE SCALERS

Use of Sickle Scalers

Sickle scalers are used to remove medium- and large-sized supragingival calculus deposits from the crowns of posterior teeth. The pointed tip provides good access to the proximal surfaces apical to the contact areas on posterior teeth. Sickle scalers are NOT recommended for use on root surfaces.

Basic Concepts

1. Tilt the lower shank slightly toward the tooth surface to establish correct face-to-tooth surface angulation.
2. Maintain adaptation of the tip-third of the cutting edge to the tooth surface.
3. Before initiating a calculus removal stroke, press down with your fulcrum finger and apply pressure against the instrument handle with the index finger and thumb to create lateral pressure against the tooth surface.
4. Activate the calculus removal stroke using wrist motion activation.
5. Relax your fingers between each calculus removal stroke.

Anterior Teeth

1. For surfaces toward, sit at 8–9:00 if you are a right-handed clinician or at 4–3:00 if you are a left-handed clinician. For surfaces away, sit at 12:00.
2. Sequence: Begin with the surfaces toward your nondominant hand. Start on the canine on the opposite side of the mouth and work toward yourself. (Right-handed clinicians start with the left canine, mesial surface. Left-handed clinicians start with the right canine, mesial surface.)

Posterior Teeth

1. For aspects toward, sit at 9:00 (or 3:00). For aspects away, sit at 10–11:00 (or 2–1:00).
2. Select the correct working-end:
   • Method 1: The lower shank is parallel to the tooth surface (Posterior = Parallel). Functional shank up and over!
   • Method 2: The inner cutting edges are used on the distal surfaces. The outer cutting edges are used on the facial, lingual, and mesial surfaces.
3. Sequence: Begin at the distofacial line angle of the posterior-most tooth in the sextant and work toward the distal surface. Reposition at the distofacial line angle and complete the facial (or lingual) and mesial surfaces of the tooth, working toward the front of the mouth.

NOTE TO COURSE INSTRUCTORS: Refer to Module 18 for instrumentation strategies and patient cases relating to calculus removal.

Student: _____

Evaluator: _____

Date: _____

Anterior Area 1 = _____

Anterior Area 2 = _____

Posterior Area 3 = _____

Posterior Area 4 = _____

DIRECTIONS FOR STUDENT: Use **Column S.** Evaluate your skill level as: **S** (satisfactory) or **U** (unsatisfactory).

DIRECTIONS FOR EVALUATOR: Use **Column E.** Indicate: **S** (satisfactory) or **U** (unsatisfactory). Each **S** equals 1 point, each **U** equals 0 points.

CRITERIA:	Area 1		Area 2		Area 3		Area 4	
	S	E	S	E	S	E	S	E
Position:								
Positioned correctly on clinician stool								
Positioned correctly with relation to patient, equipment, and treatment area								
Establishes correct patient head position								
Dental Mirror:								
Uses correct grasp and establishes secure rest with mirror								
Uses the mirror correctly for retraction and/or indirect vision								
Modified Pen Grasp with Dominant Hand:								
Thumb and index finger pads positioned opposite one another on handle; fingers not touching or overlapped.								
Pad of middle finger rests lightly on shank; touches the ring finger								
Handle rests between the 2nd knuckle of the index finger and the "V" of hand								
Intraoral Fulcrum:								
Ring finger is straight and supports weight of hand								
Fulcrums on same arch, near tooth being instrumented								
Technique with Sickle Scaler:								
Establishes and maintains correct face-to-tooth surface angulation								
Maintains correct adaptation; rolls handle when needed for adaptation								
Uses controlled supragingival calculus removal strokes in a coronal direction								
Applies appropriate stroke pressure in a coronal direction								
Uses correct sequence in the sextant								
Uses overlapping strokes (1) at midline of anterior teeth, (2) under the contact area, (3) at line angles of posterior teeth								
OPTIONAL GRADE PERCENTAGE CALCULATION Total **S**'s in each E column.								

Sum of **S**'s _____ divided by Total Points Possible (**64**) equals the Percentage Grade _____

SKILL EVALUATION MODULE 14   SICKLE SCALERS

Student: _____

EVALUATOR COMMENTS

_____

_____

_____

_____

_____

_____

_____

_____

_____

_____

_____

_____

_____

_____

_____

_____

_____

_____

_____

Box for sketches pertaining to written comments.

Universal Curets

Module Overview

This module presents the design characteristics of universal curets and step-by-step instructions for using universal curets to remove small- or medium-sized calculus deposits from the anterior and posterior teeth. *Module 13, Concepts in Periodontal Debridement, should be completed before beginning this module.*

Module Outline

Key Terms

Universal curet
Face at 90 degrees to the lower shank

Learning Objectives

1. Identify the design characteristics of universal curets.

2. Discuss the advantages and limitations of the design characteristics of universal curets.

3. Name the uses of universal curets.

4. Describe how the clinician can use visual clues to select the correct working-end of a universal curet on anterior and posterior teeth.

5. Explain why the lower shank of a universal curet should be tilted slightly toward the tooth surface being instrumented to obtain correct angulation.

6. Using a universal curet, demonstrate correct adaptation and use of calculus removal strokes on the anterior teeth.

7. Using a universal curet, demonstrate correct adaptation and use of calculus removal strokes on the posterior teeth.

8. Using a universal curet, demonstrate horizontal calculus removal strokes at the distofacial line angles of posterior teeth and at the midlines on the facial and lingual surfaces of anterior teeth.

Section I
Universal Curets

GENERAL DESIGN CHARACTERISTICS

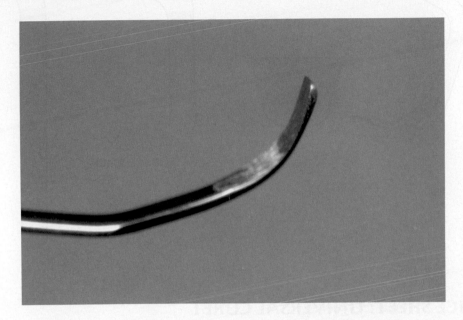

A universal curet is a periodontal instrument used to remove small- and medium-sized calculus deposits from the crowns and roots of the teeth. A universal curet usually is a double-ended instrument with paired, mirror image, working-ends.

1. Universal curets are one of the most frequently used and versatile of all the calculus removal instruments.
   a. This type of curet is called "universal" because it can be applied to both anterior and posterior teeth. In other words, it is used universally throughout the entire mouth.
   b. Universal curets can be used both supragingivally and subgingivally—on crown and root surfaces—for removal of small- to medium-sized calculus deposits.
2. The working-end of a universal curet has several unique design characteristics:
   a. A rounded back
   b. A rounded toe
   c. Semicircular in cross section
   d. Two cutting edges per working-end
   e. The face is at a 90-degree angle to the lower shank and as a result, the two cutting edges are level with one another
3. The following are some examples of universal curet instruments: the Columbia 2R/2L; Columbia 13/14; Rule 3/4; Barnhart 1/2; Barnhart 5/6; Younger-Good 7/8; Indiana University 13/14; HU 1/2; Bunting 5/6; Mallery 1/2; Langer 1/2; Langer 3/4; Langer 5/6, and Langer 17/18

WORKING-END DESIGN

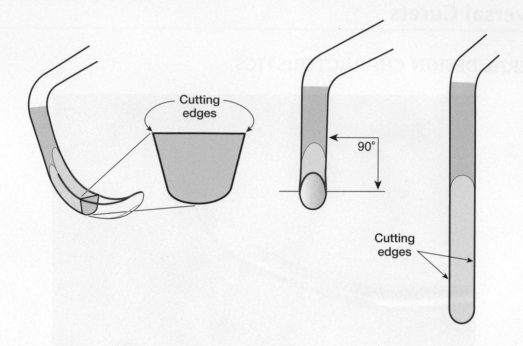

Cutting edges

90°

Cutting edges

REFERENCE SHEET: UNIVERSAL CURET

TABLE 15-1. Universal Curet	
Cross Section	Semicircular cross section; this design allows it to be used both supragingivally and subgingivally
Working-End	Rounded back and toe
	Two working cutting edges per working-end
Face	Face is at a 90-degree angle to the lower shank and as a result, the two cutting edges on a working-end are level with one another
	Because the face is perpendicular to the lower shank, *the lower shank must be tilted slightly toward the tooth surface to establish correct angulation*
Cutting Edges	Two parallel cutting edges meet in a rounded toe
Application	Universal use—one double-ended instrument can be used on both anterior and posterior teeth
Primary Functions	Debridement of crown and root surfaces
	Removal of small- to medium-sized calculus deposits

Section 2
Selecting a Universal Curet

To select a universal curet, consider its design characteristics. These photographs compare two universal curets, demonstrating how design characteristics make an impact on instrument selection.

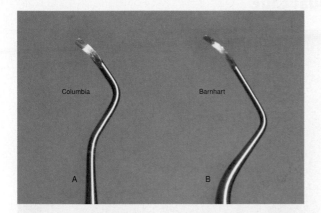

Two Universal Curet Designs:

A, The Columbia 13/14 has a short lower shank and working-end.

B, The Barnhart 1/2 has a long lower shank and working-end.

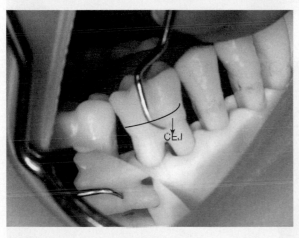

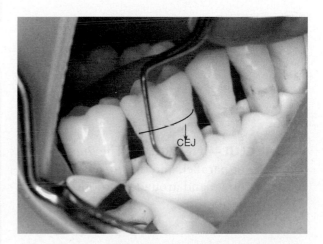

Comparison of Shank Length. A. The Columbia curet is limited to use within normal sulci or shallow pockets. **B.** The Barnhart can be used to instrument root surfaces within deep pockets.

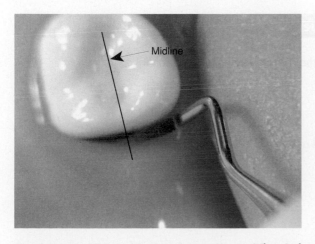

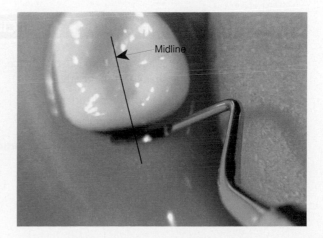

Comparison of Working-End Length. A. The Columbia curet with its shorter working-end does not reach the midline. **B.** The Barnhart curet with its longer working-end is a better choice for instrumenting the proximal surfaces of posterior teeth.

Section 3
Technique Practice: Posterior Teeth

CHOOSING THE CORRECT WORKING-END
Method 1: The Lower Shank as a Visual Clue

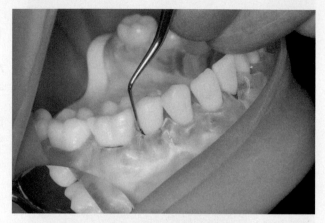

VISUAL CLUE—CORRECT: The *lower shank* is parallel to the proximal surface, and the *functional shank* goes "up and over the tooth."

Correct Working-End

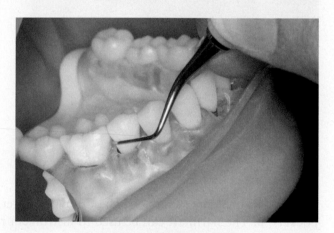

VISUAL CLUE—INCORRECT: The *lower shank* is not parallel, and the *functional shank* is "down and around the tooth."

Incorrect Working-End

Box 15-1. The Lower Shank as a Visual Clue

When the working-end is adapted to the distal surface, the correct working-end has the following relationship between the shank and the tooth:

- Lower shank is parallel to the distal surface
- Functional shank goes up and over the tooth

Think: **Posterior = Parallel. Functional shank up and over!**

Method 2: The Inner and Outer Cutting Edges as Visual Clues

There is a second method that you can use to choose the correct working-end of a universal curet. For this method, the cutting edges provide the visual clues. It is not important whether you use Method 1 or Method 2 to select the working-end. Use the method that is easiest for you.

Method 2: Each of the working-ends has two cutting edges, an inner and an outer cutting edge:

1. The outer cutting edges are *farther* from the instrument handle.
2. The inner cutting edges are *closer* to the instrument handle.

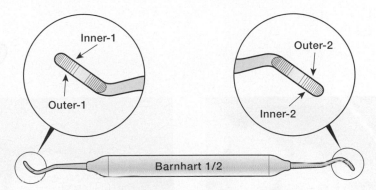

The Cutting Edges as Visual Clues. Each of the two working-ends of a universal curet has two cutting edges, an inner and an outer cutting edge.

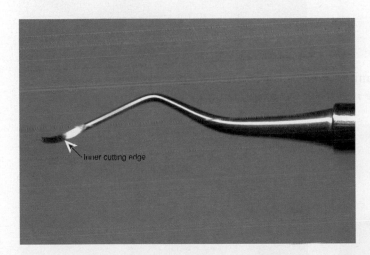

Inner Edge. To identify the cutting edges, hold the instrument so that you are looking at the face of the working-end.

Box 15-2. The Inner and Outer Cutting Edges as Visual Clues

The inner cutting edges are used to instrument the distal surfaces.

The outer cutting edges are used to instrument the facial (lingual) and mesial surfaces.

ESTABLISHING 70- TO 80-DEGREE ANGULATION

Working-End Design. In establishing correct angulation, it is important to remember that on a universal curet *the face of the working-end is at a 90° angle to the lower shank.*

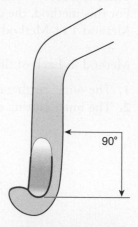

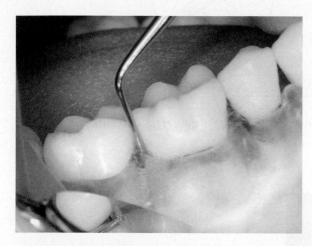
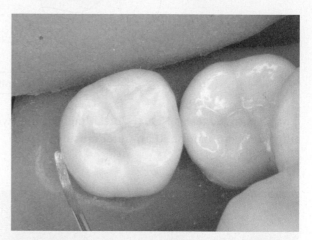

Incorrect angulation. Because the lower shank is at a 90-degree angle to the face, *positioning the lower shank parallel to the tooth surface results in an angulation of 90 degrees.*

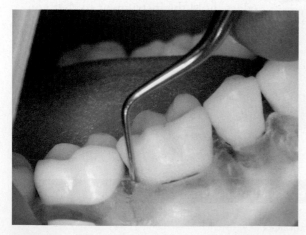
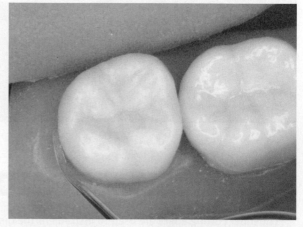

Correct angulation. Correct angulation is *achieved by tilting the lower shank slightly toward the tooth surface* to be instrumented. In this position, the face-to-tooth surface angulation is between 70 and 80 degrees.

APPLICATION OF THE CUTTING EDGES

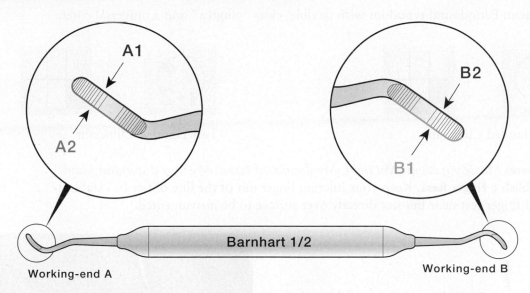

Cutting Edges. A universal curet has two working-ends. Both cutting edges on working-end **A** and on working-end **B** are used to instrument the posterior teeth.

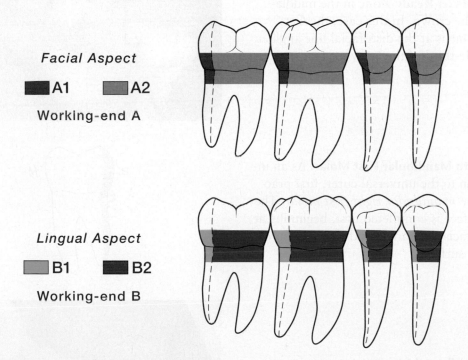

Facial Aspect

■ A1   ■ A2

Working-end A

Lingual Aspect

■ B1   ■ B2

Working-end B

Application to Posterior Surfaces. The illustration indicates how the cutting edges of a universal curet are applied to the posterior tooth surfaces.

STEP-BY-STEP TECHNIQUE ON MANDIBULAR FIRST MOLAR

Equipment: Periodontal typodont with flexible, clear "gingiva" and a universal curet.

Right-Handed Clinicians   Left-Handed Clinicians

1. **Prepare:** *Me. My patient. My light. My dominant hand. My non-dominant hand.*
2. **Establish a Finger Rest.** Keep your fulcrum finger **out of the line of fire** by establishing a finger rest near but not directly over surface to be instrumented.

3. **Get Ready.** Turn the toe of the working-end toward the distal surface. Place the working-end in the Get Ready Zone in the middle-third of the crown. In this case, the Get Ready Zone is at the distofacial line angle in the middle-third of the crown.

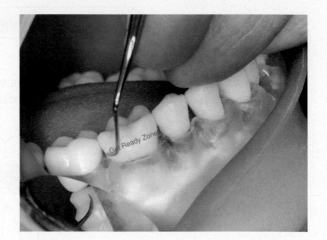

4. **Begin With Mandibular First Molar.** As an introduction to the universal curet, first practice on the *mandibular right first molar*. The distal surface is completed first, beginning at the distofacial line angle and working onto the distal surface.

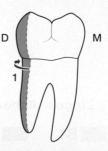

5. **Lower Handle and Insert.**
   - Lower the instrument handle and establish a 0-degree angulation.
   - Gently slide the working-end beneath the gingival margin and onto the distal surface of the root.

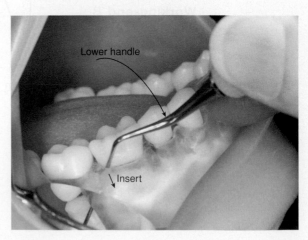

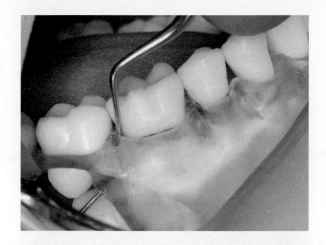

6. **Establish Angulation and Lock Toe-Third.**
   - Establish an 80-degree face-to-root surface angulation *by tilting the lower shank slightly toward the distal surface.*
   - Adapt the toe-third of the working-end to the distal surface of the root. *Imagine "locking" the toe-third against the tooth surface.*

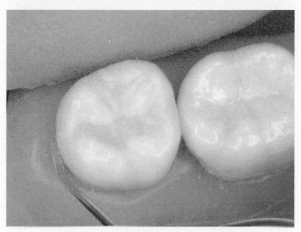

7. **Technique Check.** This photograph shows an "aerial view" looking down at the occlusal surface. The curet's face should be at a 70 to 80-degree angulation to the distal surface. To obtain this angulation, the lower shank will be tilted toward the distal surface.

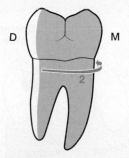

D   M

2

8. **Instrumentation of the Facial Surface.** You are now ready to instrument the facial and mesial surfaces of the tooth, beginning at the disto-facial line angle.

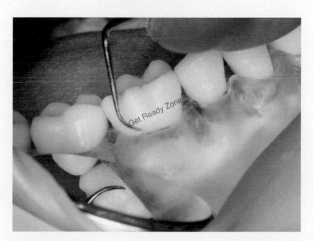

Get Ready Zone

9. **Get Ready for Facial Aspect.**
   - Turn the working-end so that the toe of the curet is "pointing toward" the front of the mouth.
   - Place the working-end in the Get Ready Zone on the middle-third of the facial surface near the line angle.

10. **Insert.**
    - Gently slide the working-end beneath the gingival margin.
    - Imagine the face sliding along the facial surface all the way to the base of the pocket.

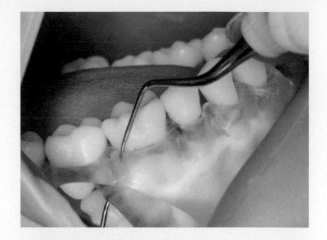

11. **Instrument the Facial Surface. Roll Handle at Line Angle.**
    - As you approach the mesiofacial line angle, roll the handle slightly to maintain adaptation.
    - Keep the toe-third "locked" against the tooth surface.

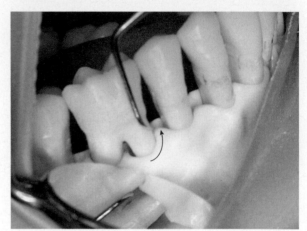

12. **Technique Check.** Make sure that your strokes extend past the midline of the mesial proximal surface.
    - Work at least halfway across the mesial surface from the facial aspect while maintaining proper angulation.
    - The other half of the mesial surface will be instrumented from the lingual aspect.

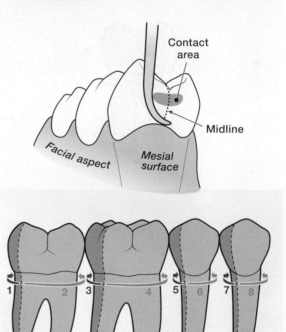

13. **Sequence for Sextant.** Next, use the sequence shown in this illustration to instrument the facial aspect of the entire sextant, beginning with the posterior-most molar. This sequence allows you to instrument the sextant in an efficient manner.

Section 4
Technique Alert: Lower Shank Position

AN UNHINDERED STROKE PATH ON FACIAL AND LINGUAL SURFACES

Adapting the working-end to the facial and lingual root surfaces of the mandibular posterior teeth is challenging for two reasons: (1) the clinician's hand position may block the view of the mandibular lingual surfaces and (2) the rounded posterior crowns make it difficult to instrument the root surfaces of these teeth.

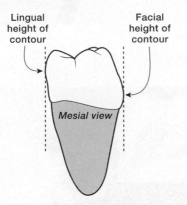

Lingual height of contour — Facial height of contour

Mesial view

Posterior Teeth "Overhang" Their Roots. This illustration shows a molar, looking at the *mesial surface.*

Note that the crown protrudes out over the root surface.

INCORRECT TECHNIQUE

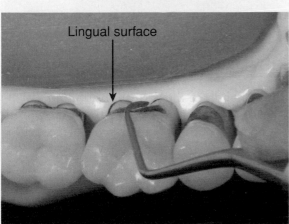

Incorrect Handle Position. Inexperienced clinicians often tilt the instrument handle down in an attempt to gain a better view of the mandibular lingual surfaces closest to them.

These are the mandibular right lingual surfaces if you are right-handed or the mandibular left lingual surfaces if you are left-handed.

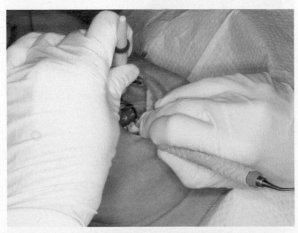

Lingual surface

INCORRECT:
Tilting the Handle Makes Instrumentation of Root Surfaces Impossible. Tilting the handle toward the clinician may make it easier to view the lingual surfaces, but it also makes calculus removal difficult.

This incorrect technique handle position causes the lower shank to touch lingual and occlusal surfaces of the crown. **In this position, it is not possible to adapt the working-end to the root surface because the root is smaller in diameter than the crown.**

INCORRECT:

This Position Causes the Lower Shank to Rock Against the Tooth. With the handle tilted, the lower shank touches the lingual and occlusal surfaces of the tooth crown. In this position, it is not possible to make an effective instrumentation stroke up the root surface. The lower shank simply rocks against the occlusal surface of the crown causing the working-end to lift off of the root surface without engaging the calculus deposit.

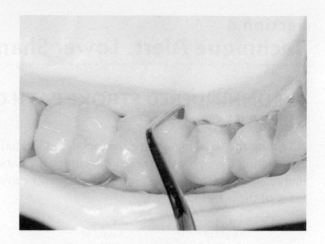

CORRECT TECHNIQUE

Correct Handle Position. When working on the lingual surfaces, keep the handle in the normal position and use the mirror for indirect vision.

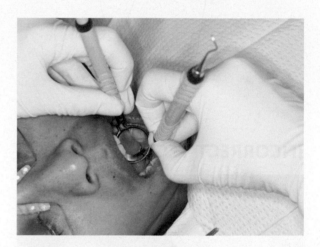

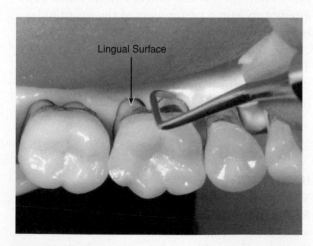

Lingual Surface

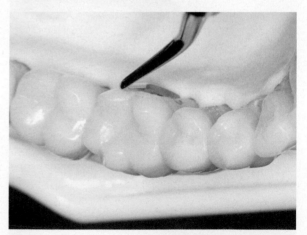

Correct Technique Produces an Unimpeded Stroke. With the handle in the correct position, the lower shank is not in contact with either the lingual or occlusal surfaces of the tooth crown. In this position, it is easy to make oblique or vertical instrumentation strokes up the root surface without rocking against the occlusal surface of the crown.

Section 5
Technique Practice: Anterior Teeth

Adapting a universal curet to the anterior teeth requires a technique that is very different from that used with any other instrument. For this reason, some clinicians prefer not to use universal curets on the anterior sextants. The complex shank design of the universal curet, however, sometimes facilitates access to the lingual root surfaces of the mandibular anterior teeth.

CHOOSING THE CORRECT WORKING-END
Method 1: The Instrument Face as a Visual Clue

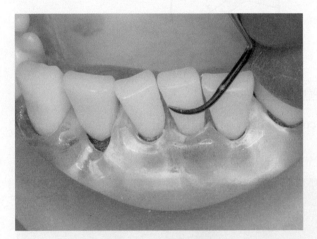

Correct Working-End

VISUAL CLUE—CORRECT: When the working-end is placed against the midline of the facial (or lingual) surface, *the instrument face* tilts toward the tooth surface. As you look down on the working-end, the face is partially hidden.

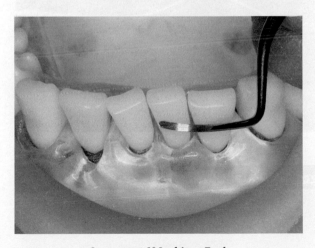

Incorrect Working-End

VISUAL CLUE—INCORRECT: When the working-end is placed against the midline of the facial (or lingual) surface, **the instrument face** tilts slightly away from the tooth surface. As you look down on the working-end, the entire face is clearly visible.

This working-end would traumatize the soft tissue if used subgingivally!

Box 15-3. The Instrument Face as a Visual Clue

When the working-end is adapted to the facial (or lingual) surface, the *face* of the correct working-end *tilts slightly toward the tooth* and is partially hidden from view.

Method 2: The Inner and Outer Cutting Edges as a Visual Clue

There is a second method that you can use to choose the correct working-end of a universal curet. For this method, the cutting edges provide the visual clue. It is not important whether you use method 1 or method 2 to select the working-end. Use the method that is easiest for you.

Method 2: Each working-end has two cutting edges, an inner and outer cutting edge:

1. The outer cutting edges are *farther* from the instrument handle.
2. The inner cutting edges are *closer* to the instrument handle.

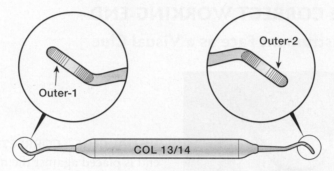

The Cutting Edges as a Visual Clue. Only the outer cutting edges of a universal curet are used on the anterior teeth.

Inner and Outer Cutting Edges. To identify the cutting edges, hold the instrument so that you are looking at the face of the working-end.

Only the outer cutting edges are used to instrument the anterior teeth.

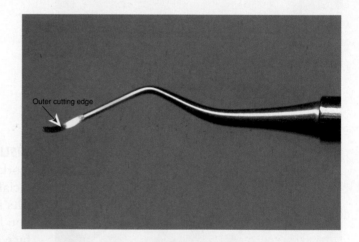

Box 15-4. The Inner and Outer Cutting Edges as Visual Clues
When using a universal curet on anterior teeth, only the *outer cutting edges* are used.

APPLICATION OF THE CUTTING EDGES

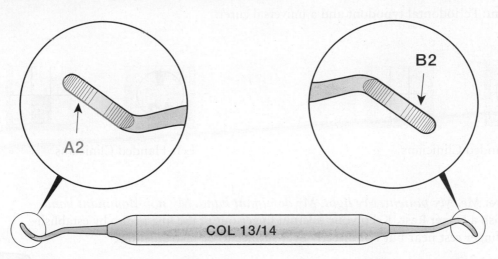

Cutting Edges. On a universal curet, only the two outer cutting edges—A2 and B2—are *used on anterior tooth surfaces.*

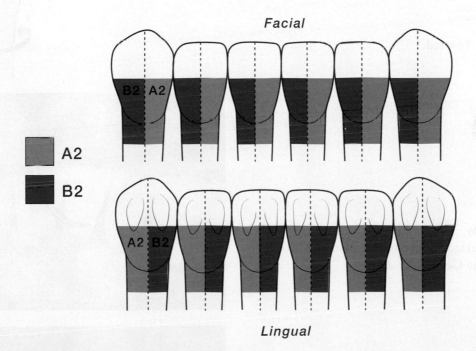

Application to Posterior Surfaces. The illustration indicates how the cutting edges of a universal curet are applied to the anterior tooth surfaces.

STEP-BY-STEP TECHNIQUE

Equipment: Periodontal typodont and a universal curet.

Right-Handed Clinicians

Left-Handed Clinicians

1. **Prepare:** *Me. My patient. My light. My dominant hand. My non-dominant hand.*
2. **Establish a Finger Rest.** Keep your fulcrum finger out of the line of fire by establishing a finger rest near but not directly over surface to be instrumented.

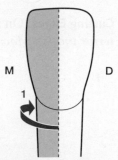

M   D

3. **Surfaces Toward.**

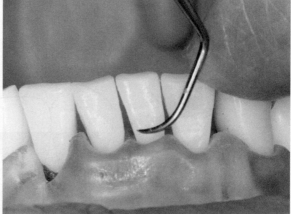

4. **Get Ready.** The toe should be aimed toward the mesial surface of the tooth. Place the working-end in the Get Ready Zone.

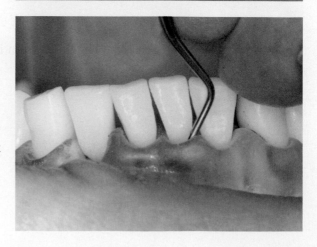

5. **Insert and Lock Toe-Third.** Gently slide the working-end beneath the gingival margin. Lock the toe-third of the working-end against the tooth surface.

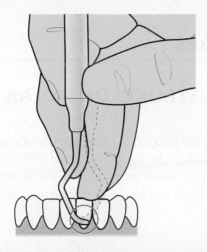

6. The Shank Provides a Visual Clue on the Proximal Surfaces.
- When using a universal curet on a mesial or distal surface, *the lower shank reaches across the facial (or lingual) surface.*
- To help you remember this, think *"anterior across"*.

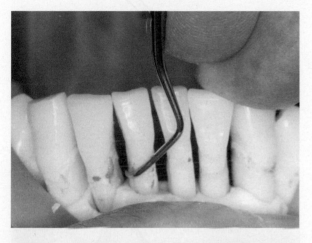

7. Roll the Instrument Handle. As you approach the mesiofacial line angle, roll the instrument handle to maintain adaptation of the toe-third of the working-end.

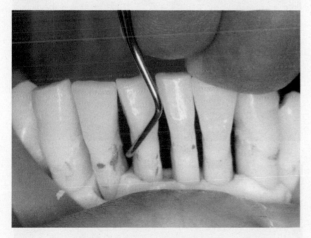

8. Instrument Under the Contact Area. Continue strokes until you work at least halfway across the mesial surface. (The other half of the mesial surface will be instrumented from the lingual aspect of the tooth.)

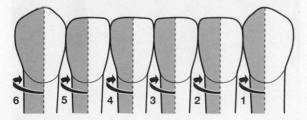

9. Sequence 1. Next, use the sequence shown in this illustration to instrument the colored tooth surfaces of the facial aspect. Begin with the left canine and end with the right canine.

Section 6
Technique Alert: Horizontal Strokes

TECHNIQUE PRACTICE 1: HORIZONTAL STROKES ON MOLAR TOOTH

Novice clinicians often fail to remove calculus deposits that are located (1) near the distofacial or distolingual line angle of posterior teeth and (2) at the midline of the facial or lingual surfaces of anterior teeth. Horizontal calculus removal strokes are extremely useful in calculus removal in these areas. Follow the directions below to practice making horizontal calculus removal strokes at the distofacial line angle of the mandibular first molar.

Horizontal Strokes. Horizontal calculus removal strokes are made in a perpendicular direction to the long axis of the tooth.

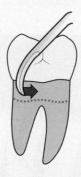

Establish Handle Position. Insert the curet slightly distal to the distofacial line angle. Lower the instrument handle until the curet working-end is oriented with the toe toward—but not touching—the base of the sulcus or pocket.

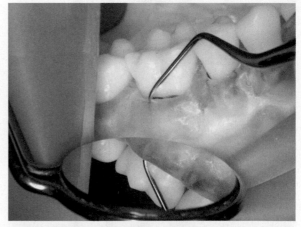

Make Several Horizontal Strokes. Begin a calculus removal stroke slightly distal to the distofacial line angle. Make several short, controlled strokes around the distofacial line angle.

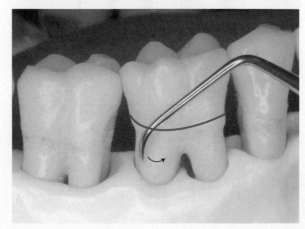

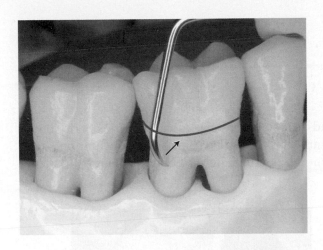

Reassume Oblique Strokes. After completing several horizontal strokes, reposition the curet with the lower shank parallel to the facial surface. Make oblique strokes across the facial surface in the usual manner.

TECHNIQUE PRACTICE 2: HORIZONTAL STROKES ON CENTRAL INCISOR

Follow the directions below to practice making horizontal strokes at the midline of the facial surface of a central incisor.

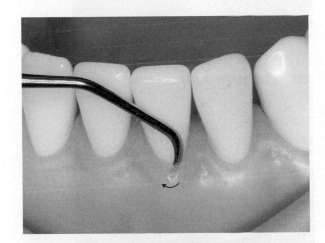

Horizontal Strokes on Facial Surface. Insert the working-end just distal to the midline. Lower the handle until the curet toe is toward—but not touching—the base of the sulcus. Make several short, controlled horizontal strokes across the midline of the facial surface.

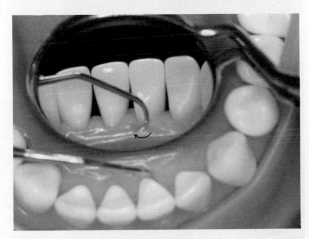

Horizontal Strokes on Lingual Surface. Lower the handle until the curet toe is toward—but not touching—the base of the sulcus. Make several short, controlled horizontal strokes across the midline of the lingual surface.

Section 7
Skill Application

PRACTICAL FOCUS

Case 1: You have been assigned to observe a second-year student, Ling, as she performs periodontal debridement on a patient. The photographs below are characteristic of Ling's instrumentation technique. What feedback could you give Ling about her instrumentation technique and instrument selection?

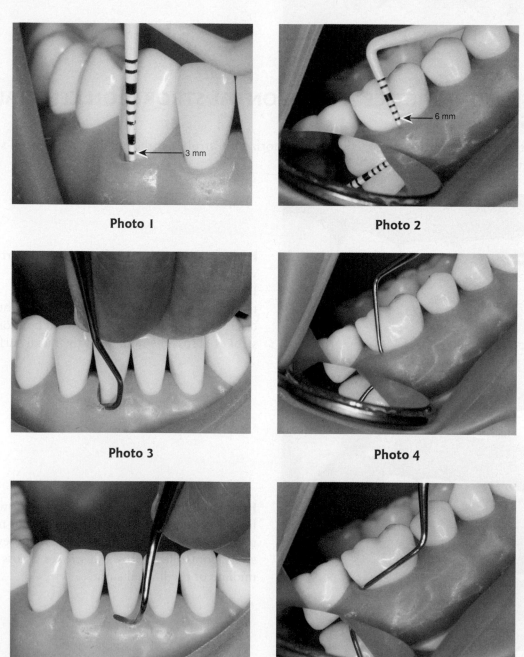

Photo 1

Photo 2

Photo 3

Photo 4

Photo 5

Photo 6

SUMMARY SHEET: UNIVERSAL CURETS

Use of Universal Curets

A universal curet is a periodontal instrument used to remove light and medium calculus deposits from the crowns and roots of the teeth.

Basic Concepts

1. Tilt the lower shank slightly toward the tooth surface to establish correct face-to-tooth surface angulation.
2. Insert the working-end beneath the gingival margin at a 0- to 40-degree angulation.
3. Maintain adaptation of the tip-third of the cutting edge to the tooth surface.
4. Before initiating a calculus removal stroke, press down with your fulcrum finger and apply pressure against the instrument handle with the index finger and thumb to create lateral pressure against the tooth surface.
5. Activate the calculus removal stroke using wrist motion activation.
6. Relax your fingers between each calculus removal stroke.

Anterior Teeth

1. For surfaces toward, sit at 8–9:00 if you are a right-handed clinician or at 4–3:00 if you are a left-handed clinician. For surfaces away, sit at 12:00.
2. Select the correct working-end:
   - Method 1: When adapted to a facial or lingual surface, the face tilts slightly toward the tooth. When adapted on a proximal surface, the lower shank goes across the tooth (Anterior = Across).
   - Method 2: Only the outer cutting edges are used to instrument the anterior teeth.
3. Sequence: Begin with the surfaces toward your nondominant hand. Start on the canine on opposite side of the mouth and work toward yourself. (Right-handed clinicians start with the left canine, mesial surface. Left-handed clinicians start with the right canine, mesial surface.)

Posterior Teeth

1. For aspects toward, sit at 9:00 (or 3:00). For aspects away, sit at 10–11:00 (or 2–1:00).
2. Select the correct working-end:
   - Method 1: The lower shank is parallel to the tooth surface (Posterior = Parallel). Functional shank up and over!)
   - Method 2: The inner cutting edges are used on the distal surfaces. The outer cutting edges are used on the facial, lingual, and mesial surfaces.
3. Sequence: Begin at the distofacial line angle of the posterior-most tooth in the sextant and work toward the distal surface. Reposition at the distofacial line angle and complete the facial (or lingual) and mesial surfaces of the tooth, working toward the front of the mouth.

NOTE TO COURSE INSTRUCTOR: Refer to Module 18 for instrumentation strategies and patient cases relating to calculus removal.

Refer to Module 22, Instruments for Advanced Root Debridement, for content on the design and use of Langer curets, Gracey designs with extended shanks and miniature working-ends, Curvettes, and OH debridement curets.

Student: _____

Evaluator: _____

Date: _____

Anterior Area 1 = _____
Anterior Area 2 = _____
Posterior Area 3 = _____
Posterior Area 4 = _____

DIRECTIONS FOR STUDENT: Use **Column S.** Evaluate your skill level as: **S** (satisfactory) or **U** (unsatisfactory).

DIRECTIONS FOR EVALUATOR: Use **Column E.** Indicate: **S** (satisfactory) or **U** (unsatisfactory). Each **S** equals 1 point, each **U** equals 0 points.

CRITERIA:	Area 1		Area 2		Area 3		Area 4	
	S	E	S	E	S	E	S	E
Position:								
Positioned correctly on clinician stool								
Positioned correctly with relation to patient, equipment, and treatment area								
Establishes correct patient head position								
Dental Mirror:								
Uses correct grasp and establishes secure rest with mirror								
Uses the mirror correctly for retraction and/or indirect vision								
Modified Pen Grasp with Dominant Hand:								
Thumb and index finger pads positioned opposite one another on handle; fingers not touching or overlapped								
Pad of middle finger rests lightly on shank; touches the ring finger								
Handle rests between the 2nd knuckle of the index finger and the "V" of hand								
Intraoral Fulcrum:								
Ring finger is straight and supports weight of hand								
Fulcrums on same arch, near tooth being instrumented								
Technique with Universal Curet:								
Establishes and maintains correct face-to-tooth surface angulation								
Maintains correct adaptation; rolls handle when needed for adaptation								
Uses controlled calculus removal strokes in a coronal direction								
Applies appropriate stroke pressure in a coronal direction								
Uses correct sequence in the sextant								
Demonstrates horizontal strokes at (1) the midlines of anterior teeth and (2) the line angles of posterior teeth								

OPTIONAL GRADE PERCENTAGE CALCULATION
Total **S**'s in each E column.

Sum of **S**'s _____ divided by Total Points Possible (**64**) equals the Percentage Grade _____

SKILL EVALUATION MODULE 15 | UNIVERSAL CURETS

Student: _____

EVALUATOR COMMENTS

_____

_____

_____

_____

_____

_____

_____

_____

_____

_____

_____

_____

_____

_____

_____

_____

_____

_____

Box for sketches pertaining to written comments.

Area-Specific Curets

Module Overview

This module presents the design characteristics of area-specific curets and step-by-step instructions for using area-specific curets to remove light calculus deposits from the anterior and posterior teeth. *Module 13, Concepts in Periodontal Debridement, should be completed before beginning this module.*

Module Outline

Key Terms

Area-specific curet
Working cutting edge

Nonworking cutting
edge

Self-angulated curet
Lower cutting edge

Traditional and
modified pairings of
Gracey curets

Learning Objectives

1. Identify the design characteristics of area-specific curets.

2. Name the uses of area-specific curets.

3. Describe how the clinician can use visual clues to select the correct working-end of an area-specific curet on anterior and posterior teeth.

4. Explain why the lower shank of an area-specific curet should NOT be tilted slightly toward the tooth surface being instrumented to obtain correct angulation.

5. Using an area-specific curet, demonstrate correct adaptation and use of calculus removal strokes on the anterior teeth.

6. Using area-specific curets, demonstrate correct adaptation and use of calculus removal strokes on the posterior teeth.

7. Using area-specific curets, demonstrate horizontal calculus removal strokes at the disto-facial line angles of posterior teeth and at the midlines on the facial and lingual surfaces of anterior teeth.

8. Given any sickle scaler, universal curet, or area-specific curet, identify its function and where it should be used on the dentition.

9. Discuss the advantages and limitations of the design characteristics of area-specific curets.

NOTE TO COURSE INSTRUCTOR: Refer to Module 23, Advanced Techniques for Root Surface Debridement, for content on the following topics and instruments:

- Anatomy of root surfaces; root concavities
- Instrumentation of bi- and trifurcated roots
- Design and use of Langer curets, Gracey designs with extended shanks and miniature working-ends, Curvettes, and OH debridement curets.

Section I
Area-Specific Curets

GENERAL DESIGN CHARACTERISTICS

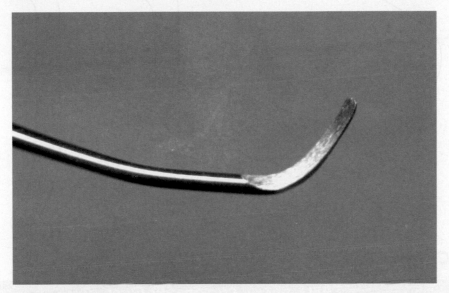

An area-specific curet is a periodontal instrument used to remove light calculus deposits from the crowns and roots of the teeth. Area-specific curets have long, complex functional shanks that make them especially suited for root surface debridement within periodontal pockets. These curets represent an important breakthrough in instrument design and have unique design characteristics.

1. The name "area-specific" signifies that each instrument is designed for use only on certain teeth and certain tooth surfaces. For this reason, several area-specific curets are required to instrument the entire mouth. Area-specific curets can be used both supragingivally and subgingivally—on crown and root surfaces—for removal of light calculus deposits.

2. Area-specific curets have only one *working* cutting edge per working-end that is used for periodontal debridement.
   a. A working cutting edge is a cutting edge that is used for periodontal debridement.
   b. The nonworking cutting edge is a cutting edge that is not used for periodontal debridement.

3. Area-specific curets are self-angulated.
   a. A self-angulated curet is a curet in which the face is tilted in relation to the lower shank. The face of an area-specific curet is tilted in relation to the lower shank.
   b. The tilted face causes one cutting edge—the working cutting edge—to be lower than the other cutting edge on each working-end.
   c. This design feature positions the working cutting edge in correct angulation to the root surface while the opposite cutting edge is angled away from the soft tissue wall of the pocket.

4. Other design features of an area-specific curet are similar to those of universal curets: a rounded back, a rounded toe, and a semicircular cross section.

5. The following are some examples of area-specific curets: the Gracey curet series, Kramer-Nevins series, Turgeon series, After Five Gracey curet series, Gracey +3 curet series, Mini Five Gracey curet series, Gracey +3 Deep Pocket series, and Vision Curvette series.

WORKING-END DESIGN

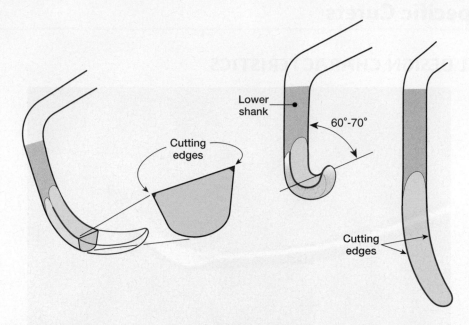

REFERENCE SHEET: AREA-SPECIFIC CURET

TABLE 16-1. Area-Specific Curet	
Cross Section	Semicircular cross section
Working-End	Rounded back and toe
	One working cutting edge per working-end
Face	Face is tilted at approximately a 70-degree angle to the lower shank; this means that the working cutting edge is lower than the nonworking cutting edge
	Tilted relationship of face to the lower shank means that the working cutting edge of an area-specific curet is self-angulated—*the working cutting edge is automatically at the correct angulation when the lower shank is parallel to the tooth surface to be instrumented.*
Cutting Edges	Curved cutting edges; the curved cutting edges and rounded toe enhance adaptation to rounded root surfaces and root concavities
Application	Area-specific, each curet is limited to use on certain teeth and certain surfaces
Primary Functions	Debridement of crown and root surfaces
	Standard curets are used to remove light calculus deposits and for deplaquing; rigid Gracey curets can remove medium-sized deposits

THE GRACEY CURET SERIES

Area-specific curets were developed through the vision of Dr. Clayton Gracey, who envisioned a periodontal instrument that would reach root surfaces within deep periodontal pockets without trauma to the pocket epithelium. In the early 1940s, Dr. Gracey worked with Hugo Friedman of Hu-Friedy Manufacturing Company to develop 14 single-ended area-specific Gracey curets. The Gracey instrument series continues to be popular today and is the basis for several other area-specific curets. The Gracey series continues to evolve and is currently available in standard, rigid, extended shank, and miniature working-end versions.

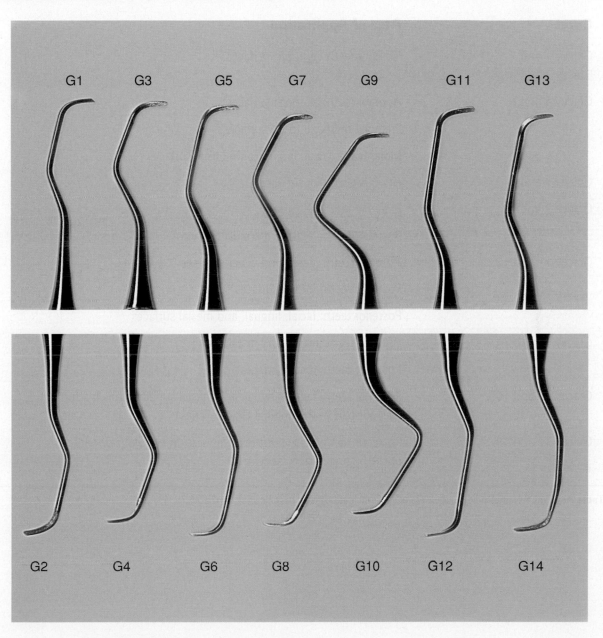

APPLICATION OF GRACEY CURETS

The original Gracey series contains 14 curets, Gracey 1–14. In practice, rarely are all 14 curets used on a single patient's mouth. Over the years, clinicians have found that they are able to instrument the mouth using a lesser number of Gracey curets. A set of three or four Gracey curets may be adequate to instrument the entire dentition.

TABLE 16-2. The Gracey Instrument Series	
Curet	**Area of Application**
Gracey 1 and 2 Gracey 3 and 4	Anterior teeth: all tooth surfaces [G]
Gracey 5 and 6	Anterior teeth: all tooth surfaces[G] Premolar teeth: all tooth surfaces[G] Molar teeth: facial, lingual, and mesial surfaces
Gracey 7 and 8 Gracey 9 and 10	Anterior teeth: all surfaces Premolar teeth: all surfaces Posterior teeth: facial and lingual surfaces[G]
Gracey 11 and 12	Anterior teeth: mesial and distal surfaces Posterior teeth: mesial surfaces[G] Posterior teeth: facial, lingual, and mesial surfaces
Gracey 13 and 14	Anterior teeth: mesial and distal surfaces Posterior teeth: distal surfaces[G]
Gracey 15 and 16	Posterior teeth: facial, lingual, and mesial surfaces (this instrument was not part of the original Gracey series)
Gracey 17 and 18	Posterior teeth: distal surfaces (this instrument was not part of the original Gracey series)

Table Key: The [G] symbol indicates the areas of application as originally designated by Dr. Gracey.

EVOLUTION IN GRACEY DESIGN
Rigid Gracey Curets

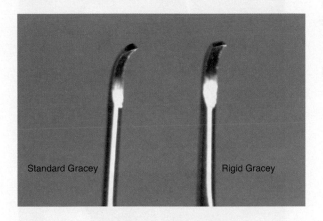

Standard Gracey   Rigid Gracey

Rigid Gracey Curets. This photograph shows a standard and a rigid Gracey curet. When compared with a standard Gracey curet, the rigid Gracey curet has a larger, stronger, less flexible working-end and shank.

Rigid Gracey curets can be used to remove medium-sized calculus deposits. The rigid shank, however, limits tactile information to the clinician's fingers.

Gracey 15/16 and 17/18 Curets
The Gracey 15/16 and 17/18 curets are modifications of the Gracey 11/12 and 13/14 curets. These curets were developed to provide superior access to the proximal surfaces of posterior teeth. The following photographs provide a comparison of the traditional Gracey 11/12 and 13/14 curets with the innovative Gracey15/16 and 17/18 curets.

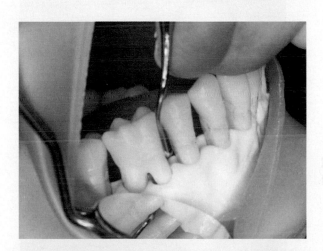

Gracey 11/12 on Mesial Surface. A finger rest close to the tooth being instrumented is needed in order to position the lower shank of the Gracey 11/12 parallel to the mesial surface.

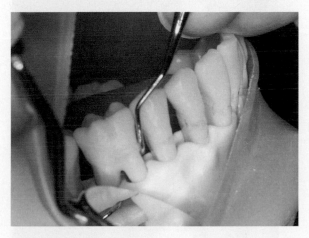

Gracey 15/16 on Mesial Surface. The finger rest can be further away from the tooth being instrumented when using the Gracey 15/16. The Gracey 15/15 can be easier to use if the patient is unable to open widely.

Gracey 13/14 on Distal Surface. Access to the distal surfaces of molar teeth with a Gracey 13/14 can be limited by the patient's ability to open widely. As shown in this photograph, it is necessary to establish a finger rest near the tooth being instrumented to adapt the Gracey 13/14.

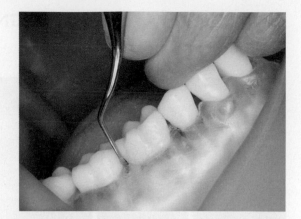

Gracey 17/18 on Distal Surface. The Gracey 17/18 is a modification of the Gracey 13/14 curet that has a longer, more angulated lower shank that minimizes interference from the teeth in the opposing arch.

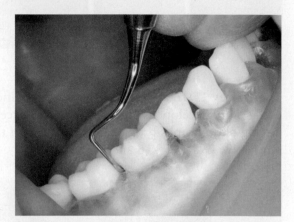

Gracey 17/18 on Distal Surface. On the Gracey 17/18, the increased angle of the lower shank bend makes it easier to position the lower shank parallel to the distal surfaces of the maxillary posterior teeth.

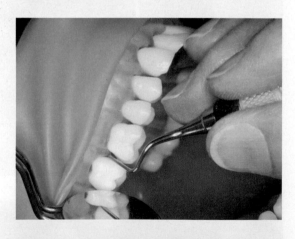

Gracey 15/16 on Mesial Surface. This photograph shows the Gracey 15/16 curet adapted to the mesial surface of the maxillary first molar. The modified shank design facilitates adaptation by allowing the clinician to establish a finger rest farther from the molar tooth.

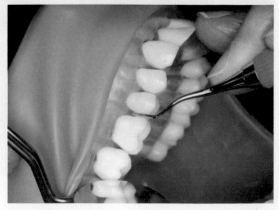

RELATION OF FACE TO LOWER SHANK

The face of an area-specific curet is titled in relation to the lower shank. The tilted face causes one cutting edge—the working cutting edge—to be lower than the other cutting edge on each working-end. The nonworking cutting edge is too close to the lower shank to be used for periodontal debridement. This design characteristic of an area-specific curet differs significantly from that of sickle scalers and universal curets.

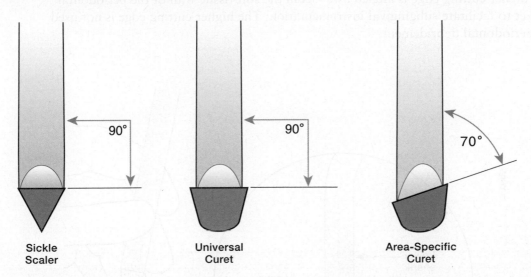

| Sickle Scaler | Universal Curet | Area-Specific Curet |

Relation of Face to the Lower Shank. The face of a sickle scaler or universal curet is at a 90° angle to the lower shank. The cutting edges on these instruments are level. The face of an area-specific curet is tilted in relation to the lower shank. The tilted face causes one cutting edge—the working cutting edge—to be lower than the other cutting edge on each working-end.

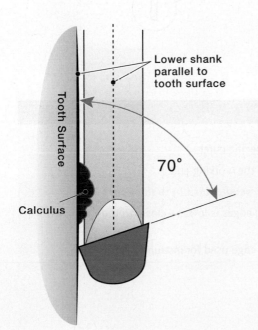

Self-Angulated Curet. The lower cutting edge of an area-specific curet is automatically at the correct angulation for periodontal debridement when the lower shank is parallel to the tooth surface to be instrumented.

IDENTIFYING THE LOWER CUTTING EDGE

Because the face of an area-specific curet is tilted in relation to the lower shank, one cutting edge is lower than the other cutting edge.

1. Only the lower cutting edge of an area-specific curet is used for periodontal debridement.

2. The higher cutting edge is angled away from the soft tissue wall of the periodontal pocket to facilitate subgingival instrumentation. The higher cutting edge is not used for periodontal debridement.

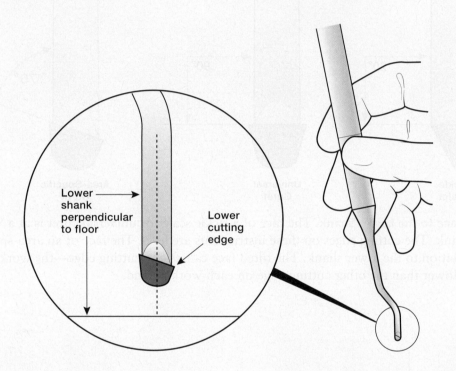

Lower shank perpendicular to floor

Lower cutting edge

Box 16-1. Identifying the Lower Cutting Edge

Follow these steps to identify the working cutting edge of an area-specific curet:

1. Hold the instrument so that you are looking directly at the *toe* of the working-end.

2. Raise or lower the instrument handle until the *lower shank is perpendicular (⊥) to the floor.*

3. Look closely at the working-end, and note that one of the cutting edges is lower—closer to the floor—than the other cutting edge.

4. The lower cutting edge is the working cutting edge—the cutting edge used for instrumentation.

Section 2
Technique Practice: Anterior Teeth

CHOOSING THE CORRECT WORKING-END
The Instrument Face as a Visual Clue

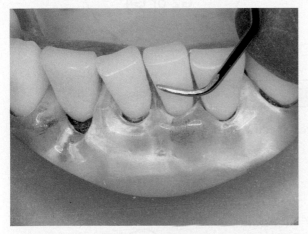

Correct Working-End

VISUAL CLUE—CORRECT: When the working-end is placed against the midline of the facial (or lingual) surface, the *instrument face* tilts toward the tooth surface. As you look down on the working-end, the face is partially hidden.

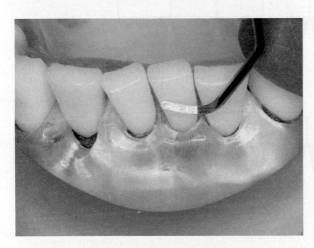

Incorrect Working-End

VISUAL CLUE—INCORRECT: When the working-end is placed against the midline of the facial (or lingual) surface, the *instrument face* tilts slightly away from the tooth surface. As you look down on the working-end, the entire face is clearly visible.

This working-end would traumatize the soft tissue if used subgingivally!

Box 16-2. The Instrument Face as a Visual Clue

When the working-end is adapted to the facial (or lingual) surface, the *face* of correct working-end *tilts slightly toward the tooth* and is partially hidden from view.

APPLICATION OF THE CUTTING EDGES TO THE ANTERIOR TEETH

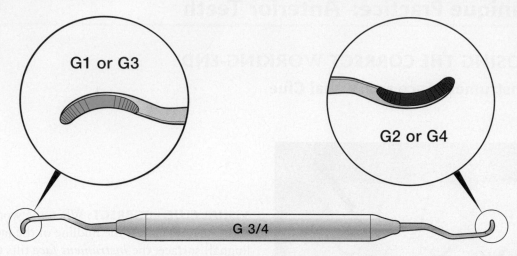

Application to Anterior Surfaces. A double-ended area-specific curet has two lower cutting edges that are used on anterior tooth surfaces.

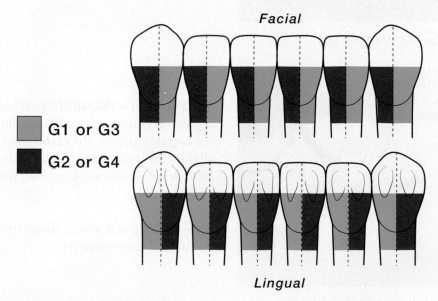

Application to Anterior Surfaces. This illustration indicates how the cutting edges of an area-specific curet are applied to the anterior tooth surfaces.

STEP-BY-STEP TECHNIQUE

Equipment: Periodontal typodont and an anterior area-specific curet.

Right-Handed Clinicians   Left-Handed Clinicians

1. **Prepare:** *Me. My patient. My light. My dominant hand. My non-dominant hand.*
2. **Establish a Finger Rest.** Keep your fulcrum finger out of the line of fire by establishing a finger rest near but not directly over surface to be instrumented.

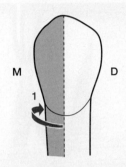

3. **Surfaces Toward.**

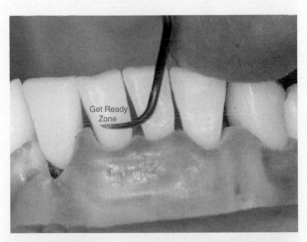

4. **Get ready.** Turn the toe of the working-end toward the distal surface. Place the working-end in the Get Ready Zone.

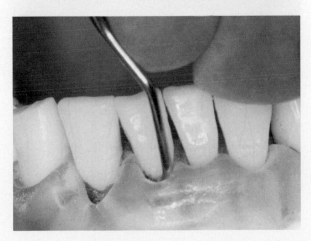

5. **Insert and lock toe.**
   - Gently slide the working-end beneath the gingival margin.
   - Adapt the toe-third of the cutting edge to the tooth surface. Imagine "locking" the toe-third against the tooth surface.

6. **Work Across the Mesial Surface.**

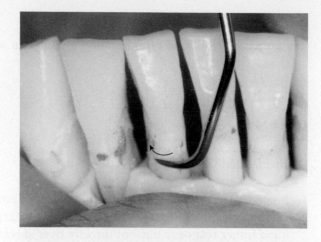

7. **Roll the Instrument Handle.** As you approach the line angle, roll the instrument handle to maintain adaptation of the toe-third of the working-end.

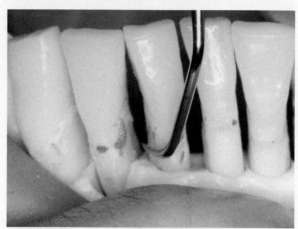

8. **Instrument Under the Contact Area.** Continue strokes until you work at least halfway across the distal proximal surface. (The other half of the distal surface will be instrumented from the lingual aspect of the tooth.)

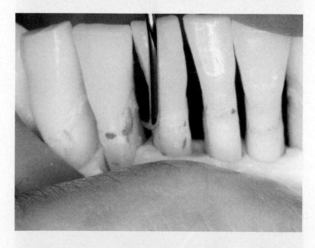

9. **Sequence.** Next, use the sequence shown in this illustration to instrument the colored tooth surfaces of the facial aspect.

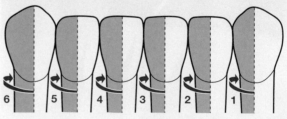

Section 3
Technique Practice: Posterior Teeth

CHOOSING THE CORRECT WORKING-END
The Lower Shank as a Visual Clue

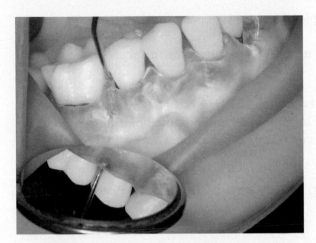

Correct Working-End

VISUAL CLUE—CORRECT: The *lower shank* is parallel to the proximal surface, and the *functional shank* goes "up and over the tooth."

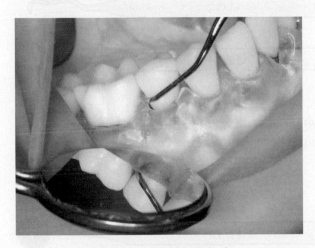

Incorrect Working-End

VISUAL CLUE—INCORRECT: The *lower shank* is not parallel, and the *functional shank* is "down and around the tooth."

Box 16-3. The Lower Shank as a Visual Clue

When the working-end is adapted to the distal surface, the correct working-end has the following relationship between the shank and the tooth:

- Lower shank is parallel to the distal surface
- Functional shank goes up and over the tooth

Think: **Posterior = Parallel. Functional shank up and over!**

APPLICATION OF THE CUTTING EDGES TO THE POSTERIOR TEETH

At least four area-specific curets—two double-ended instruments—are needed to debride the posterior teeth. Commonly, four to six curets are used to instrument the posterior teeth. For example:

1. The Gracey 11, 12, 13, and 14 might be selected for the posterior teeth.
2. The Gracey 15, 16, 17, and 18 curets could make up a set of curets for the posterior teeth.
3. The Gracey 9, 10 11, 12, 13, and 14 is an example of a set of six curets for the posterior teeth.
4. The Gracey 7, 8, 15, 16, 17, and 18 could make up a set of six curets for the posterior teeth.

Traditional Pairings: Gracey 11/12, 13/14, and 15/16, 17/18

The Gracey 11, 12, 13, and 14 curets are available in **traditional and modified pairings** on double-ended instruments. The Gracey 15, 16, 17, and 18 curets are paired as the Gracey 15/16 and 17/18 instruments.

Example: Use of Traditional Pairings on the Mandibular Right Posterior Sextant

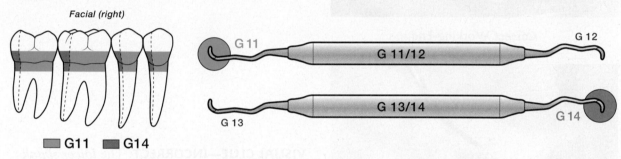

Traditional Pairings on Facial Aspect of Mandibular Right Sextant. With a traditional pairing of Gracey curets, two double-ended instruments are required to complete the facial aspect of the mandibular right posterior sextant:

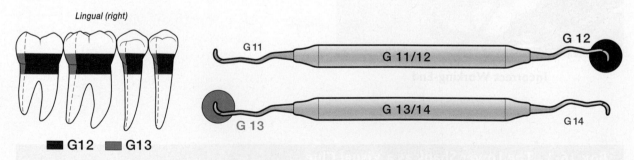

Traditional Pairing on Lingual Aspect of Mandibular Right Sextant. With a traditional pairing of Gracey curets, two double-ended instruments are required to complete the lingual aspect of the mandibular right posterior sextant:

Modified Pairing: Gracey 11/14 and 12/13

The Gracey 11, 12, 13, and 14 curets also are available in a modified pairing as the Gracey 11/14 and Gracey 12/13 instruments. Many clinicians find the modified pairing to be more convenient because an entire aspect of a posterior sextant can be completed without changing instruments. For example, the facial aspect of the mandibular right posterior sextant can be completed with the G11/14 curet (without having to use the G12/13 curet).

When using the G11/14, G12/13 instruments:

1. The clinician uses one instrument—G11/14—to complete the entire facial aspect of the mandibular right posterior sextant.
2. The clinician would use the other instrument—G12/13—to complete the lingual aspect of the mandibular right posterior sextant.

Example: Use of Modified Pairing on the Mandibular Right Posterior Sextant

Facial (right)

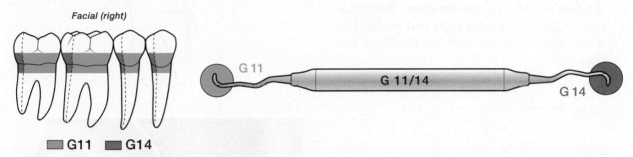

■ G11 ■ G14

Modified Pairing on Facial Aspect of Mandibular Right Sextant. With the modified pairing of Gracey curets, only one double-ended instrument—the G11/14—is required to complete the facial aspect of the mandibular right posterior sextant.

Lingual (right)

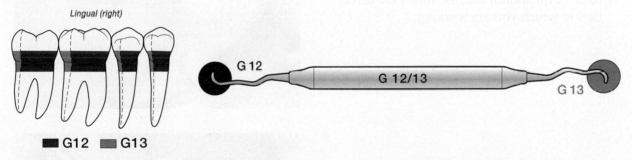

■ G12 ■ G13

Modified Pairing on Lingual Aspect of Mandibular Right Sextant. With the modified pairing of Gracey curets, only one double-ended instrument—the G12/13—is required to complete the lingual aspect of the mandibular right posterior sextant.

STEP-BY-STEP TECHNIQUE ON MANDIBULAR FIRST MOLAR

Equipment: A periodontal typodont and a set of area-specific curets. Examples of Gracey sets for this sextant include: (1) G11 and G14, (2) G15 and G18, (3) G7, G11, G14, (4) G9, G11, G14, (5) G7, G15, and G18, or (5) G7, G15, and G18.

Right-Handed Clinicians   Left-Handed Clinicians

Instrumenting the Distal Surface

1. **Begin With the Distal Surfaces.** As an introduction to the area-specific curet, first practice on the mandibular right first molar. *Use a distal area-specific curet on the distal surface.*

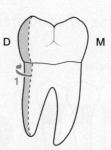

2. **Get Ready.** The toe should aim toward the back of the mouth because this is the direction in which you are working.

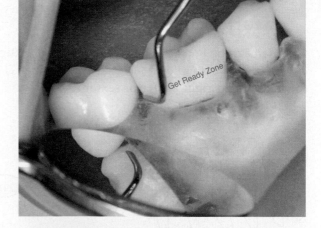

3. **Insert.** Lower handle and gently slide the working-end beneath the gingival margin.

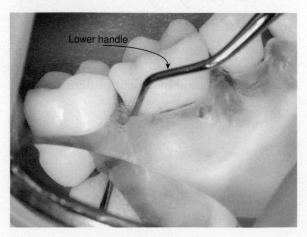

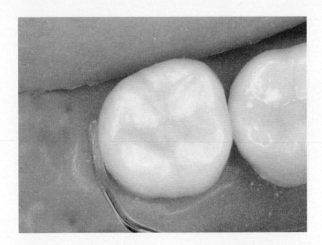

4. **Technique Check.** If the lower shank of the area-specific curet is parallel to the distal surface, then the instrument face-to-tooth surface angulation will be 70-degrees.

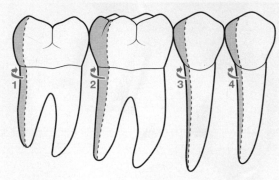

5. **Sequence for Distal Surfaces.** Use the sequence shown in this illustration to debride the distal surfaces in the sextant. It is easier to begin with the posterior-most molar and move forward toward the first premolar because of the pressure exerted against your hand by the patient's cheek.

Instrumenting the Facial and Mesial Surfaces

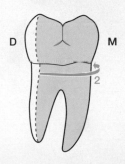

6. **Instrument of the Facial and Mesial Surfaces.** *Use a facial or mesial curet to debride the facial surface of the tooth, beginning at the distofacial line angle.*

7. **Get Ready.**

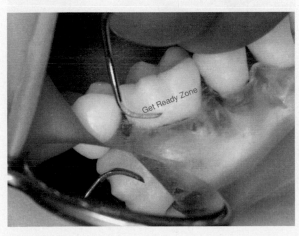

8. **Insert.** Lower the instrument handle and gently slide the working-end beneath the gingival margin.

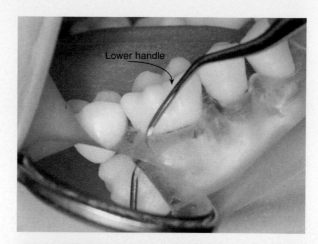

9. **Roll the Handle.** As you approach the mesiofacial line angle, roll the handle slightly to maintain adaptation.

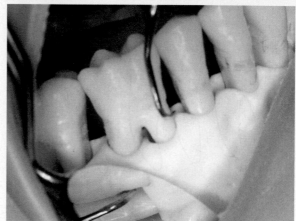

10. **Technique Check.** Make sure that your strokes extend past the midline of the mesial proximal surface.
    • Work at least halfway across the mesial surface from the facial aspect.
    • The other half of the mesial surface will be instrumented from the lingual aspect.

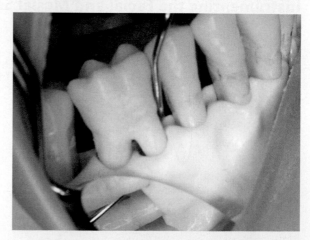

11. **Sequence for Facial and Mesial Surfaces.** Use the sequence shown in this illustration to debride the facial and mesial surfaces in the sextant.

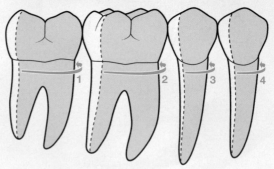

Section 4
Horizontal Strokes

Horizontal strokes are extremely useful in removing calculus deposits that are located (1) near the distofacial or distolingual line angle of posterior teeth and (2) at the midline of the facial or lingual surfaces of anterior teeth.

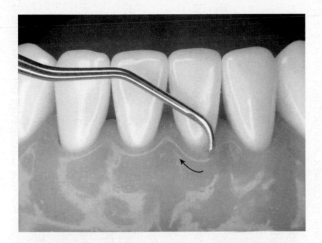

Anterior Teeth. The technique for making horizontal strokes with an area-specific curet is similar to that used with a universal curet.

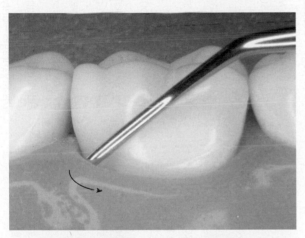

Posterior Teeth. Horizontal calculus removal strokes are very effective in removing deposits from the line angle region of posterior teeth.

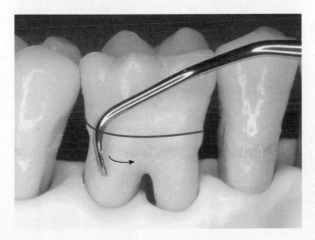

Technique Check. The gingiva has been removed from the typodont in this photograph to provide a view of the working-end of an area-specific curet during a horizontal stroke.

Section 5
Design Analysis of Scalers and Curets

TABLE 16-1. **Design Analysis of Sickle Scalers and Curets**

Instruments	Characteristic	Critique
Sickle	Back pointed	Advantage—strong, "bulky" working-end
		Disadvantage—cannot be used subgingivally
Universal & Area-specific	Back rounded	Advantage—used subgingivally without tissue trauma
		Disadvantage—none
Sickle	Tip (pointed)	Advantage—provides good access to proximal surfaces on anterior crowns and enamel surfaces apical to contact areas of posterior teeth
		Disadvantage—sharp point can gouge cemental surfaces
Universal & Area-specific	Toe (rounded)	Advantage—adapts well to convex, rounded root surfaces and root concavities
		Disadvantage—is wider than a pointed tip and, therefore, more difficult to adapt to proximal surfaces of anterior crowns
Sickle	Cutting edge straight	Advantage—none
		Disadvantage—adapts poorly to rounded root surfaces and root concavities
Area-specific	Cutting edge curves up at the toe	Advantage—enhances adaptation to rounded root surfaces and root concavities
		Disadvantage—none
Sickle & Universal	Face perpendicular to lower shank	Advantage—efficient, two cutting-edges per working-end, both of which can be used for calculus removal
		Disadvantage—level cutting edges mean that the lower shank must be tilted slightly toward the tooth for correct angulation
Area-specific	Face tilts in relation to lower shank	Advantage—working cutting edge is self-angulated
		Disadvantage—only one working cutting edge per working-end means frequent instrument changes

Section 6
Skill Application

PRACTICAL FOCUS
Periodontal Debridement Case: Mr. Smithfield

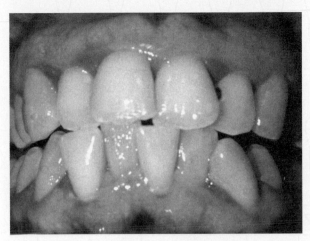

Mr. Smithfield: Intraoral Photograph

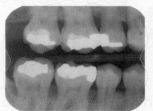

Mr. Smithfield: Right Bitewings

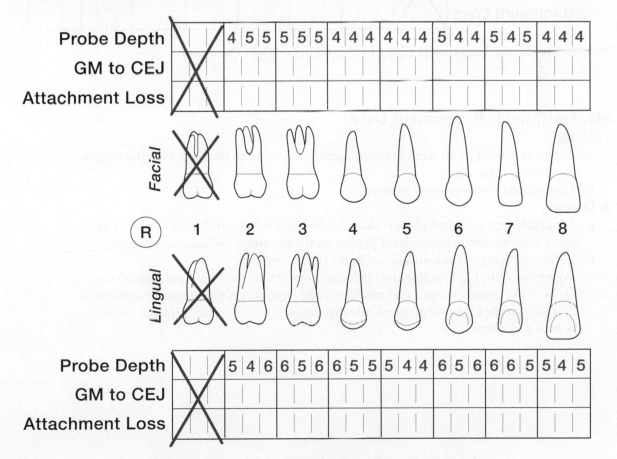

Mr. Smithfield: Periodontal Chart for Maxillary Right Quadrant

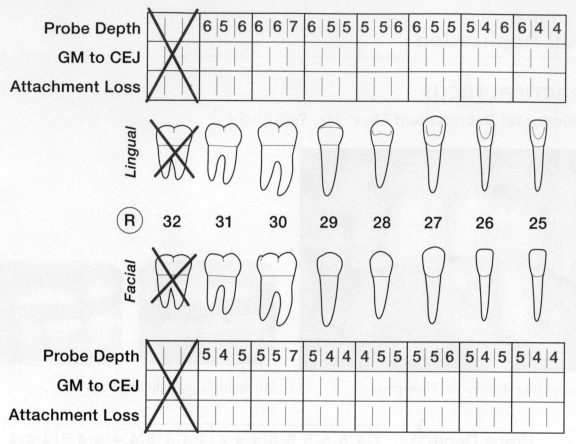

Probe Depth			6	5	6	6	6	7	6	5	5	5	5	6	6	5	5	5	4	6	6	4	4
GM to CEJ																							
Attachment Loss																							

(R)	32	31	30	29	28	27	26	25

Probe Depth			5	4	5	5	5	7	5	4	4	4	5	5	5	5	6	5	4	5	5	4	4
GM to CEJ																							
Attachment Loss																							

Mr. Smithfield: Periodontal Chart for Mandibular Right Quadrant

Mr. Smithfield: Assessment Data

1. Tissue
   a. Gingival margin of all teeth in this quadrant is level with the CEJ. Probing depths are noted on the chart.
   b. Generalized bleeding upon probing.
2. Deposits
   a. Moderate supragingival plaque on all teeth. Light subgingival plaque on all surfaces with moderate subgingival plaque on the proximal surfaces on all teeth.
   b. Light supragingival calculus deposits on all the teeth.
   c. Posterior teeth: Light subgingival calculus deposits on the facial and lingual surfaces of the posterior teeth and medium-sized deposits on the proximal surfaces. Anterior teeth: Light subgingival calculus deposits on all surfaces (facial, lingual, mesial and distal).

Mr. Smithfield: Case Questions

1. Does the assessment data indicate healthy sulci or periodontal pockets? Explain which data you used to determine the presence of sulci or pockets?

2. How effective is Mr. Smithfield's self-care (daily plaque control)? Explain which data helped you evaluate the effectiveness of his self-care?

3. After obtaining the probing depths, which type of explorer would you select to explore the teeth in this quadrant?

4. Which of the following instruments would you select for calculus removal on the anterior teeth in this quadrant: sickle scalers, universal curets, and/or area-specific curets? Explain your rationale for instrument selection.

5. Which of the following instruments would you select for calculus removal on the posterior teeth in this quadrant: sickle scalers, universal curets, and/or area-specific curets? Explain your rationale for instrument selection.

SUMMARY SHEET: AREA-SPECIFIC CURETS

Use of Area-Specific Curets

An area-specific curet is a periodontal instrument used to remove light calculus deposits from the crowns and roots of the teeth and to deplaque (remove plaque from) the root surfaces.

Basic Concepts

1. Insert the working-end beneath the gingival margin at a 0- to 40-degree angulation.
2. Maintain adaptation of the tip-third of the cutting edge to the tooth surface.
3. Before initiating a calculus removal stroke, press down with your fulcrum finger, and apply pressure against the instrument handle with the index finger and thumb to create lateral pressure against the tooth surface.
4. Activate the calculus removal stroke using wrist motion activation. Use digital activation in areas where movement is restricted, such as furcation areas and narrow, deep pockets.
5. Relax your fingers between each calculus removal stroke.

Anterior Teeth

1. For surfaces toward, sit at 8–9:00 if you are a right-handed clinician or at 4–3:00 if you are a left-handed clinician. For surfaces away, sit at 12:00.
2. Select the correct working-end:
   • Use only the lower cutting edges for periodontal debridement.
   • The lower shank is parallel to the tooth surface being instrumented.
3. Sequence: Begin with the surfaces toward your nondominant hand. Start on the canine on opposite side of the mouth and work toward yourself. (Right-Handed clinicians start with the left canine, mesial surface; Left-Handed clinicians start with the right canine, mesial surface.)

Posterior Teeth

1. For aspects toward, sit at 9:00 (or 3:00). For aspects away, sit at 10–11:00 (or 2–1:00).
2. Select the correct working-end:
   • Use only the lower cutting edges for periodontal debridement.
   • The lower shank is parallel to the tooth surface.
   • Use a distal curet for distal surfaces. Use a mesial curet for mesial surfaces. For facial and lingual surfaces, a mesial curet or the G7, G8, G9, G10 curets may be used.
3. Sequence: Complete all distal surfaces first; next, instrument the facial and mesial surfaces (or the lingual and mesial surfaces).

NOTE TO COURSE INSTRUCTOR: Refer to Module 18 for instrumentation strategies and patient cases relating to calculus removal.

Refer to Module 23, Advanced Techniques for Root Surface Debridement, for content on the design and use of Langer curets, Gracey designs with extended shanks and miniature working-ends, Curvettes, and OH debridement curets.

Student: _____

Evaluator: _____

Date: _____

Anterior Area 1 = _____
Anterior Area 2 = _____
Posterior Area 3 = _____
Posterior Area 4 = _____

DIRECTIONS FOR STUDENT: Use **Column S.** Evaluate your skill level as: **S** (satisfactory) or **U** (unsatisfactory).

DIRECTIONS FOR EVALUATOR: Use **Column E.** Indicate: **S** (satisfactory) or **U** (unsatisfactory). Each **S** equals 1 point, each **U** equals 0 points.

CRITERIA:	Area 1		Area 2		Area 3		Area 4	
	S	E	S	E	S	E	S	E
Position:								
Positioned correctly on clinician stool								
Positioned correctly with relation to patient, equipment, and treatment area								
Establishes correct patient head position								
Dental Mirror:								
Uses correct grasp and establishes secure rest with mirror								
Uses the mirror correctly for retraction and/or indirect vision								
Modified Pen Grasp with Dominant Hand:								
Thumb and index finger pads positioned opposite one another on handle; fingers not touching or overlapped								
Pad of middle finger rests lightly on shank; touches the ring finger								
Handle rests between the 2nd knuckle of the index finger and the "V" of hand								
Intraoral Fulcrum:								
Ring finger is straight and supports weight of hand								
Fulcrums on same arch, near tooth being instrumented								
Technique with Area-Specific Curet:								
Establishes and maintains correct face-to-tooth surface angulation								
Maintains correct adaptation; rolls handle when needed for adaptation								
Uses controlled calculus removal strokes in a coronal direction								
Applies appropriate stroke pressure in a coronal direction								
Uses correct sequence in the sextant								
Demonstrates horizontal strokes at (1) the midlines of anterior teeth and (2) the line angles of posterior teeth								

OPTIONAL GRADE PERCENTAGE CALCULATION
Total **S's** in each E column.

Sum of **S's** _____ divided by Total Points Possible (**64**) equals the Percentage Grade _____

SKILL EVALUATION MODULE 16 | AREA-SPECIFIC CURETS

Student: _____

EVALUATOR COMMENTS

_____

_____

_____

_____

_____

_____

_____

_____

_____

_____

_____

_____

_____

_____

_____

_____

_____

Box for sketches pertaining to written comments.

Periodontal Files

Module Overview

This module presents the design characteristics and technique for use of periodontal files. The periodontal file is restricted in its use, serving only as a supplement to other periodontal instruments.

Module Outline

Key Terms

Periodontal file
Two-point contact

Learning Objectives

1. Identify the design characteristics of periodontal files.

2. Describe the uses and limitations of periodontal files.

3. Describe two-point contact with a periodontal file.

4. Using a periodontal file, demonstrate correct adaptation and use of calculus removal strokes on the anterior and posterior teeth.

Section I
Periodontal Files

GENERAL DESIGN CHARACTERISTICS

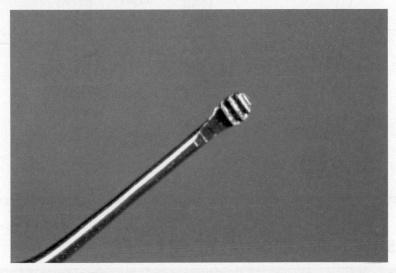

A periodontal file is a periodontal instrument that is used to prepare calculus deposits before removal with another instrument. A periodontal file is used to crush or roughen a heavy calculus deposit so that it can be removed with a sickle scaler or curet.

1. Each file is designed for use only on a certain tooth surface; therefore, a set of files is needed to instrument the entire mouth.
2. The working-end of a periodontal file has several unique design characteristics:
   a. The working-end has a series of cutting edges lined up on a base.
   b. The cutting edges are at a 90- to 105-degree angle to the base.
   c. The base may be round, rectangular, or oblong.
   d. The back is round to permit subgingival use.
   e. The shank is rigid and transmits limited tactile information to the clinician's fingers.
   f. A file with a base that is small in circumference is best for subgingival use.
3. Periodontal files are restricted in use, serving only as a supplement to sickle scalers or curets.
   a. They are used to crush large, tenacious subgingival calculus deposits that are not accessible to the sickle scalers usually used to remove heavy calculus deposits. After the deposit has been crushed, it is removed by a curet.
   b. Files are used to roughen the surface of burnished calculus deposits to facilitate removal of these deposits with a curet.
   c. Periodontal files can be used to smooth overhanging amalgam restorations.
   d. Files are limited to use on enamel surfaces or the outer surface of a calculus deposit. The flat base and straight cutting edges do not adapt well to curved root surfaces.
4. Because of their design limitations, periodontal files have been replaced to a great extent by ultrasonic instruments. Ultrasonic instruments are very effective at removing large calculus deposits.
5. Examples of periodontal files include the following: Hirschfeld 3/7, 5/11, and 9/10 files and the Orban 10/11 and 12/13 files.

WORKING-END DESIGN

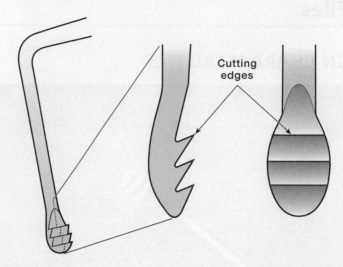

Cutting edges

Design Characteristics. The working-end of a file has multiple straight cutting edges.

REFERENCE SHEET: PERIODONTAL FILE

TABLE 17-1. Periodontal File	
Working-End	Thin in width and round, rectangular, or oblong in shape
Face	Has a series of cutting edges lined up on a base
Cutting Edges	Multiple, at a 90- to 105-degree angulation to the base
Application	Each working-end designed for single-surface use; a set of files is required to instrument the entire mouth
Primary Functions	Crush large calculus deposit
	Roughen burnished calculus deposit
	Smooth overhanging amalgam restoration
	Limited to use on enamel surfaces or the outer surface of a calculus deposit; the flat base does not adapt well to curved root surfaces

TABLE 17-2. Use of Periodontal Files	
Design Advantages	**Design Limitations**
1. The strong working-end and rigid shank enable the file to crush or fracture large calculus deposits.	1. The rigid shank provides limited tactile information to the clinician's fingers.
2. The thin, flat working-end can be used to remove large deposits that are inaccessible to the sickle scalers. For example, a periodontal file can be used subgingivally, where a sickle scaler should not be used.	2. Because of the large base circumference, subgingival use may cause excessive stretching of the soft tissue wall. If the file does not insert easily, trauma to the soft tissue results. Use of a file at the very base of a pocket can traumatize the junctional epithelium.

INSTRUMENTATION PRINCIPLES

1. **Grasp and Fulcrum.** A modified pen grasp is used in combination with a secure intraoral finger rest. Firm instrumentation strokes are needed to crush or roughen calculus deposits with these instruments.
2. **Insertion.**
   a. The file is inserted beneath the calculus deposit, and a two-point contact is established.
   b. A file should be used subgingivally only if it inserts easily beneath the gingival margin. Forcing the working-end beneath the gingival margin results in excessive stretching and trauma to the soft tissue wall of the pocket. Files should not be inserted to the very base of a pocket because the large base can traumatize the junctional epithelium.
3. **Adaptation.**
   a. Two-point contact is (1) adaptation of the working-end to a calculus deposit while (2) resting the lower shank against the tooth. This two-point contact provides the additional stability and leverage needed when making an instrumentation stroke with a file.
   b. The *entire face* of the working-end should be flat against the calculus deposit (parallel to the root surface). The face should not be applied at an angle to the tooth surface; in this position, the sharp corners on one side of the cutting edges can gouge the cementum whereas the sharp corners on the opposite end can traumatize the soft tissue.
4. **Instrumentation Stroke.**
   a. Firm lateral pressure is applied to the deposit as a pull stroke is activated in a vertical direction.
   b. The instrumentation stroke is most effective when firm, consistent pressure is applied throughout the entire stroke.
   c. Strokes are repeated until the deposit has been crushed sufficiently to be removed with a curet.

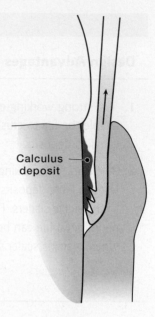

Calculus deposit

Cross Section of a File in Use. The face of the working-end should be flat against the calculus deposit so that the corners of the straight cutting edges do not gouge the root surface or the soft tissue.

Use of a file at the very base of a pocket can traumatize the junctional epithelium.

FILE SELECTION

Each periodontal file is designed for use only on certain tooth surfaces; therefore, a set of files is needed to instrument the entire mouth. One of the most versatile series of files is the Hirschfeld series. A set of Hirschfeld periodontal files includes the Hirschfeld 9/10, 3/7, and 5/11 files. Another common file series is the Orban series. There are two Orban files—the Orban 10/11 and 12/13.

TABLE 17-3.	Application of Periodontal File
File	**Area of Application**
Hirschfeld 9/10	Facial and lingual surfaces of the anterior teeth
Hirschfeld 3/7	Facial and lingual surfaces of the posterior teeth
Hirschfeld 5/11	Mesial and distal surfaces of the posterior teeth
Orban 10/11	Facial and lingual surfaces of the posterior teeth
Orban 12/13	Mesial and distal surfaces of the posterior teeth

Section 2
Technique Practice: Posterior Teeth

When using periodontal files, two double-ended instruments are required for use on the posterior teeth.

APPLICATION OF THE CUTTING EDGES

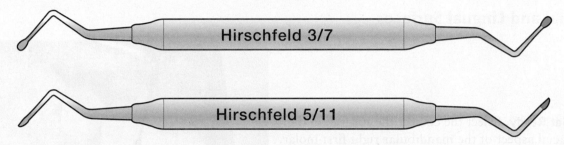

Application of Hirschfeld Files to Posterior Surfaces. Two files are used on the posterior teeth. The H 3/7 for facial and lingual surfaces and the H5/11 for the proximal surfaces.

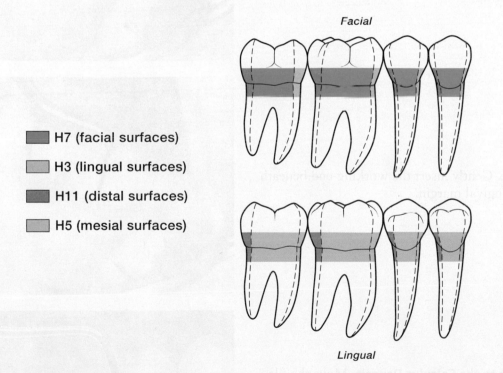

H7 (facial surfaces)
H3 (lingual surfaces)
H11 (distal surfaces)
H5 (mesial surfaces)

Application to Posterior Surfaces. This illustration indicates how the Hirschfeld files are applied to the posterior tooth surfaces.

TECHNIQUE ON MANDIBULAR FIRST MOLAR

Equipment: A periodontal typodont and a set of periodontal files.

Right-Handed Clinicians   Left-Handed Clinicians

Facial and Lingual Surfaces

1. **Get Ready.** Select the correct file for use on the facial aspect of the mandibular right first molar. In preparation for insertion, place the working-end against the facial surface.

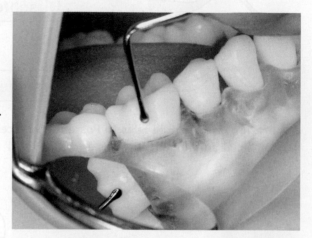

2. **Insert.** Gently insert the working-end beneath the gingival margin.

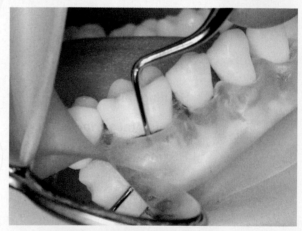

3. **Adapt to the Calculus Deposit.** Move the file along the root surface until it is adapted to the calculus deposit.
   • *Remember to establish a two-point contact with the working-end and the lower shank.*
   • Activate pull strokes in a vertical direction.

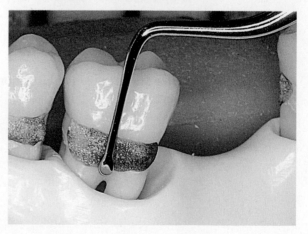

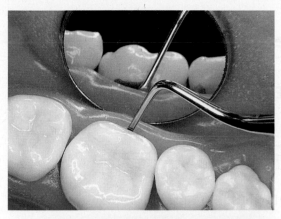

4. **Lingual Surface.** Select the correct file for use on the lingual surface. Gently slip the working-end beneath the gingival margin. Establish two-point contact. Use indirect vision to check the placement of the periodontal file.

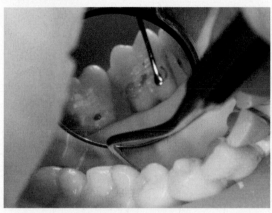

5. **Adapt to the Calculus Deposit.** Move the file along the root surface until it is adapted to the calculus deposit. Activate pull strokes in a vertical direction.

Mesial and Distal Surfaces

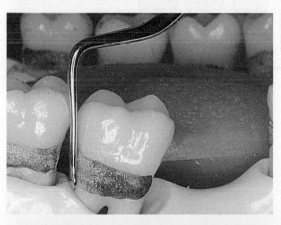

6. **Distal Surface.** Select the correct file for the distal surface. Insert the file beneath the gingival margin and position it on the calculus deposit. Activate pull strokes in a vertical direction.

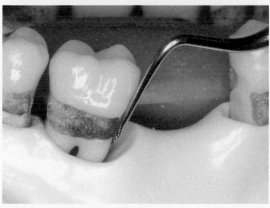

7. **Mesial Surface.** Using the correct file for the mesial surface, position the working-end on the calculus deposit. Remember to maintain two-point contact. Activate pull strokes in a vertical direction.

Section 3
Technique Practice: Anterior Teeth

APPLICATION OF THE CUTTING EDGES

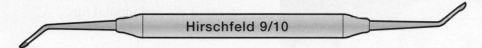

Application of a Hirschfeld File to Anterior Teeth. The Hirschfeld 9/10 file is used to instrument the anterior teeth.

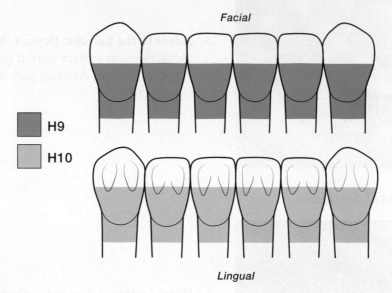

Application to Anterior Surfaces. This illustration indicates how the 9/10 Hirschfeld file is applied to the anterior tooth surfaces.

TECHNIQUE ON ANTERIORS

1. Equipment: an anterior periodontal file
2. Position yourself for the sextant shown in the icons below.

Right-Handed Clinicians

Left-Handed Clinicians

3. Remember: "Me, My Patient, My Light, My Dominant Hand, My Nondominant Hand, My Finger Rest, My Adaptation."

Facial and Lingual Surfaces

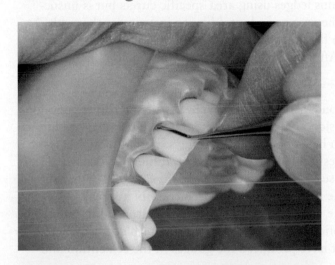

4. **Facial Surfaces.** Select the correct file for the facial surface, and place it on the calculus deposit. Activate pull strokes in a vertical direction.

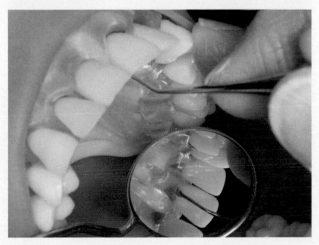

5. **Lingual Surfaces.** Insert the correct file beneath the gingival margin. Adapt to the calculus deposit, and activate a series of pull strokes in a vertical direction.

Section 4
Skill Application

PRACTICAL FOCUS

Case 1: You have been assigned to observe a second-year student, LaWanda, as she performs periodontal debridement on a patient. You observe LaWanda using a periodontal file on the facial aspect of the maxillary right first molar. She is working within a periodontal pocket. LaWanda makes several vertical strokes with the file and then uses an area-specific curet to remove a calculus deposit. What reason would LaWanda have to use both a file and an area-specific curet on the facial aspect of this molar?

Case 2: You have been assigned to work as a team with a second-year student, Henry, to provide care for Mr. Wilson. Mr. Wilson has ledges of subgingival calculus throughout his mouth. The calculus deposits are located in 5- to 6-mm pockets. Today, the mandibular left posterior quadrant will be instrumented. Henry tries to remove the calculus ledges using area-specific curets but is unsuccessful because the deposits are so tenacious, so he uses periodontal files to instrument the teeth. At this point, Henry says that you should be able to finish instrumentation on this quadrant. What do you expect to find when you explore the teeth? After exploring the teeth, what do you plan to do next?

Case 3: You have been assigned to observe a second-year student, Wynne, as she performs periodontal debridement on a patient. Wynne spends considerable time instrumenting the maxillary right second molar with an area-specific curet. This tooth has a pocket and Wynne says that there is a ledge of calculus that she just cannot budge. You suggest that she try a periodontal file. As you and Wynne walk to the clinic dispensary to obtain a set of periodontal files, Wynne confesses that she has never used a file on a patient. Wynne uses the file in the area and is successful in breaking up the calculus ledge. When she checks the facial surface with an explorer, Wynne is surprised to find several long gouges in the root surface. You also notice that the soft tissue began to bleed heavily after Wynne used the file. What technique error might have produced the gouges in the cementum and traumatized the tissue wall of the pocket?

SKILL EVALUATION MODULE 17	PERIODONTAL FILES

Student: _____

Evaluator: _____

Date: _____

Area 1 = _____
Area 2 = _____
Area 3 = _____
Area 4 = _____

DIRECTIONS FOR STUDENT: Use **Column S.** Evaluate your skill level as: **S** (satisfactory) or **U** (unsatisfactory).

DIRECTIONS FOR EVALUATOR: Use **Column E.** Indicate: **S** (satisfactory) or **U** (unsatisfactory). Each **S** equals 1 point, each **U** equals 0 points.

CRITERIA:	Area 1		Area 2		Area 3		Area 4	
	S	E	S	E	S	E	S	E
Position:								
Positioned correctly on clinician stool								
Positioned correctly with relation to patient, equipment, and treatment area								
Establishes correct patient head position								
Dental Mirror:								
Uses correct grasp and establishes secure rest with mirror								
Uses the mirror correctly for retraction and/or indirect vision								
Modified Pen Grasp with Dominant Hand:								
Thumb and index finger pads positioned opposite one another on handle; fingers not touching or overlapped								
Pad of middle finger rests lightly on shank; touches the ring finger								
Handle rests between the 2nd knuckle of the index finger and the "V" of hand								
Intraoral Fulcrum:								
Ring finger is straight and supports weight of hand								
Fulcrums on same arch, near tooth being instrumented								
Technique with Periodontal Files:								
Selects the correct file for the tooth surface								
Establishes two-point contact								
Uses vertical strokes								
Applies appropriate stroke pressure in a coronal direction								
OPTIONAL GRADE PERCENTAGE CALCULATION Total **S**'s in each E column.								

Sum of **S**'s _____ divided by Total Points Possible (**56**) equals the Percentage Grade _____

SKILL EVALUATION MODULE 17   PERIODONTAL FILES

Student: _____

EVALUATOR COMMENTS

_____

_____

_____

_____

_____

_____

_____

_____

_____

_____

_____

_____

_____

_____

_____

_____

_____

_____

_____

Box for sketches pertaining to written comments.

Instrumentation Strategies and Patient Cases

Module Overview

This module introduces the concepts of appointment planning and instrument sequencing for calculus removal. The Practical Focus section contains patient cases for practice in appointment planning for multiple calculus removal appointments.

Module Outline

Key Terms

Pellicle

Full-mouth debridement

Full-mouth disinfection

Gross scaling

Circuit scaling

Abscess of the periodontium

Learning Objectives

1. Name the three modes of calculus attachment to tooth surfaces.

2. Describe how calculus attachment to cementum differs from calculus attachment to enamel.

3. Describe how the mode of calculus attachment influences the ease of calculus removal.

4. Define full-mouth debridement, and discuss the advantages of this approach to calculus removal.

5. Discuss the various approaches for dividing up the work when multiple appointments are planned for calculus removal.

6. Discuss the disadvantages of gross calculus removal.

7. Select calculus removal instruments based on the size and location of the calculus deposits.

8. Using the multiple appointment approach, plan a series of calculus removal appointments based on the patient's assessment data.

Section 1
Modes of Calculus Attachment

Dental calculus attaches to tooth surfaces through several modes; different attachment mechanisms can exist in the same calculus deposit (Table 18-1).

1. **Attachment by Means of Pellicle.**
   a. Calculus deposits attached to the pellicle. The pellicle is a thin coating of salivary proteins that attaches to the tooth surface within minutes after a professional cleaning. The pellicle acts like double-sided adhesive tape, adhering to the tooth surface on one side and providing a sticky surface for attachment of calculus on the other side.
   b. Calculus deposits attached to the pellicle are removed easily because the attachment is on the surface of the tooth (and not locked into the tooth surface).
   c. This mode of attachment occurs most commonly on enamel tooth surfaces.
2. **Attachment to Irregularities in the Tooth Surface.**
   a. Calculus deposits are attached to microscopic irregularities in the tooth surface, such as (1) cracks, (2) tiny openings in root surface left where periodontal ligament fibers are detached, and (3) grooves in cemental surfaces as the result of overinstrumentation during previous calculus removal procedures.
   b. Calculus that is attached in tooth irregularities is difficult to remove because the deposits lie sheltered in these tooth defects.
   c. This mode of attachment occurs most commonly on root surfaces.
3. **Attachment by Direct Contact of the Calcified Component and the Tooth Surface.**
   a. In this mode of attachment, the matrix of the calculus deposit is interlocked with the inorganic crystals of the tooth.
   b. These deposits are difficult to remove because they are firmly interlocked in the tooth surface.
   c. This mode of attachment occurs most commonly on root surfaces.

TABLE 18-1. Calculus Attachment Modes		
Tooth Surface	**Attachment Mode**	**Attachment Strength**
Enamel surfaces	To pellicle	Weak
Root surfaces	In microscopic surface irregularities	Strong
Root surfaces	Interlocked with organic crystals of tooth	Extremely strong

Section 2
Planning for Calculus Removal

Clinicians should be aware that philosophies for planning calculus removal appointments have changed over the years. Two common approaches to appointment planning for calculus removal are (1) full-mouth debridement and (2) sextant or quadrant debridement. Traditionally, calculus removal has been accomplished a sextant or quadrant at a time during multiple appointments. *Recent research findings suggest that the best response to periodontal debridement is obtained when calculus removal is completed in a single appointment or in two appointments within a 24-hour period.* Sextant or quadrant debridement, however, may be most appropriate for student clinicians.

FULL-MOUTH DEBRIDEMENT

Full-mouth debridement is defined as calculus removal that is completed in a single appointment or in two appointments within a 24-hour period. [1-4]

1. Because periodontal disease is an infection, the full-mouth approach to periodontal debridement is based on the assumption that the pathogenic bacteria in untreated areas of the mouth can re-infect the treated areas.
2. In some research studies, the full-mouth debridement procedure was combined with the use of topical antimicrobial therapy. Full-mouth disinfection is full-mouth debridement with the use of professionally applied topical antimicrobial therapy. It is unclear, however, whether the antimicrobial therapy actually contributed to the improved results derived from the full-mouth periodontal debridement alone.
3. Full-mouth debridement is best accomplished by the dental hygienist working with an assistant.
4. Initially, patients may be resistant to the concept of scheduling one or two long appointments for the purpose of periodontal debridement. One or two long appointments, however, may in reality be less disruptive to an individual's work schedule than two to six 1-hour appointments over a period of several weeks. In addition, the dental hygienist should explain the rationale behind full-mouth debridement.

SEXTANT OR QUADRANT DEBRIDEMENT

Full-mouth debridement of difficult patient cases is not a realistic goal for beginning student clinicians. In this instance, calculus removal completed in sextants or quadrants over multiple appointments is appropriate.

1. The multiple-appointment approach to calculus removal is based on the concept of *complete calculus removal on the teeth treated at each appointment.*
2. If periodontal debridement is completed over multiple appointments, at each appointment the clinician should treat only as many *teeth, sextants, or quadrants* as he or she can thoroughly debride of calculus during that appointment. For example, the student clinician may complete a single sextant (facial and lingual aspects) on a patient with periodontitis or complete two quadrants (half the mouth) on a patient with gingivitis.

PLANNING MULTIPLE APPOINTMENTS FOR CALCULUS REMOVAL

When multiple appointments are needed for calculus removal, the student clinician must decide how to divide the work. The following approaches are recommended:

1. **Complete several teeth.**
   a. For extremely difficult cases, the student clinician may complete only a few teeth (both facial and lingual aspects).
   b. In most instances, however, the clinician is able to complete the facial and lingual aspects of a sextant or quadrant.
2. **Complete one sextant or quadrant.**
   a. Usually it is possible to complete one sextant or quadrant at an appointment.
   b. For example, the clinician might begin by treating the facial and lingual aspects of a posterior sextant. Treatment can end here for the appointment, or, if time permits, the adjacent anterior teeth are completed to the midline of the arch (resulting in completion of the quadrant).
3. **Complete two quadrants on the same side of the mouth.**
   a. When two quadrants are completed at one appointment, treatment of a *maxillary and mandibular quadrant on the same side of the mouth* is recommended (rather than treating the entire maxillary arch or the entire mandibular arch).
   b. Completing a maxillary and mandibular quadrant on one side of the mouth is preferred for several reasons.
      1) This approach gives the patient an untreated side on which to chew comfortably.
      2) Completing quadrants on one side of the mouth usually divides the work more evenly because the maxillary arch is more difficult for most clinicians.
      3) When local anesthesia is indicated for two quadrants, it is recommended that a maxillary and mandibular quadrant on the same side of the mouth be selected.

GROSS CALCULUS REMOVAL—AN HISTORICAL PERSPECTIVE

In the past, a common method of planning multiple calculus removal appointments involved removing only the large-sized calculus deposits from the entire mouth at the first appointment. This intentional incomplete removal of calculus is commonly known as gross scaling. This approach to calculus removal was common in the '60s and '70s but is *no longer recommended*. Gross scaling is discussed here because clinicians may encounter patients who have undergone gross scaling procedures as well as clinicians who still use this method of appointment planning for calculus removal.

1. The gross scaling approach involved devoting the first calculus removal appointment to removal of large-sized *supragingival* calculus deposits from the entire mouth.
2. The initial calculus removal appointment was followed by several additional appointments for calculus removal.
3. Usually, the entire mouth is treated at each appointment, "whittling away" the calculus deposits bit by bit. This approach of incomplete removal of deposits from the entire mouth at each appointment was known as **circuit scaling** (because the clinician goes around and around the mouth at appointment after appointment).

4. The gross scaling approach is *not recommended* because of the undesirable consequences that can result from incomplete calculus removal:

a. **Proliferation of Microorganisms.** Gross scaling leaves behind partially removed deposits that are rough, irregular, and covered with bacterial plaque. As the marginal tissue shrinks, it closes off the entrance to the pocket, providing a protected environment within the pocket in which the microorganisms continue to multiply.

b. **Abscess Formation.** Incomplete calculus removal has been implicated in the formation of an abscess of the periodontium. An abscess of the periodontium is a localized collection of pus in the periodontal tissues.

1) Abscesses usually occur on teeth with a deep probing depth in which a gross scaling removes only the calculus deposits located above and slightly beneath the gingival margin.

2) It is theorized that this incomplete calculus removal allows the gingival margin to tighten around the tooth like a drawstring pouch, preventing drainage of bacterial waste products from the pocket.

3) Medically compromised individuals—such as those with uncontrolled diabetes—and those with deep periodontal pockets are especially prone to abscess formation.

c. **Difficult Instrumentation.** Insertion beneath the gingival margin is often more difficult at appointments that follow the initial gross scale appointment because the gingival margin is more closely adapted to the tooth surface.

d. **Decreased Patient Motivation for Treatment.** Many patients are motivated to seek treatment for esthetic (appearance) reasons. Removal of the visible *supra*gingival deposits combined with the improved appearance of the gingival tissues may influence the patient to forego further treatment. It is hard for patients to recognize that "what they can't see can hurt them."

e. **Patient Frustration.** When the patient undergoes multiple appointments at which the entire mouth is instrumented, he or she begins to feel that nothing is being accomplished by the treatment. All he knows is that the clinician goes around and around his mouth at each appointment, seemingly without end. ("I thought you cleaned all of my teeth at the LAST appointment!")

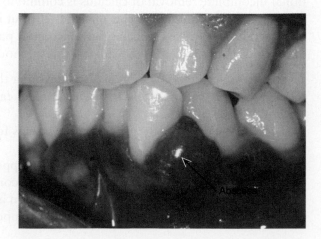

Typical Clinical Appearance of an Abscess of the Periodontium. Note that the swelling is very localized. When palpated, this swelling feels like a fluid-filled sac.

Section 3
Sequence and Instrument Selection

SEQUENCE FOR CALCULUS REMOVAL

Different instrument classifications are required for the removal of large- versus small-sized calculus deposits.

1. Large-sized calculus deposits most commonly are located above the gingival margin and can be removed using sickle scalers.
2. Small- or medium-sized calculus deposits usually are located below the gingival margin and can be removed using either universal or area-specific curets.
   a. Small- or medium-sized deposits on root surfaces located within sulci or shallow periodontal pockets can be removed with a universal curet.
   b. Small- or medium-sized deposits located on root surfaces within deep periodontal pockets can be removed with area-specific curets.
   c. Tenacious and large-sized deposits can be removed with rigid curets, ultrasonic instruments, or sonic instruments. Ultrasonic and sonic instrumentation is discussed in Module 24, Ultrasonic and Sonic Instrumentation.

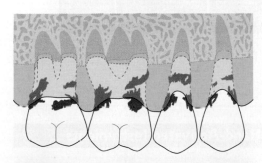

Deposit Size and Location. Large-sized calculus deposits typically are located above the gingival margin. Subgingival deposits usually are medium or small in size.

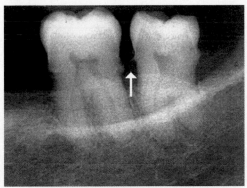

Dental Calculus. Large interproximal calculus deposits are visible on this radiograph.
(From Nield-Gehrig, J.S. and Willmann, D.E., Foundations of periodontics for the dental hygienist, 2003. Philadelphia: Lippincott Williams & Wilkins, p. 207.)

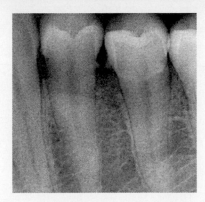

Dental Calculus. Large interproximal calculus deposits are visible on the proximal surfaces of the premolar teeth in this radiograph.

INSTRUMENT SELECTION FOR CALCULUS REMOVAL

For calculus removal, periodontal instruments are selected based on the size and location of the calculus deposits.

1. **Size.** Calculus deposits may be light, medium, or heavy in size.
2. **Location.**
   a. Supragingival, above the gingival margin
   b. Subgingival deposits located on the cervical-third of the root
   c. Subgingival deposits located on the middle- or apical-third of the root

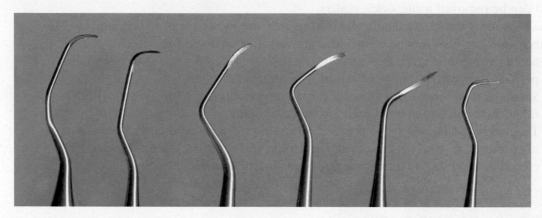

Calculus Removal Instruments. An important component of periodontal debridement is selecting the correct instrument for the task.

TABLE 18-2.	General Guide for Selection of Hand-Activated Instruments	
Type of Deposit	**Location of Deposit**	**Instrument**
Large-sized deposits	Above the gingival margin	Sickle scalers
Medium-sized deposits	Above and below the gingival margin	Universal curets
Small-sized deposits	Above the gingival margin	Universal curets
Small-sized deposits	On cervical-third of root	Universal curets
Small-sized deposits	On middle- or apical-third of root	Area-specific curets

SUMMARY SHEET: USE OF HAND-ACTIVATED INSTRUMENTS

TABLE 18-3.   Use of Hand-Activated Instruments

Classification	Purpose
Calibrated Probe	Measurement of pocket depths, clinical attachment level, width of attached gingiva, gingival recession, and intraoral lesions. Evaluation of gingival tissue for consistency and presence of bleeding or exudate.
Furcation Probe	Detection of furcation involvement in multirooted teeth. (Refer to Module 21.)
Explorer	Detection of calculus deposits, tooth surface irregularities, defective margins on restorations, decalcified areas, and carious lesions.
Sickle Scaler	Removal of medium- to large-sized calculus deposits from enamel surfaces. Provides good access to proximal surfaces on anterior crowns and enamel surfaces apical to contact areas of posterior teeth. Usually confined to supragingival use; should NOT be used for root surface debridement.
Periodontal File	Used to crush large calculus deposits and prepare burnished calculus before removal with another instrument.
Universal Curet	Debridement of crown and root surfaces. Removal of light- to medium-sized supra- and subgingival calculus deposits. Some designs have long functional shanks that allow access to the cervical and middle-thirds of root surfaces.
Area-Specific Curet	Debridement of crown and root surfaces. Removal of light supra- and subgingival calculus deposits. These curets have extended shanks that allow access to the middle- and apical-thirds of root surfaces.

SAMPLE DEBRIDEMENT PLANS

Although it is critical for the clinician to develop a calculus removal plan that will meet the needs of each individual patient, beginning clinicians often find it helpful to review an example of a typical plan for calculus removal. On this and the next pages are two patient profiles and examples of a typical calculus removal plan. Each calculus removal plan shown simply provides an example of one approach to calculus removal—other acceptable plans for calculus removal can be developed.

Box 18-1.   Patient Assessment Data: Patient 1

This patient has the following characteristics:

- Twenty-eight teeth (third molars have not erupted)

- Gingival margin is at the cemento-enamel junction on all teeth; probing depths vary between 2 and 3 mm

- Supragingival deposits—heavy deposits above the gingival margin on the lingual surface of the mandibular anterior teeth and the facial aspect of the maxillary molars

- Subgingival deposits—small-sized deposits generalized on all teeth

TABLE 18-4.   Calculus Removal Plan

Treatment Area	Instrument(s)—Listed in the order of use
Appt. 1: Mandibular right quadrant and maxillary right quadrant	1. Anterior sickle for supragingival deposits on anterior teeth
	2. Posterior sickle for supragingival deposits on posterior teeth
	3. Universal curet for light-sized deposits
Appt. 2: Mandibular left quadrant and maxillary left quadrant	1. Anterior sickle for supragingival deposits on anterior teeth
	2. Posterior sickle for supragingival deposits on posterior teeth
	3. Universal curet for light-sized deposits

Box 18-2. Patient Assessment Data: Patient 2

This patient has the following characteristics:

- Twenty-eight teeth (third molars have not erupted)
- Gingival margin is at the cemento-enamel junction on all teeth; probing depths vary between 4 and 5 mm
- **Supragingival deposits**—heavy deposits above the gingival margin on the lingual surface of the mandibular anterior teeth and the facial aspect of the maxillary molars
- **Subgingival deposits**—medium-sized deposits on the cervical-third of the roots of all teeth; small-sized deposits generalized on all teeth

TABLE 18-5. Calculus Removal Plan

Treatment Area	Instrument(s)—Listed in the Order of Use
Appt. 1: Mandibular anterior sextant	1. Anterior sickle for supragingival deposits 2. Universal curet for medium-sized deposits 3. Area-specific curets for small-sized deposits
Appt. 2: Mandibular right posterior sextant	1. Universal curet for medium-sized deposits 2. Area-specific curets for small-sized deposits
Appt. 3: Maxillary right posterior sextant	1. Posterior sickle for supragingival deposits on molar teeth 2. Universal curet for medium-sized deposits 3. Area-specific curets for small-sized deposits
Appt. 4: Maxillary anterior sextant	1. Universal curet for medium-sized deposits 2. Area-specific curets for small-sized deposits
Appt. 5: Maxillary left posterior sextant	1. Posterior sickle for supragingival deposits on molar teeth 2. Universal curet for medium-sized deposits 3. Area-specific curets for small-sized deposits
Appt. 6: Mandibular left posterior sextant	1. Universal curet for medium-sized deposits 2. Area-specific curets for small-sized deposits

Section 4
Practical Focus: Patient Cases

Instruments for Patient Cases

For the patient cases in this section, you may select calculus removal instruments from (1) your school's instrument kit or (2) the list below.

> Anterior sickle scaler
> Posterior sickle scaler
> Columbia universal curet
> Barnhart universal curet
> Gracey 3/4 curets
> Gracey 9/10 curets
> Gracey 11/12 curets
> Gracey 13/14 curets
> Hirschfeld 3/7 file
> Hirschfeld 5/11 file
> Hirschfeld 9/10 file

Case Questions

Directions: Photocopy the CALCULUS REMOVAL PLAN form on the next page of this module (or create a similar form yourself on tablet paper).

For each patient case, develop a Calculus Removal Plan:

1. Determine how many appointments you will need for calculus removal.

2. List the treatment area(s) to be completed at each appointment. For example, at a single appointment, can you complete the (1) entire mouth, (2) the maxillary and mandibular right quadrants (half the mouth), (3) the mandibular right quadrant (half the mandibular arch), (4) the mandibular right sextant, or (5) the mandibular anterior sextant?

3. Select appropriate instruments for use at each appointment. Indicate the sequence in which the instruments will be used and the use of each instrument.

4. On the back of the form, explain your rationale for instrument selection and sequence.

Calculus Removal Plan	
Treatment Area	**Instrument(s)—Listed in the order of use**
Appt. 1:	
Appt. 2 (if needed):	
Appt. 3 (if needed):	
Appt. 4 (if needed):	
Appt. 5 (if needed):	
Appt. 6 (if needed):	

PERIODONTAL DEBRIDEMENT CASE 1: MISS MARKUS

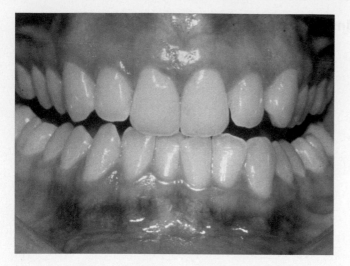

Miss Markus: Intraoral Photograph

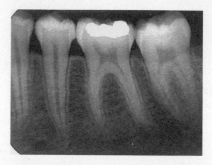

Miss Markus: Radiograph Mandibular Left

1	1	1	1	1	1	1	2	2	2	2	2	3	2	3	3	2	3	3	2	3				**Probing Depth**

GM to CEJ

Attachment Loss

24	23	22	21	20	19	18	17

Lingual

Ⓛ   *Facial*

1	1	1	1	1	1	1	1	2	2	2	2	2	2	2	2	2	3	3	2	3			**Probing Depth**

GM to CEJ

Attachment Loss

Miss Markus: Periodontal Chart for Mandibular Left Quadrant

Probe Depth			4	3	4	4	3	4	4	3	4	4	3	3	3	2	3	3	3	3	3	3	3	2	2
GM to CEJ																										
Attachment Loss																										

Facial

(R) 1 2 3 4 5 6 7 8

Lingual

Probe Depth			4	4	4	4	4	4	4	4	4	4	3	4	4	3	3	3	3	3	3	3	3	3	3
GM to CEJ																										
Attachment Loss																										

Mrs. Rose: Periodontal Chart for Maxillary Right Quadrant

Mrs. Rose: Assessment Data

1. Gingival Margin—the gingival margin of all teeth is level with the cemento-enamel junction. Probing depths are noted on the chart.
2. Supragingival Deposits.
   a. Moderate supragingival deposits above the gingival margin on the lingual aspect of the mandibular anteriors
   b. Moderate supragingival deposits on the facial and lingual aspects of all teeth
3. Subgingival Deposits.
   a. Small-sized deposits on the proximal surfaces of all anterior teeth
   b. Medium-sized deposits on the proximal surfaces of all posterior teeth

PERIODONTAL DEBRIDEMENT CASE 3: MR. JENKINS

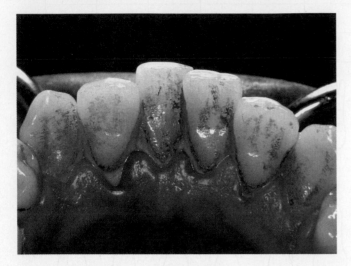

Mr. Jenkins: Intraoral Photograph

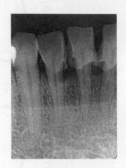

Mr. Jenkins: Anterior Radiograph

Probe Depth	8	8	9							8	7	6	6	6	5	5	5	5	5	5	5	5	5	5
GM to CEJ																								
Attachment Loss																								

Lingual

(R) 32   31   30   29   28   27   26   25

Facial

Probe Depth	8	7	7							7	5	6	6	5	5	5	5	5	5	5	5	5	5	5
GM to CEJ																								
Attachment Loss																								

Mr. Jenkins: Periodontal Chart for Mandibular Right Quadrant

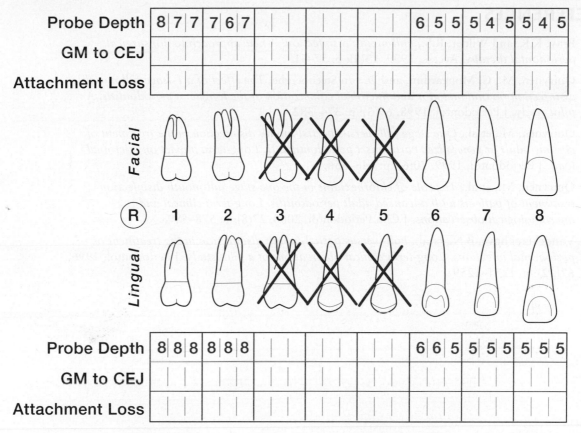

Probe Depth	8	7	7	7	6	7								6	5	5	5	4	5	5	4	5
GM to CEJ																						
Attachment Loss																						

Probe Depth	8	8	8	8	8	8								6	6	5	5	5	5	5	5	5
GM to CEJ																						
Attachment Loss																						

Mr. Jenkins: Periodontal Chart for Maxillary Right Quadrant

Mr. Jenkins: Assessment Data

1. Gingival Margin—the gingival margin on the mandibular anteriors is slightly apical to the cemento-enamel junction. The gingival margin on the remaining teeth is level with the cemento-enamel junction. Probing depths are noted on the chart.
2. Supragingival Deposits.
   a. Moderate supragingival deposits on the lingual aspect of all mandibular teeth
   b. Moderate supragingival deposits on the facial aspect of all maxillary teeth
3. Subgingival Deposits.
   a. Medium-sized deposits on the proximal surfaces of all teeth
   b. Small-sized deposits on the facial and lingual surfaces of all teeth

REFERENCES

1. Bray, K.K. and Wilder, R.S., *Full-mouth disinfection: A new approach to nonsurgical periodontal therapy*. Access, 1999. **13**(8): p. 57–61.

2. Quirynen, M., C. Mongardini, and D. van Steenberghe, *The effect of a 1-stage full-mouth disinfection on oral malodor and microbial colonization of the tongue in periodontitis. A pilot study*. J Periodontol, 1998. **69**(3): p. 374–382.

3. Quirynen, M., et al., *One stage full- versus partial-mouth disinfection in the treatment of chronic adult or generalized early-onset periodontitis. II. Long-term impact on microbial load*. J Periodontol, 1999. **70**(6): p. 646–656.

4. Quirynen, M., et al., *The role of chlorhexidine in the one-stage full-mouth disinfection treatment of patients with advanced adult periodontitis. Long-term clinical and microbiological observations*. J Clin Periodontol, 2000. **27**(8): p. 578–589.

5. Vandekerckhove, B.N., et al., *Full- versus partial-mouth disinfection in the treatment of periodontal infections. Long-term clinical observations of a pilot study*. J Periodontol, 1996. **67**(12): p. 1251–1259

Problem Identification:
Difficulties in Instrumentation

Module Overview

This module provides solutions for the most common instrumentation problems encountered by beginning clinicians. These problems are divided into seven cate-

Box 19-1. Directions for Use of the Problem Charts

1. First select the category *that most closely describes the problem* that you are having. Turn to the problem chart for that category.

2. The "Cause" column lists possible causes of the problem. In each category, the causes are listed in order from the most likely cause to the least likely cause.

3. Read the "Solution" column for suggestions on how to correct the problem.

Problem Chart 1: Can't See the Treatment Area!

Cause	Solution
Clinician seated in wrong "clock position" for treatment area	Refer to Positioning Summary Sheets
Patient positioned too high	Lower patient chair until the patient's mouth is below your elbow when you hold your arms against your side.
Patient head position	Mandibular arch = chin down
	Maxillary arch = chin up
	Aspect toward = turned slightly away
	Aspect away = turned toward
Not using indirect vision	A combination of direct vision and indirect vision is required in most treatment areas.
Using mirror, but still can't see	Be sure that you are using the mirror to fully retract the tongue or cheek away from the treatment area.
	If you can't see the treatment area in the mirror's reflecting surface, try rotating the mirror head slightly.
	Move mirror farther away from treatment area. For mandibular lingual aspects, move mirror toward midline of the mouth. For maxillary anteriors, move mirror closer to the mandibular arch.
Finger rest too close to surface to be instrumented	Move rest slightly forward in the mouth so that your finger isn't covering up the surface to be instrumented.
Hand is blocking view	Swivel or pivot your hand and arm until you can see the treatment area.

Problem Chart 2: Can't Locate the Calculus!

Cause	Solution
Middle finger not resting on shank	You will receive more tactile information if your finger is resting on the shank.
Using middle finger to hold the instrument (index finger is just "going along for the ride" rather than holding the handle)	Using the middle finger to hold the handle prevents it from detecting vibrations. The thumb and index finger should be across from one another. You should be able to lift your middle finger off of the shank and not drop the instrument.
Using "death grasp" on handle	Relax your fingers and grasp the handle as lightly as possible. Try working on a typodont without wearing gloves—if your fingers are blanched, you are holding the handle too tightly.
Not beginning strokes at the junctional epithelium	Be sure to insert the working-end to the base of the sulcus or pocket before initiating an assessment stroke. If you can't tell where the base is, get an instructor to help you.
Too few strokes, not overlapping strokes	When working subgingivally, use instrumentation zones and overlapping strokes to cover the entire root surface.
Not detecting calculus at line angles on posterior teeth	Position the working-end distal to the line angle with the explorer tip aimed toward the junctional epithelium (but NOT touching the junctional epithelium), and make short horizontal strokes *around* the line angle toward the front of the mouth.
Not detecting calculus at midlines of anterior teeth	Make small, controlled horizontal strokes at the midline on facial or lingual surfaces.

Problem Chart 3: Poor Illumination of Treatment Area!

Cause	Solution
Unit light too close to mouth	Positioning the light close to the patient's mouth creates excessive shadowing and actually makes it harder to see. Light should be an arm's length above or in front of the clinician.
Patient's head positioned incorrectly for treatment area	Mandibular arch = chin down Maxillary arch = chin up Aspect toward = turned slightly away Aspect away = turned toward
Not using mirror for indirect illumination	Use mirror to direct light onto the treatment area.

Problem Chart 4: Can't Adapt Cutting Edge to Tooth Surface!

Cause	Solution
Trying to adapt the middle-third of cutting edge	Usually only the tip-third or toe-third of the cutting edge can be adapted.
Using the wrong cutting edge for the tooth surface	Review the visual guidelines for the cutting edge selection for the instrument in question.
Using the wrong instrument for the task or area of the mouth	Review uses and applications of instrument classifications.
Finger rest too far away	Establish a finger rest near the tooth to be instrumented.
Lower shank not parallel to facial or lingual surface of posterior tooth	On posterior teeth, the lower shank should be parallel to the tooth surface, but not touching it at any point.

Problem Chart 5: Can't Maintain Adaptation!

Cause	Solution
Incorrect grasp; not rolling instrument handle	Sloppy technique with grasp makes it difficult to control the instrument. As you work around the circumference of the tooth, roll the handle between your index finger and thumb to maintain adaptation.
Split grasp	Keep fingers together in the correct grasp position.
Fulcrum too close to or too far away from tooth to be instrumented	Finger rest should be near (but not on) the tooth to be instrumented.
Fulcrum finger lifts off of the tooth as stroke is made	Fulcrum finger should be maintained in a straight, upright position throughout the stroke (acting as a support beam). Press down against the tooth with your fulcrum finger so finger can act as a brake to stop the stroke.
Tilting the instrument face away from the tooth surface during stroke (so lateral surface or back of working-end contacts tooth)	Maintain correct face-to-tooth surface angulation as you use a pull stroke to move the working-end in a coronal direction. Handle position should stay parallel to the tooth surface as you make strokes (it should not tilt away from the tooth surface).
Not pivoting on finger rest	On posterior teeth, pivot at line angles to maintain adaptation. In anterior sextants, as you work toward yourself, your hand and arm should gradually pivot closer to your body.

Problem Chart 6: Uncontrolled or Weak Calculus Removal Stroke!

Cause	Solution
Instrument handle is supported solely by index finger and thumb	Handle should rest against the index finger or hand for support.
Split grasp—fingers not in contact	Keep fingers together in correct grasp position for control of strokes.
"Death grip" on handle	Use a firm grasp, but not a choking grasp.
Fulcrum finger lifts off of the tooth as stroke is made	Press down against the tooth with your fulcrum finger so finger can act as a brake to stop the stroke.
Fulcrum finger is relaxed and bent	Fulcrum finger should be straight and apply pressure against rest point on tooth (acting as a support beam).
Stroke not stabilized; no lateral pressure with cutting edge against tooth surface	During a work stroke, the index finger and thumb should apply equal pressure against the instrument handle, and the fulcrum finger applies pressure against the tooth surface.
Wrist and arm not in neutral position	Assess patient position, clinician position, and arm position.
Using a push-pull stroke	Apply lateral pressure only with the pull stroke, away from the junctional epithelium.
Working too rapidly, strokes too fast	Pause briefly after each stroke. Make slow, controlled strokes.
On posterior teeth, lower shank not parallel—shank rocks on height of contour	On posterior teeth, the lower shank should be parallel to the facial or lingual surface but not touching it at any point.

Problem Chart 7A: Missed Calculus Deposits!
Deposits Missed at Midlines of Anterior Teeth

Cause	Solution
Not using horizontal strokes at midline of facial or lingual surface	Position the curet to the side of the midline with the toe aiming toward the junctional epithelium (but not touching the junctional epithelium). Make a series of short controlled horizontal strokes.
Not overlapping vertical strokes at midline	Position the working-end so that strokes overlap for surfaces toward and away.
Not using a specialized instrument when indicated	Use an area-specific curet with a miniature working-end at midlines.

Problem Chart 7B: Missed Calculus Deposits!
Deposits Missed at Line Angles of Posterior Teeth

Cause	Solution
Not using horizontal strokes at the line angles	Position the curet distal to the line angle with the toe aiming toward the junctional epithelium (but not touching the junctional epithelium). Make a series of short strokes around the line angle.
Not rolling handle to maintain adaptation to line angle	As you work around a line angle, it is necessary to roll the instrument handle between the index finger and thumb to maintain adaptation.

Problem Chart 7C: Missed Calculus Deposits!
Deposits Missed on Proximal Surfaces

Cause	Solution
Not using indirect vision	Beginning clinicians often have trouble learning to use indirect vision; therefore, try to view all surfaces directly. Use of indirect vision is vital for proximal surfaces.
Not rotating reflecting surface to view proximal surfaces	This problem is common on lingual surfaces of anterior teeth. First, angle the mirror to view the surfaces toward you, and then turn the mirror to view the surfaces away from you.
Strokes not extended under contact area	Instrument at least one-half of a proximal surface from the facial and lingual aspects. Place curet between the papilla and the tooth surface. Adapt the working-end to the tooth surface and insert it into the junctional epithelium. (Do not "trace" papilla with working-end.)
Not rolling handle to maintain adaptation	As you work around a line angle and onto the proximal surface, make small, continuous adjustments in adaptation by rolling the handle.
Working-end not aimed toward surface to be instrumented	For distal surfaces of posterior teeth, the toe should aim toward the back of the mouth. Don't try to "back the working-end" onto the distal surface.

Instrument Sharpening

Module Overview

This module discusses the importance and advantages of using sharp instruments. Topics include methods for evaluating sharpness and how to reestablish sharp cutting edges without altering the original design characteristics of the working-end. Skill practice sections provide experience in positioning the instrument and stone. Step-by-step instructions are provided in the moving stone and moving instrument techniques for sharpening sickle scalers, universal curets, and area-specific curets.

Module Outline

Key Terms

Sharp cutting edge	Sharpening test stick	Straight cutting edge
Pointed junction	Sharpening stones	Curved cutting edge
Dull cutting edge	Lubricant	Rotating the stone
Rounded surface	Limited use-life	Recontouring
Visual evaluation	Position of the face	Metal burs
Tactile evaluation	Stone angulation	Wire edge

Learning Objectives

1. State the goal of instrument sharpening and the advantages of sharp instruments.

2. Define sharp cutting edge and dull cutting edge.

3. Demonstrate two methods of evaluating sharpness.

4. Describe important design characteristics to be maintained when sickle scalers and universal and area-specific curets are sharpened.

5. Describe common sharpening errors.

6. Demonstrate correct sharpening technique with sickle scalers and universal and area-specific curets to produce a sharp cutting edge by removing a minimum amount of metal and maintaining the original design characteristics.

7. Describe the types of sharpening stones and explain care of stones.

8. Value sharp instruments and the practice of sharpening at the first sign of dullness.

Section I
Introduction to Sharpening Concepts

ADVANTAGES OF SHARP INSTRUMENTS

Effective periodontal debridement with hand-activated instruments is possible only with properly maintained sharp cutting edges. New periodontal instruments have precise, sharp cutting edges and working-ends that have been carefully designed to facilitate calculus removal. *It is impossible to overemphasize the importance of mastering the techniques for instrument sharpening.* Instrument sharpening is a skill needed on a daily basis. Effective periodontal debridement cannot be achieved with dull periodontal instruments.

Calculus removal involves the use of firm lateral pressure against the tooth surface. As an instrument is used, metal is worn away from the working-end, resulting in a dull rounded surface. A sharp cutting edge allows:

1. **Easier calculus removal**
   a. A sharp cutting edge "bites into" the calculus deposit, removing it in an efficient manner.
   b. A dull cutting edge slides over the calculus deposit and may burnish it.
2. **Improved stroke control**
   a. A dull cutting edge must be pressed with greater force against the tooth surface to achieve calculus removal.
   b. Excessive force used with a dull cutting edge increases the likelihood of losing control of the stroke. The clinician is more likely to slip or sustain an instrument stick when using a dull instrument.
3. **Reduced number of strokes**
   a. It takes fewer strokes to remove a calculus deposit with a sharp cutting edge.
   b. Sharp instruments reduce the overall treatment time.
4. **Increased patient comfort and satisfaction**
   a. More lateral pressure must be exerted against the tooth when using a dull instrument. A sharp instrument allows the clinician to use less force; this makes the instrumentation process more comfortable for the patient.
   b. A sharp cutting edge permits the clinician to make fewer and better-controlled instrument strokes. Therefore, sharp instruments decrease the time required for calculus removal. Patients appreciate shorter appointments.
5. **Reduced clinician fatigue**
   a. A dull cutting edge requires greater stroke pressure and more instrumentation strokes for calculus removal.
   b. The excessive lateral pressure and extra number of strokes needed with a dull instrument places unnecessary strain on the clinician's musculoskeletal system.

GOAL OF INSTRUMENT SHARPENING

The goal of instrument sharpening is to restore a fine sharp cutting edge to a dull instrument. To be successful, a sharpening technique should remove a minimum amount of metal from the instrument and maintain the original design characteristics of the working-end.

THE CUTTING EDGE

Correct sharpening technique requires knowledge of the design characteristics of sickle scalers and curets. It is important to understand the cross-sectional design of sickle scalers and curets and to recognize that the relationship of the face to the lateral surface is the same for all these instruments. On all sickle scalers and curets, a sharp cutting edge is a fine line formed by the pointed junction of the instrument face and lateral surface. A dull cutting edge results when metal is worn away from the cutting edge until the junction between the face and the lateral surface becomes a rounded surface rather than a fine line.

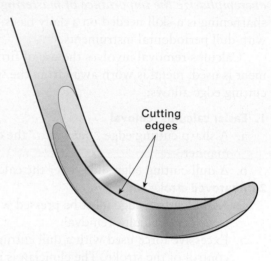

The Sharp Cutting Edge. A sharp cutting edge is a line. It has length, but no width.

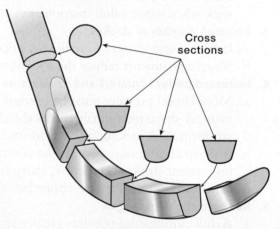

Working-End Cross Section. The key to understanding the cutting edge of an instrument is the ability to visualize the working-end in cross section.

A cutting edge is formed by the junction of the instrument face and the lateral surface.

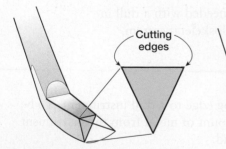
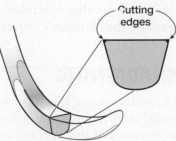
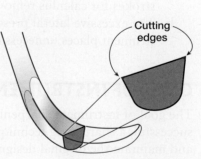

Cross Section. For all sickle scalers and curets, a cutting edge is formed by the junction of the instrument face and lateral surface.

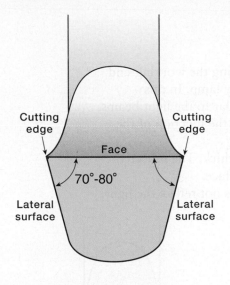

The Cutting Edge. The internal angle formed by the junction of the face and the lateral surface of a universal curet is between 70° and 80°.

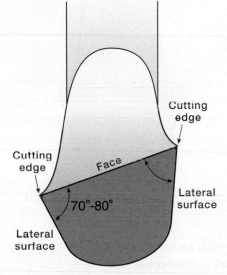

The Cutting Edge. The relationship of the face to the lower shank is unique for area-specific curets. Just as for a universal curet, however, the internal angle formed by the junction of the face and the lateral surface of an area-specific curet is between 70° and 80°.

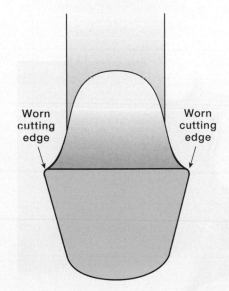

The Dull Cutting Edge. With use against the tooth surface, metal is worn away from the cutting edge until it becomes a *rounded surface* instead of a fine line.

A dull cutting edge is a rounded junction between the instrument face and the lateral surface.

EVALUATING SHARPNESS

A dull cutting edge can be detected by visual or tactile evaluation.

1. **Visual evaluation.** A cutting edge is evaluated visually by holding the working-end under a light source, such as the dental light or a high-intensity lamp. In this method, the instrument face is held approximately perpendicular to the light beams. The working-end is slowly rotated while the clinician looks at the junction of the face and the lateral surface.
   a. A dull cutting edge reflects light because it is rounded and thick. The reflected light appears as a bright line running along the edge of the face.
   b. A sharp cutting edge is a line—with no thickness—and does not reflect the light.

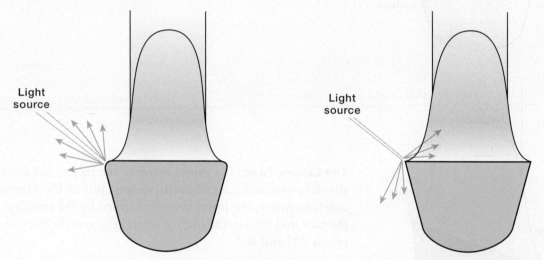

Light source   Light source

Visual Detection. The rounded surface of a dull cutting edge reflects light. A sharp cutting edge has no thickness and therefore does not reflect light.

2. **Tactile evaluation.** Another method of evaluating sharpness is with tactile means by testing the cutting edge against a plastic or acrylic rod known as a sharpening test stick.
   a. A dull cutting edge slides over the surface of the stick.
   b. A sharp cutting edge scratches the surface of the test stick.

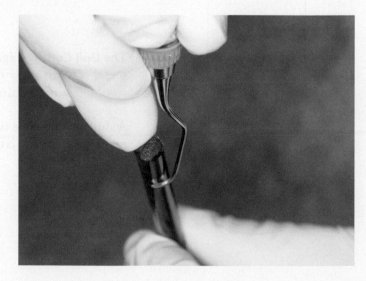

Sharpening Test Stick. Sharpness can be evaluated using a test stick. A test stick is a cylindrical rod made of plastic or acrylic. Sharpening test sticks are autoclavable.

Section 2
Planning for Instrument Maintenance

WHEN TO SHARPEN

Sickle scalers, curets, and periodontal files should be sharpened at the *first sign of dullness.*

1. **Sharpening during treatment**
   a. Depending on the extent of calculus deposits present, instruments may have to be sharpened during treatment.
   b. Sharpening stones should be a part of each instrument cassette so that sterile sharpening stones are always available. If instrument cassette tray setups are not used, sharpening stones should be kept in sealed sterilized packages until needed.
2. **Sharpening immediately after treatment**
   a. Each sickle scaler or curet used during the appointment should be sharpened.
   b. Instruments that were not used do not need to be sharpened; modern stainless steel instruments are not dulled by autoclaving.

TABLE 20-1. Frequency of Sharpening	
Immediate Sharpening	**Infrequent Sharpening**
Maintained cutting edges need only a few light sharpening strokes and minor recontouring	Dull, neglected cutting edges require many firm sharpening strokes and extensive recontouring
Calculus removal is easier for both clinician and patient	Calculus removal is difficult and tiring for both clinician and patient
Instruments have a long use-life	Instruments have a short use-life

WORK AREA AND EQUIPMENT

A sharpening work area must be a part of every treatment room so that debridement instruments can be sharpened at the first sign of dullness. The right work area is important in ensuring an efficient and safe sharpening procedure.

1. A stable work surface is essential for good sharpening technique. A countertop in the treatment room makes a good surface. A bracket table or other unstable surface is not appropriate for the sharpening procedure.
2. The work area should be disinfected and covered with a barrier such as plastic wrap or an impervious-backed paper. The barrier should cover both the top and the edge of the countertop.
3. A good light source, such as the dental unit light or a high-intensity lamp, should illuminate the sharpening work area.
4. All equipment required for sharpening should be sterile and ready for use in the treatment room (Box 20-1).

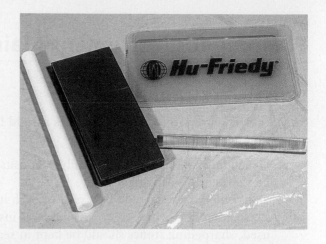

Sharpening Kit. The supplies for sharpening include a rectangular sharpening stone, cylindrical sharpening stone, text stick, and a magnifying lens.

Synthetic sharpening stones are recommended because they require only water for lubrication.

Box 20-1. Sharpening Equipment

Rectangular and cylindrical sharpening stones
Sharpening test stick
Magnifying lens or loupes
Gauze
Lubricant
Personal protective equipment: protective eyewear, gloves, and mask

SHARPENING STONES

Sharpening stones are made of abrasive particles that are harder than the metal of the instruments to be sharpened (Table 20-2). Sharpening stones may be made from natural stone or from synthetic, man-made materials. The grain—or abrasiveness—is an important characteristic of sharpening stones. Fine-grain stones—400 grit or higher—produce significantly sharper cutting edges that stay sharper longer.

TABLE 20-2. Types of Sharpening Stones

Stone Type	Grain	Use	Lubrication
Composition synthetic stones	Coarse	Extensive reshaping of improperly sharpened or extremely dull, worn cutting edges	Water
India synthetic stones	Medium	Reshaping of dull cutting edges	Water or oil
Arkansas natural stones	Fine	Routine sharpening of well-maintained cutting edges Finishing after use of coarse or medium grain stones	Oil
Ceramic synthetic stones	Fine	Routine sharpening of well-maintained cutting edges Finishing after use of coarse or medium grain stones	Water

LUBRICATION AND CARE OF STONES

1. Lubrication

a. A lubricant is a substance such as water or oil, which is applied to the surface of a sharpening stone to reduce friction between the stone and the instrument.

b. Lubrication helps to prevent the metal shavings from sticking to the surface of the stone. These metal shavings can become embedded in the surface of the sharpening stone and reduce its effectiveness.

c. Lubrication reduces frictional heat between the metal instrument and the stone. Stones that are used without lubrication need to be replaced more frequently than stones used with lubricant.

d. A synthetic stone that can be lubricated with water is recommended for use when sharpening instruments during patient treatment.

e. A natural stone that must be lubricated with oil is not recommended for use when sharpening during patient treatment because the oil cannot be effectively sterilized.

2. Care

a. The sharpening stone should be cleaned in an ultrasonic cleaner or scrubbed with a brush and hot water to remove metal particles from the surface of the stone.

b. After cleaning, the stone should be dried on a paper towel and placed in an autoclave bag or on an instrument cassette to be sterilized.

INSTRUMENT REPLACEMENT

It is important to recognize that sickle scalers and curets have a limited use-life and must eventually be discarded. Frequent sharpening that preserves the working-end design combined with care during handling and sterilization prolongs an instrument's use-life. Eventually, however, every instrument needs to be replaced. When a working-end becomes thin from use and sharpening, the instrument should be discarded. One research study reports that a 20 percent reduction in size results in a significant reduction in working-end strength. [1]

BROKEN INSTRUMENT TIPS

The instrument's working-ends should be carefully inspected under magnification after each use.

1. Instruments with thin working-ends should be discarded, whereas improperly sharpened working-ends should be resharpened or discarded.

   a. Thin or improperly sharpened working-ends can break when lateral pressure is applied against the tooth surface.

   b. Frequent sharpening, correct sharpening technique, and discarding of instruments with thin or poorly sharpened working-ends minimizes the possibility of a broken tip.

2. Breaking a working-end during instrumentation creates a serious problem.

   a. If not removed, the metal fragment can cause tissue inflammation and abscess formation.

   b. If the tip is aspirated (inhaled) into the lungs, a serious infection is likely to develop.

   c. If swallowed, the tip probably will pass harmlessly through the gastrointestinal system.

   d. If the tip cannot be located in the mouth, the patient should be referred for a chest x-ray to ensure that the tip has not been aspirated into a lung.

   e. Refer to Box 20-2 for the procedure for finding and retrieving a broken instrument tip.

Box 20-2. Retrieving a Broken Instrument Tip

1. Remain calm and do not alarm the patient by informing him or her of the problem.

2. Maintain retraction and patient head position.
   a. Do NOT use compressed air to attempt to locate the metal fragment. Compressed air could move the metal fragment around the mouth or drive it into the soft tissues.
   b. Do NOT use suction to attempt to remove the metal fragment. Suction could remove the tip but also eliminates the ability to confirm that the metal fragment has been removed.

3. Examine the location where the fracture occurred, the mucobuccal fold, and the floor of the mouth. If the metal fragment is located on the surface of the tissue, blot the area with a gauze square. The metal fragment will catch in the gauze material for easy removal.

4. If the metal fragment cannot be located on the outer surfaces of the tissues, examine the sulci or pockets in the area.
   a. Insert a curet into the sulcus at the distofacial or distolingual line angle, and move slowly forward until the fragment is located.
   b. Once located, use the curet like a scoop to remove the tip from beneath the gingival margin, and catch it with a gauze square.

5. If the metal fragment cannot be located, take a periapical radiograph of the area. If located, use a curet as described above to remove the tip. If this fails, refer the patient to a periodontist for surgical removal of the metal fragment.

6. If the metal fragment still cannot be located in the mouth, the patient should be referred for a chest x-ray to ensure that the tip has not been aspirated into a lung. After referral, it is important to follow up with the patient to confirm that a chest x-ray was obtained.

Section 3
Reestablishing Sharpness

SHARPENING METHODS

As the working-end is used against the tooth surface, over time, the metal of the cutting edge is worn away to form a rounded surface. Two sharpening methods exist for reestablishing the pointed junction of the face and lateral surfaces (Table 20-3).

1. The first method is to *grind metal from the face* of the instrument. **This method is not recommended because it results in a thin, weak working-end that could easily break during calculus removal.**
2. The second method is to *grind metal from the lateral surfaces* of the working-end. Removing metal from the lateral surfaces is the recommended sharpening method because it restores a sharp cutting edge while preserving the strength of the working-end.

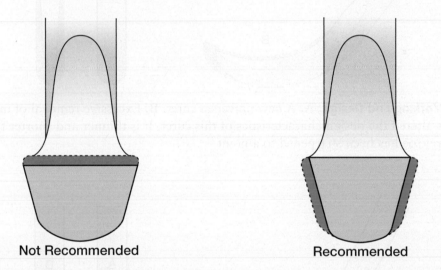

Not Recommended   Recommended

TABLE 20-3.	Comparison of Sharpening Methods	
	Metal Removed From Face	**Metal Removed From Side**
Advantages	Sharpens both cutting edges at one time	Preserves strength of instrument
		Provides longest instrument use-life
Disadvantages	Decreases strength of the instrument	Requires knowledge of the correct angulation for sharpening
	Shortens instrument use-life	

COMMON SHARPENING ERRORS

A clinician who is not knowledgeable about working-end design can radically alter an instrument's design characteristics with incorrect sharpening technique. An incorrectly sharpened instrument will be ineffective for calculus removal and may fracture easily.

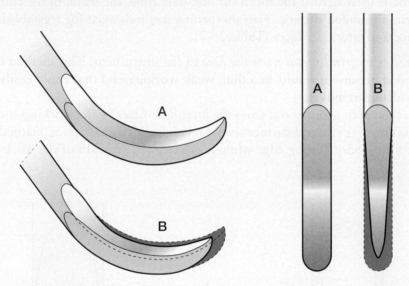

Alteration of Working-End Design. A. A new universal curet. **B.** Excessive removal of metal during sharpening has altered the design characteristics of this curet. It is thinner and shorter than the original and the curet toe has been sharpened to a point.

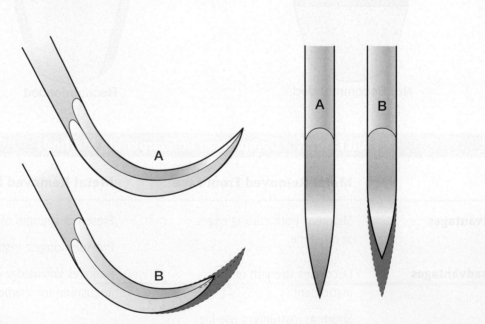

Unnecessary Metal Removal. A. A new sickle scaler. **B.** The working-end of this scaler has been excessively shortened in length by sharpening.

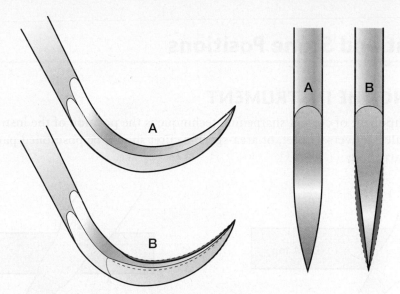

Altered Shape. A. A new sickle scaler. **B.** Only the tip- and middle-thirds of this cutting edge were sharpened, thus destroying the shape of the working-end. The entire length of the cutting edge should be sharpened even if only a portion of the edge is dull. In addition, incorrect sharpening technique resulted in straight cutting edges, whereas the cutting edges on the original sickle were curved (flame-shaped).

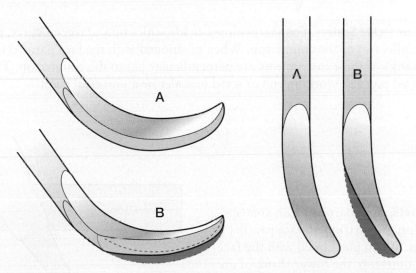

Flattened Cutting Edge. A. A new area-specific curet with curved cutting edges. **B.** The *nonworking* cutting edge of this area-specific curet was sharpened by mistake; only the lower cutting edge should be sharpened. In addition, incorrect sharpening technique created a straight lateral surface and a pointed tip.

Section 4
Instrument and Stone Positions

POSITIONING THE INSTRUMENT

An important component of correct sharpening technique is the **position of the instrument face.** The face of a sickle scaler, universal curet, or area-specific curet should be positioned parallel to the countertop for sharpening.

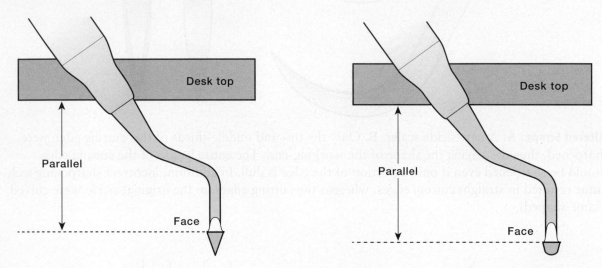

Universal Curets or Sickle Scalers. For sharpening a sickle scaler or a universal curet, position the instrument face parallel (=) to the countertop. When positioned with the face parallel to the countertop, the lower shanks of these instruments are perpendicular (⊥) to the countertop. Two cutting edges are sharpened on each working-end of a sickle scaler or a universal curet.

Area-Specific Curets. For sharpening an area-specific curet, position the instrument face parallel (=) to the countertop. When positioned with the face parallel to the countertop, the lower shank of an area-specific curet is NOT perpendicular to the countertop. One cutting edge, the working cutting edge, is sharpened on each area-specific curet.

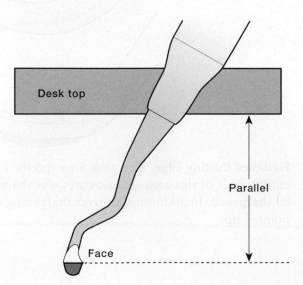

Visualize for Easier Instrument Positioning. A visualization technique for improved instrument positioning is to imagine that the working-end is a spoon filled with red, sticky cough syrup. The spoon must be held level, or the red syrup will spill. Likewise, correct sharpening technique calls for the instrument face to be level with the countertop.

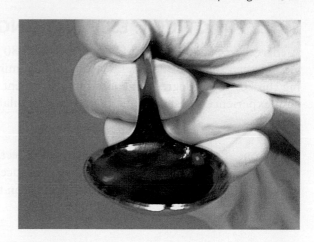

Box 20-3. Principle for Positioning the Instrument

Position the working-end of a sickle scaler, universal curet, or area-specific curet so that the **face** is **parallel (=) to the countertop**.

POSITIONING THE SHARPENING STONE

A sharp cutting edge is restored by removing metal from the lateral surface while maintaining the 70° to 80° internal junction between the face and lateral surface.

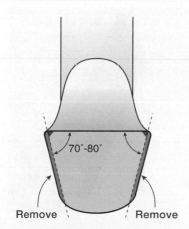

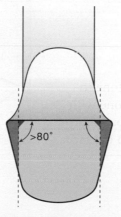

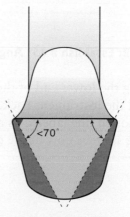

Correct Angulation. The angle between the face and lateral surface is between 70° and 80°.

Angulation Greater than 80°. This working-end would require the use of heavy lateral pressure and would be difficult to adapt.

Angulation Less than 70°. This weakened working-end would fracture easily; the cutting edge will dull very easily.

SKILL PRACTICE 1: ESTABLISHING CORRECT STONE ANGULATION

A correct stone angulation of between 70 and 80 degrees is needed to recreate the ideal pointed angle between the face and lateral surfaces. Beginning clinicians often experience difficulty in visualizing the 70- to 80-degree angle used in instrument sharpening. Follow the directions on this page to gain experience in establishing the correct angulation between the sharpening stone and the instrument face.

Directions. For this Skill Practice, you need a rectangular sharpening stone and the illustrations on the next page. Use the first illustration to practice adapting the stone to the right cutting edge of a universal curet. Next, use the second illustration to practice adapting to the left cutting edge.

Step 1: Establish a 90° Angle.

Place your sharpening stone on the dotted line labeled as a 90° angle. Your sharpening stone is now positioned at a 90° angle to the instrument face.

This position gives you a visual starting point from which to establish the correct angulation.

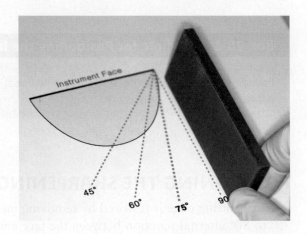

Step 2: Establish a 75° Angle.

Swing the lower end of the sharpening stone toward the instrument back. Align your stone with the dotted line labeled as a 75° angle. Your sharpening stone is now at the proper angle to the face.

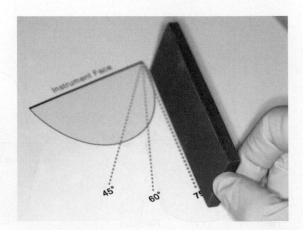

Instrument Face

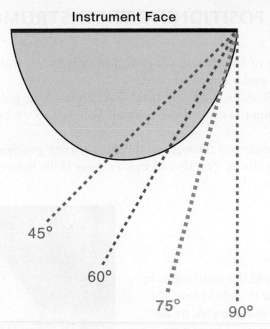

45°

60°

75°

90°

Angle for Right Cutting Edge

Instrument Face

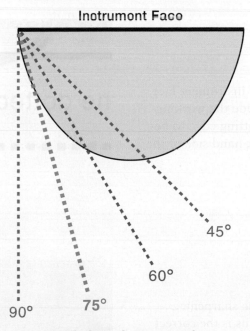

45°

60°

75°

90°

Angle for Left Cutting Edge

SKILL PRACTICE 2: POSITIONING THE INSTRUMENT AND STONE

Directions:

1. Equipment: a photocopy of Sharpening Guide R and Sharpening Guide L from Section 6 of this module and a universal curet.
2. Fold Sharpening Guide R along the heavy black line. Position the guide so that the heavy black line falls along the edge of the counter. Secure it to the counter with masking tape.
3. This Skill Practice will guide you through establishing correct positioning of the instrument and sharpening stone. You should master these skills before continuing with this module.

4. **Grasp the Instrument.** Hold the instrument in your *left hand* using your thumb against the handle, as shown in this photograph, to stabilize the instrument. Rest your hand on a stable surface.

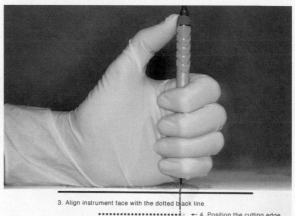

3. Align instrument face with the dotted black line.

← 4. Position the cutting edge to be sharpened here.

5. **Position the Face.** Align the instrument face with the fine dotted line. Slide the working-end to the right until the cutting edge to be sharpened is at the far right-hand side of the dotted line.

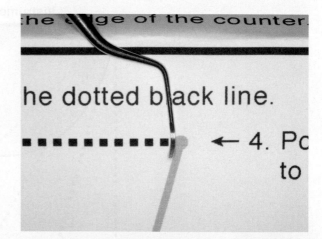

6. **Position the Stone.** Align the sharpening stone with the solid line. This is the correct angulation for sharpening sickle scalers, universal curets, and area-specific curets.

Use Sharpening Guide L to practice positioning the instrument face and sharpening stone for sharpening the left cutting edge.

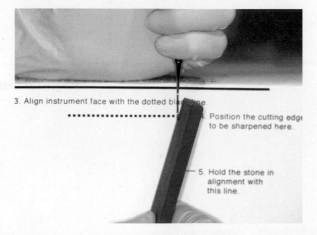

3. Align instrument face with the dotted black line.

Position the cutting edge to be sharpened here.

5. Hold the stone in alignment with this line.

Section 5
Preserving Instrument Design

Preserving the original design characteristics of the working-end is an essential goal of instrument sharpening. In addition to the 70- to 80-degree internal angle of the working-end, the design of the lateral surfaces, back, toe, and tip must be maintained.

THE LATERAL SURFACES

Because some cutting edges are curved, *it is best to make a habit of sharpening the cutting edges of any instrument in sections.* Sharpening the cutting edges in sections is a strategy that preserves the design characteristics of any working-end, regardless of whether it has straight or curved cutting edges. If you make a habit of consistently sharpening the cutting edge in sections, you will never destroy a curved cutting edge by flattening the edge. On the other hand, sharpening a straight cutting edge in sections still results in a straight cutting edge.

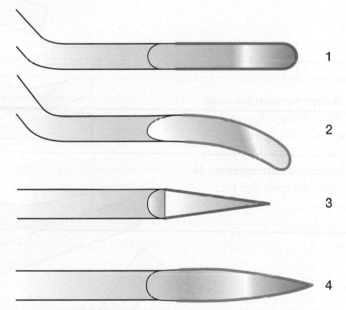

Straight Versus Curved Cutting Edges. The working-end may have straight cutting edges or curved cutting edges.

This design feature refers to the lateral surfaces being either straight or curved in design—not to whether the instrument has a rounded toe or pointed tip. To determine whether the cutting edges are straight or curved, look down at the working-end from a bird's eye view.

1. **Instrument 1** is a universal curet with straight, parallel cutting edges.
2. **Instrument 2** is an area-specific curet with curved working and nonworking cutting edges.
3. **Instrument 3** is a sickle scaler with straight cutting edges.
4. **Instrument 4** is a sickle scaler with curved cutting edges. This type of sickle scaler often is referred to as a flame-shaped sickle scaler.

Cutting Edge Sections. Divide the cutting edge into three imaginary sections for sharpening.

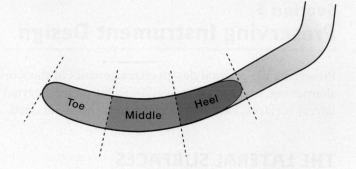

Sharpen in Sections. Adapt the cutting edge to only a portion of the cutting edge at a time to maintain a curved cutting edge. Sharpen the (1) heel-third, (2) middle-third, and (3) toe or tip-third of the cutting edge. If the instrument is a curet, sharpen the toe.

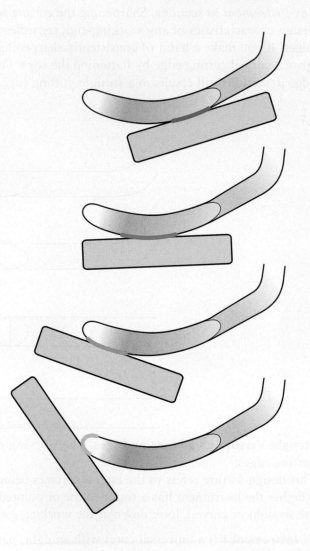

SKILL PRACTICE 3: ROTATING THE STONE TO SHARPEN IN SECTIONS

After sharpening the heel-third of the cutting edge, a technique of rotating the stone is used to adapt to the middle-third. After sharpening the middle-third, the stone is rotated again to adapt to the toe- or tip-third of the cutting edge. For this technique, the stone is rotated away from the palm of the hand *while maintaining correct angulation of the stone to the instrument face.*

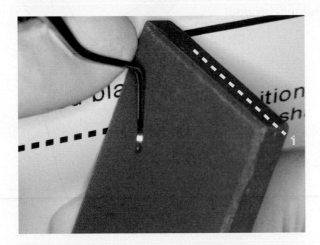

Step 1—Sharpen the Heel-Third. Begin by adapting the stone to the heel-third of the cutting edge. Note that the middle and toe-thirds of the cutting edge are not in contact with the sharpening stone. Use a Sharpening Guide to establish a 75-degree angle with the sharpening stone.

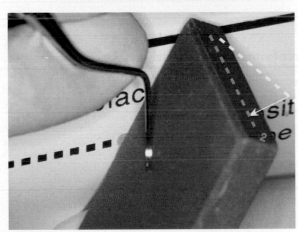

Step 2—Sharpen the Middle-Third. While maintaining correct angulation, rotate the stone away from the palm of your hand slightly. The stone is now positioned to sharpen the middle-third of the cutting edge.

- The *yellow dotted line* on the photograph indicates the position of the sharpening stone when sharpening the *heel-third.*
- The stone is rotated away from the palm of the hand to the position indicated by the *orange dotted line* for sharpening the *middle-third.*

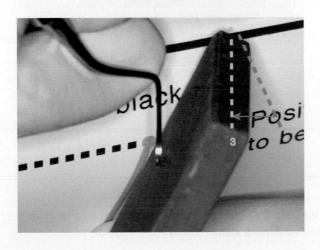

Step 3—Sharpen the Toe-Third. Rotate the stone away from the palm of your hand again. Sharpen the toe-third of the cutting edge.

- The *green dotted line* on the photograph indicates the position of the sharpening stone when sharpening the *toe-third.*

ROUNDED BACKS AND TOES

The rounded toes and backs of curets must be recontoured. Recontouring is the process of removing metal from the back and toe to restore the curved surfaces of a curet.

Recontouring the Toe. With a curet, sharpening continues around the toe to maintain the rounded contour.

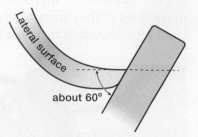

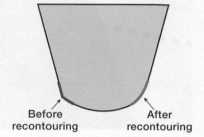

Recontouring the Back. The back of a curet must be recontoured slightly to maintain a smooth rounded back.

Before recontouring   After recontouring

METAL BURS

Sharpening can produce minute **metal burs** that project from the cutting edge.

1. A cutting edge with metal burs is sometimes termed a wire edge because the metal burs are like tiny wire projections. The use of a wire edge on the root surfaces can result in gouging of the cementum.
2. The metal burs are impossible to see with the naked eye but can be seen using magnification.
3. Burs can be avoided by finishing with a down stroke toward the cutting edge.
4. Burs can easily be seen under magnification and removed using a light stroke with a cylindrical sharpening stone.

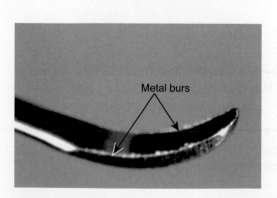

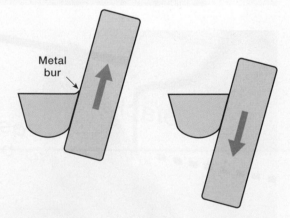

Metal Burs. Sharpening can produce minute metal burs that project from the cutting edge. Burs can be prevented by finishing with a down stroke of the sharpening stone toward the cutting edge.

Section 6
Sharpening Guides

SHARPENING GUIDES R AND L

Directions: Photocopy Sharpening Guide R and Sharpening Guide L and place them back-to-back in a single plastic page protector or have them laminated. Another way to use a photocopied sharpening guide is to tape it to the countertop and cover it with a piece of plastic wrap.

Use Sharpening Guide R for:

- The right cutting edge of a universal curet or sickle scaler
- For ODD-numbered Gracey curets, such as a G11 and G13

Sharpening Guide - R

1. Fold this page in half along the solid black line.
2. Place the folded edge on a countertop so that the black line is aligned along the edge of the counter.

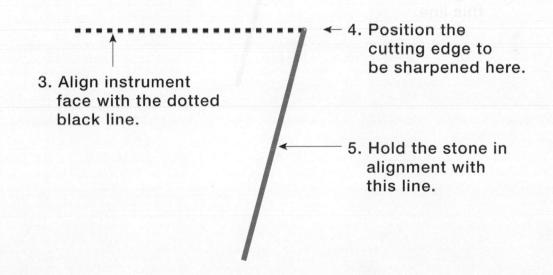

4. Position the cutting edge to be sharpened here.

3. Align instrument face with the dotted black line.

5. Hold the stone in alignment with this line.

Use **Sharpening Guide L** for:

- The left cutting edge of a universal curet or sickle scaler
- For EVEN-numbered Gracey curets, such as a G12 and G14

Sharpening Guide - L

1. Fold this page in half along the solid black line.
2. Place the folded edge on a countertop so that the black line is aligned along the edge of the counter.

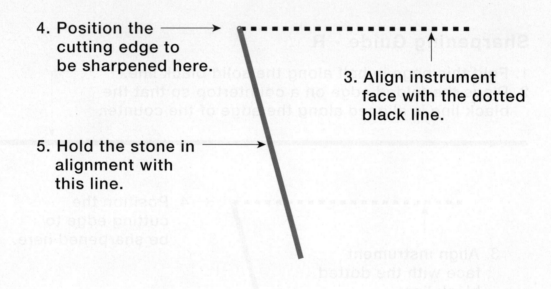

4. Position the cutting edge to be sharpened here.

3. Align instrument face with the dotted black line.

5. Hold the stone in alignment with this line.

Section 7
Moving Stone Technique

SHARPENING UNIVERSAL CURETS

As the name suggests, the moving stone technique is a method of removing metal from the working-end by moving a sharpening stone over the working-end of a stabilized instrument.

1. Cover the top and front surfaces of the counter with a barrier such as plastic wrap. Secure the barrier to the countertop with autoclave or masking tape.
2. Place Sharpening Guide R on the counter so that the heavy black line falls along the edge of the counter. Secure the guide to the countertop with autoclave or masking tape. Begin by sharpening the *right cutting edge of a universal curet.*

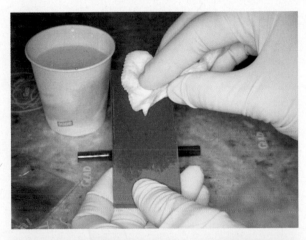

3. **Lubricate the stone.** If the stone is synthetic, lubricate it on both sides with a few drops of water. Synthetic stones are recommended for sharpening during treatment. If the stone is natural, lubricate it on both sides with a few drops of oil.

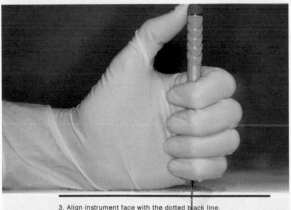

3. Align instrument face with the dotted black line.
··············· ← 4. Position the cutting e

4. **Grasp the instrument.** Grasp the instrument handle in the palm of your *left hand*. Rest your hand and arm on the countertop. Stabilize the instrument handle with your thumb.

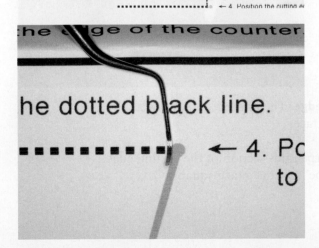

the edge of the counter.

he dotted black line.

■ ■ ■ ■ ■ ■ ■ ■ ■ ■ ← 4. Po
to

5. **Position the instrument face.** Align the instrument face with the dotted line on the sharpening guide. This positions the working-end so that the face is parallel (=) to the countertop.

Keeping the face aligned with the dotted line, slide your left hand over until the cutting edge to be sharpened is positioned *at the far right-hand side* of the dotted line.

6. **Grasp the sharpening stone with your right hand.** Hold the stone on the edges so that your fingers do not get in the way when sharpening.

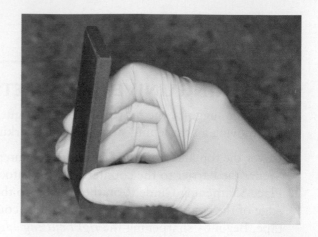

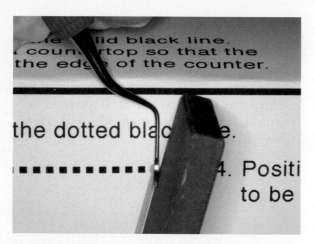

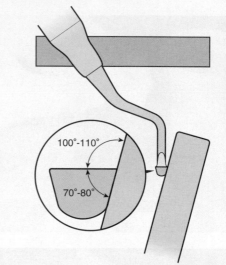

7. **Position the sharpening stone.** Align the sharpening stone with the solid line. This is the correct angulation for sharpening.

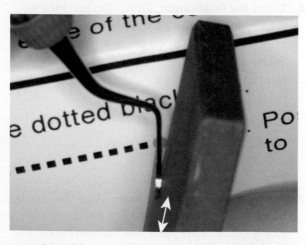

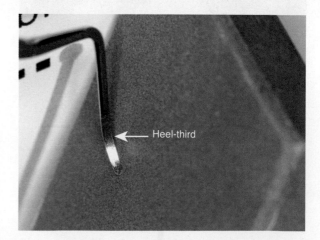

Heel-third

8. **Adapt the stone to the heel-third of the cutting edge.** The photographs show a bird's-eye view looking down at the instrument face.

Make several short up and down strokes to sharpen this section of the cutting edge. If a metal sludge forms on the working-end, wipe it with a gauze square.

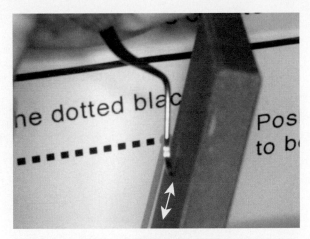

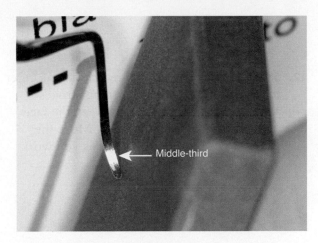

Middle-third

9. **Sharpen the middle-third of the cutting edge.** When the heel section is sharp, rotate the stone so that it is in contact with the middle-third of the cutting edge. Make several short up- and-down strokes to sharpen this section of the cutting edge.

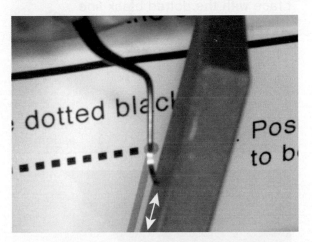

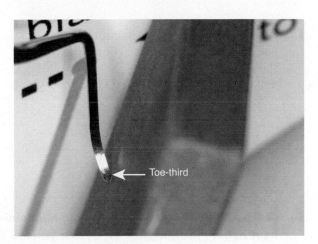

Toe-third

10. **Sharpen the toe-third of the cutting edge.** Rotate the stone so that it is in contact with the toe-third of the cutting edge. Make several short up-and-down strokes to sharpen this section of the cutting edge.

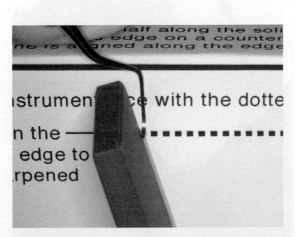

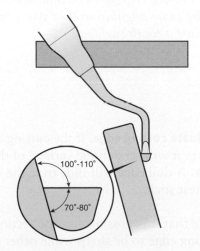

100°-110°

70°-80°

11. **Sharpen the left cutting edge on the same working-end.** Use **Sharpening Guide L.** Hold the instrument in your right hand and the stone in your left hand.

12. **Sharpen the curet toe.** To recontour the curet toe, make a series of sharpening strokes around the toe. Be careful to keep the face parallel (=) to the countertop. Move the stone in up-and-down strokes as you work your way around the toe.

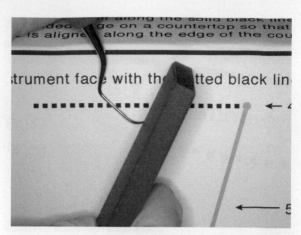

13. **Recontour the back.** To recontour the back, use semicircular strokes around the back of the curet.

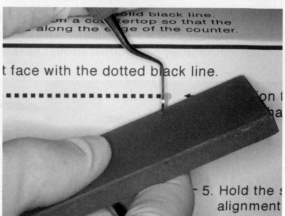

14. **Grasp a sharpening test stick in your nondominant hand.** Position the stick so that you are looking down on the top. Adapt the cutting edge at a 70- to 80-degree angle to the stick.

    The cutting edge must be adapted to the stick at the same angulation that you would use against a tooth surface.

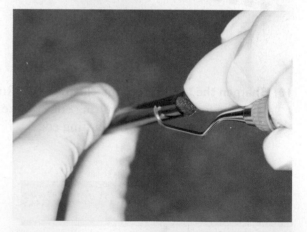

15. **Evaluate cutting edge.** If the cutting edge is sharp, it will scratch the surface of the test stick. A dull edge will slide over the surface of the test stick.

    Note that it is possible for one section of the cutting edge to be sharp while other sections are dull.

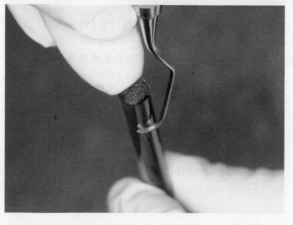

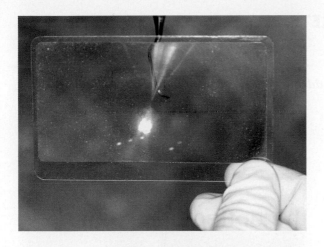

16. **Check under magnification.** Use a magnifying glass or loops to examine the working-end. Evaluate the working-end to ensure that its original design has been preserved, and check the cutting edge for the presence of metal burs.

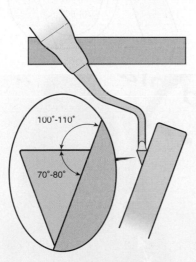

17. **Use a cylindrical stone for bur removal.** If metal burs are present, remove them with a cylindrical stone using gentle sharpening strokes on the instrument face.

SHARPENING SICKLE SCALERS

Sickle scalers are sharpened in the same manner as universal curets. Sickle scalers usually have pointed tips and backs; therefore, no recontouring of the toe or back is required. Some sickle scalers have rounded backs; in this case, the back would need to be recontoured.

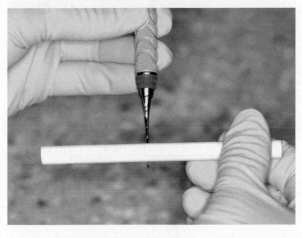

Instrument and Stone Placement. Position of the instrument face and sharpening stone when sharpening a sickle scaler is identical to that used for a universal curet.

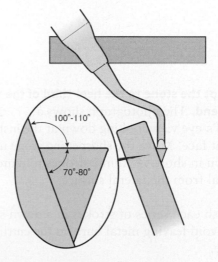

SHARPENING AREA-SPECIFIC CURETS

Directions:

1. Prepare the sharpening work area.
2. Use Sharpening Guide R when sharpening an *odd-numbered area-specific curet,* such as a Gracey 11.

3. **Position the instrument face and stone.** Align the instrument face with the dotted line on the sharpening guide. This will position the working-end so that the face is parallel (=) to the countertop.

   Align the sharpening stone with the solid line. This is the correct angulation for sharpening.

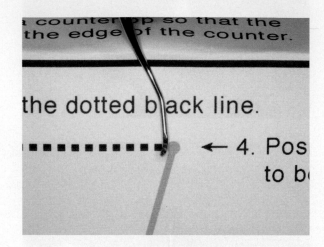

4. **Check your positioning.** Pause for a moment to check that the face of the area-specific curet is parallel (=) to the countertop and that the stone is positioned at the correct angulation.

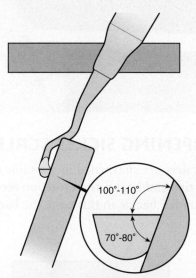

5. **Adapt the stone to the heel-third of the working-end.** The photograph shows a bird's-eye view looking down at the instrument face. Move the sharpening stone up and down in short, rhythmic strokes to remove metal from the lateral surface.

   Finish each series of strokes in a down stroke to avoid leaving metal burs on the cutting edge.

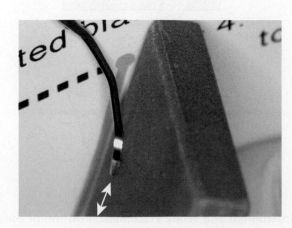

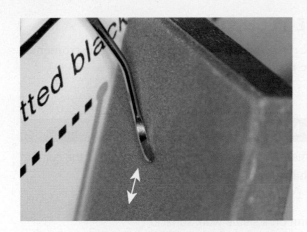

6. **Sharpen the middle-third of the cutting edge.** Reposition the stone so that it is in contact with the middle-third of the cutting edge. Sharpen this section of the cutting edge, ending with a down stroke.

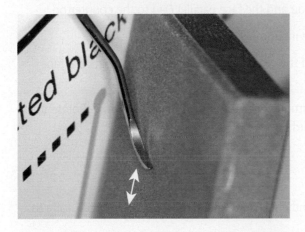

7. **Sharpen the toe-third of the cutting edge.** Reposition the stone so that it is in contact with the toe-third of the cutting edge. Sharpen this section of the cutting edge.

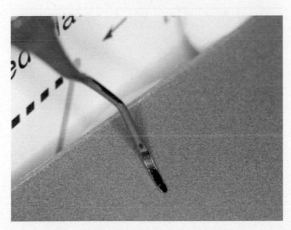

8. **Recontour the curet toe and back.** Recontour the toe and back using the same technique as for a universal curet.

9. Use **Sharpening Guide L** to sharpen the working cutting edge of EVEN-numbered Gracey curets, such as the Gracey 12.

REFERENCE SHEET—MOVING STONE TECHNIQUE

Suggestion: Photocopy this page and use it for a quick reference guide when sharpening instruments. Place the photocopied summary sheet in a plastic page protector or laminate.

TABLE 20-4. Reference Sheet: Moving Stone Technique

1. Prepare the sharpening work area and assemble equipment. If using a sharpening guide, select the correct one for the cutting edge. For Gracey curets, use **Sharpening Guide R** for ODD-numbered curets. Use **Sharpening Guide L** for EVEN-numbered Gracey curets.

2. Grasp the instrument handle and rest your hand and arm on a stable work surface.

3. Position the instrument with the toe (or tip) toward you and the face parallel (=) to the countertop.

4. Place the sharpening stone at a 90-degree angle to the instrument face.

5. Swing the lower end of the stone closer to the back of the working-end until the stone meets the face at about a 75-degree angle.

6. Activate a few light strokes on the heel-third of the cutting edge, ending with a down stroke. Rotate the stone to sharpen the middle-third, then the toe/tip-third.

7. For curets, recontour the toe and back.

8. Use a sharpening test stick to test for sharpness.

9. Use magnification to evaluate design characteristics and check for metal burs. Use a cylindrical stone to remove burs, if necessary.

Section 8
Powered Sharpening Device

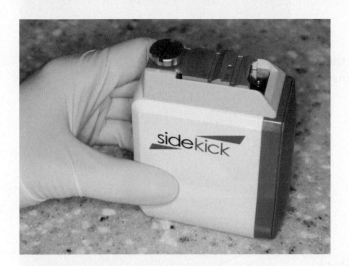

The Sidekick Sharpening Device. The Sidekick—Hu-Friedy Mfg. Co. Inc—is a battery powered sharpening device that is very user-friendly.

SIDEKICK GUIDEPLATE PARTS

The sharpening device has several parts that are used in sharpening: (1) two guideplate channels, (2) two vertical backstops, (3) two terminal shank guides, and (4) a toe guide for use with curets.

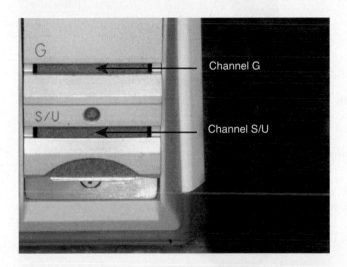

Channel G

Channel S/U

Guideplate Channels. The guideplate has two channels:

- **S/U**—for sickle and universal curets
- **G**—for Gracey curets

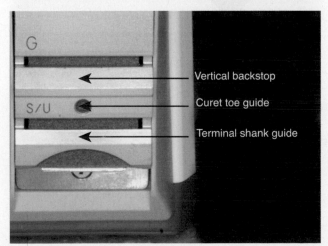

Vertical backstop

Curet toe guide

Terminal shank guide

Channel Features. Each channel has the following features:

- Vertical Backstop
- Terminal Shank Guide
- Toe Guide (for use only with curets)

SHARPENING TECHNIQUE: SICKLES AND UNIVERSAL CURETS

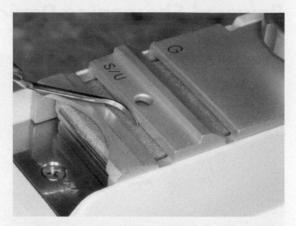

1. **Position working-end in S/U channel.** Place the middle of the back of the working-end against the *Vertical Backstop of the S/U channel.*

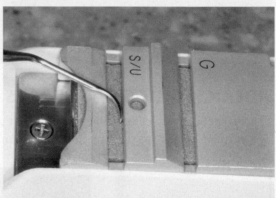

2. **Rest the lower shank against the Terminal Shank Guide.**
   * The positioning of the working-end is the same for a curved or straight cutting edge.
   * Turn on the sharpening device.

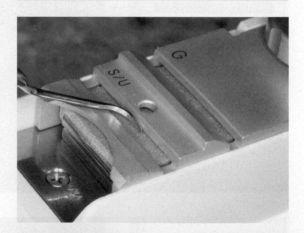

3. **Move the cutting edge against the stone with light pressure.**
   * Maintain contact with both the Vertical Backstop and Terminal Shank Guide during the sharpening process.
   * Move the cutting edge over the stone 2–3 times. Check for sharpness using a plastic test stick.
   * *Repeat this procedure for the other cutting edge on the working-end.*

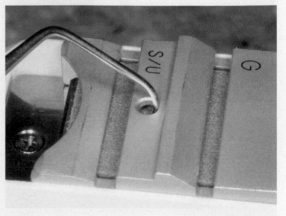

4. **Sharpen the toe of a curet.**
   * *If sharpening a universal curet,* direct the toe into the Toe Guide.
   * Keep the back of the working-end against the rim of the hole.
   * Move the toe side to side 2–3 times.

SHARPENING TECHNIQUE: AREA-SPECIFIC CURETS

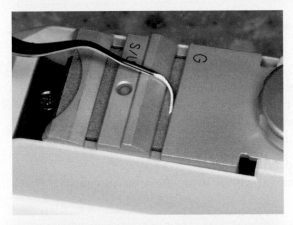

1. **Position working-end in G channel.** Place the middle of the back of the working-end against the *Vertical Backstop of the G channel.*

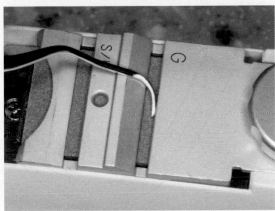

2. **Rest the lower shank against the Terminal Shank Guide.**

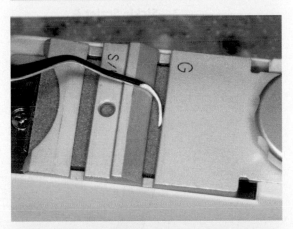

3. **Move the cutting edge against the stone with light pressure.**
   - Maintain contact with both the Vertical Backstop and Terminal Shank Guide during the sharpening process.
   - Move the cutting edge over the stone 2–3 times. Check for sharpness using a plastic test stick.

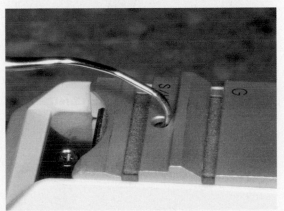

4. **Sharpen the toe.**
   - Direct the toe into the Toe Guide.
   - Keep the back of the working-end against the rim of the hole.
   - Move the toe side to side 2–3 times.

Section 9
Skill Application

PRACTICAL FOCUS

Nola has asked you to evaluate her instrumentation technique because she says that all her patients complain that she is "so rough." Nola hopes that you can tell her what she is doing wrong. Nola is about to begin periodontal debridement on a patient with moderate-sized supragingival and subgingival calculus deposits. The working-ends of her instruments are pictured below.

- Evaluate each working-end; if problems are found, identify them.
- How efficient and effective do you think calculus removal will be using these instruments?
- What recommendations would you give Nola?

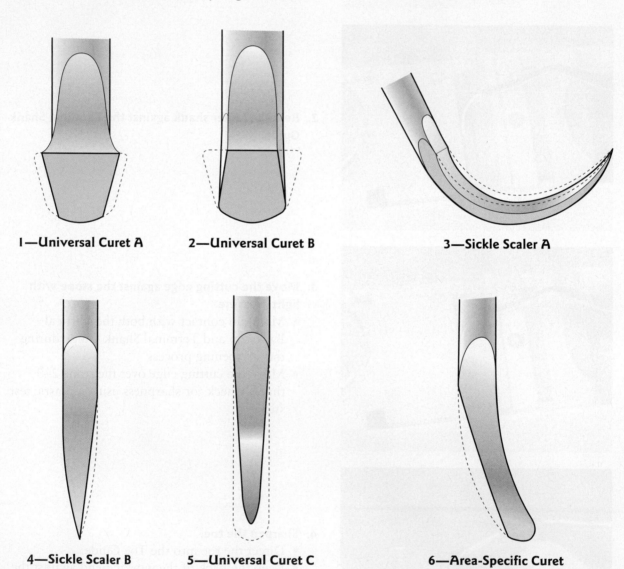

1—Universal Curet A   2—Universal Curet B   3—Sickle Scaler A

4—Sickle Scaler B   5—Universal Curet C   6—Area-Specific Curet

SKILL EVALUATION MODULE 20	INSTRUMENT SHARPENING

Student: _____

Evaluator: _____

Date: _____

Instrument 1 = _____

Instrument 2 = _____

Instrument 3 = _____

Instrument 4 = _____

DIRECTIONS FOR STUDENT: Use **Column S.** Evaluate your skill level as: **S** (satisfactory) or **U** (unsatisfactory).

DIRECTIONS FOR EVALUATOR: Use **Column E.** Indicate: **S** (satisfactory) or **U** (unsatisfactory). Each **S** equals 1 point, each **U** equals 0 points.

	1		2		3		4	
CRITERIA:	S	E	S	E	S	E	S	E
Lubricates sharpening stone								
Grasps the instrument handle and rests arm and hand on stable surface								
Identifies the cutting edge to be sharpened								
Positions the instrument with the face parallel to the countertop								
Grasps the lower third of the sharpening stone								
Establishes stone angulation between 70 and 80 degrees								
Beginning with the heel third, activates light strokes, ending with a down stroke								
Rotates the stone and, in turn, sharpens the middle- and toe/tip-thirds, ending in a down stroke and for curets, sharpens the toe and back of curet								
Evaluates sharpness of entire length of cutting edge and, if necessary, sharpens any remaining dull sections of the cutting edge								
Uses magnification to evaluate design characteristics; describes the design characteristics and indicates if the design has been preserved successfully								
OPTIONAL GRADE PERCENTAGE CALCULATION Total **S**'s in each E column.								

Sum of **S**'s _____ divided by Total Points Possible (**40**) equals the Percentage Grade _____

| SKILL EVALUATION MODULE 20 | INSTRUMENT SHARPENING |

Student: _____

EVALUATOR COMMENTS

_____

_____

_____

_____

_____

_____

_____

_____

_____

_____

_____

_____

_____

_____

_____

_____

_____

Box for sketches pertaining to written comments.

Advanced Probing Techniques

Module Overview

The clinical periodontal assessment is one of the most important functions performed by dental hygienists. This module begins with a review of the periodontal attachment system in health and attachment loss in disease. Other module sections describe techniques for advanced assessments with periodontal probes including (1) measuring oral deviations, (2) assessing tooth mobility, (3) determining the gingival margin level, (4) calculating clinical attachment levels, (5) determining the width of attached gingiva, and (6) assessing furcation involvement.

Module Outline

Key Terms

Periodontal attachment system	Periodontal assessment	Edema	Width of attached gingiva
Junctional epithelium	Furcation area	Gingival recession	Furcation
Fibers of the gingiva	Mobility	Clinical attachment level	Bifurcation
Periodontal ligament fibers	Horizontal tooth mobility	Clinical attachment loss	Trifurcation
Alveolar bone	Vertical tooth mobility	Attached gingiva	Furcation area
Loss of attachment	Mobility-rating scales		Furcation involvement
			Furcation probe

Learning Objectives

1. Discuss the uses of calibrated and furcation probes in performing a periodontal assessment.

2. Describe the rationale for assessing tooth mobility.

3. Demonstrate the technique for assessing tooth mobility, and use a mobility rating scale to classify the extent of mobility.

4. Describe the rationale and technique for determining the level of the gingival margin.

5. Describe the consequences of loss of attachment to the tooth.

6. Given the probing depth measurements and gingival margin levels for a tooth, compute the clinical attachment loss.

7. Describe the rationale for furcation detection.

8. Demonstrate correct technique for use of a furcation probe on a periodontal typodont, and classify furcation involvement according to severity.

9. Use advanced probing techniques to accurately assess a student partner's periodontium.

10. For simulated patient cases, use periodontal measurements to differentiate a healthy periodontium from periodontitis, and record these findings on a periodontal chart.

Section 1
The Periodontal Attachment System

ATTACHMENT IN HEALTH

The periodontal attachment system is a group of structures that work together *to attach* the teeth to the skull. To remain in the oral cavity, each tooth must be attached by the following:

1. Junctional epithelium—the epithelium that attaches the gingiva to the tooth.
2. Fibers of the gingiva—a network of fibers that brace the free gingiva against the tooth and unite the free gingiva with the tooth root and alveolar bone.
3. Periodontal ligament fibers—the fibers that surround the root of the tooth. These fibers attach to the bone of the socket on one side and to the cementum of the root on the other side.
4. Alveolar bone—the bone that surrounds the roots of the teeth. It forms the bony sockets that support and protect the roots of the teeth.

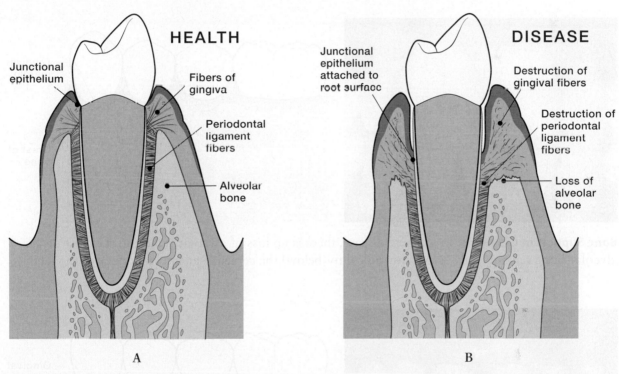

Cross Section of the Periodontal Attachment System. A, The periodontal attachment system in health. **B,** Destruction of the periodontal attachment system in disease.

LOSS OF ATTACHMENT IN DISEASE

Loss of attachment (LOA) is damage to the structures that support the tooth. LOA occurs in periodontitis and is characterized by (1) relocation of the junctional epithelium to the tooth root, (2) destruction of the fibers of the gingiva, (3) destruction of the periodontal ligament fibers, and (4) loss of alveolar bone support from around the tooth. The changes that occur in the alveolar bone in periodontal disease are significant because loss of bone height can eventually result in tooth loss (Table 21-1).

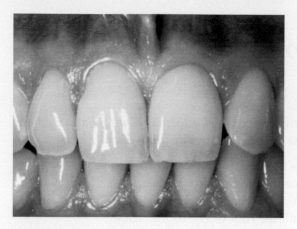
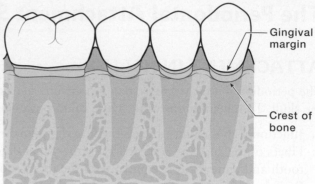

Bone Support in Health. In health, most of the tooth root is surrounded in bone. The crest of the alveolar bone is located very close to the crowns, only 1 to 2 mm apical to (below) the cemento-enamel junctions of the teeth.

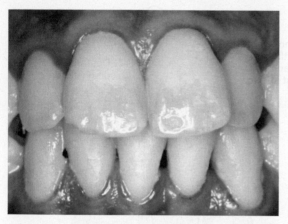
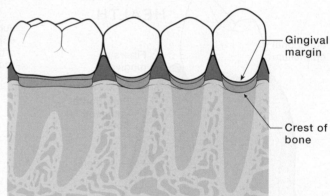

Bone Support in Gingivitis. In gingival disease, there is no loss of alveolar bone and the crest of the alveolar bone remains only 1 to 2 mm apical to (below) the cemento-enamel junctions of the teeth.

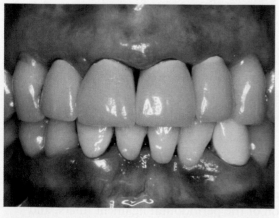
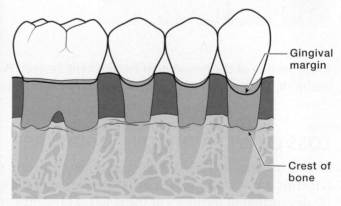

Bone Loss and Pocket Formation in Periodontitis. In periodontitis, bone is destroyed and the teeth are not well supported in the arch. In this example of bone loss, the gingival margin has remained near the cemento-enamel junction, creating deep periodontal pockets.

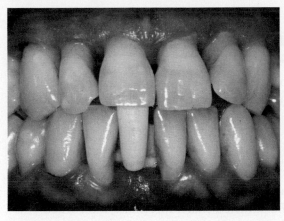

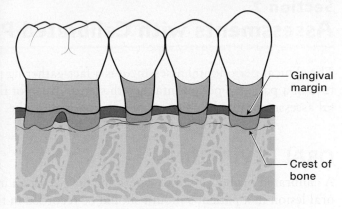

- Gingival margin

- Crest of bone

Loss of Bone and Gingival Recession in Periodontitis. In this example of periodontitis, the gingival margin has receded, and the tooth roots are visible in the mouth. Note that the alveolar bone is at the same level in this example and the one before—only the level of the gingival margin differs in these two examples.

BLEEDING ON GENTLE PROBING

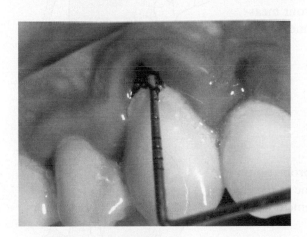

Bleeding on Gentle Probing. Bleeding on gentle probing is a sign of inflammation. Bleeding can be visible immediately when a site is probed, or it may not be evident until about 10 seconds after a site is probed.

Most periodontal charts have a row of boxes that are used to document sites that bleed; bleeding is indicated with a red dot.

TABLE 21-1. Attachment Structures in Health and Disease	
Attachment in Health	**Attachment in Disease**
• Junctional epithelium attaches to enamel at base of sulcus	• Junctional epithelium attaches to cementum at base of periodontal pocket
• Fibers brace the tissue against the crown	• Fiber destruction, tissue lacks firmness
• Many fibers attach root to bone of socket	• Fewer fibers remain to hold tooth in socket
• Most of the root is surrounded by bone; the tooth is firmly held in its socket	• Part of the root is surrounded by bone; the tooth may be movable in its socket

Section 2
Assessments with Calibrated Probes

The clinical periodontal assessment is a fact-gathering process designed to provide a complete picture of a patient's periodontal health status. Much of the information collected during the periodontal assessment involves the use of a periodontal probe.

ORAL DEVIATIONS

A calibrated probe is used to determine the size of an intraoral lesion or deviation. The finding of an oral lesion in a patient's mouth should be recorded in the patient's chart. Information recorded should include the (1) date, (2) size, (3) location, (4) color, and (5) character of the lesion as well as (6) any information provided by the patient (e.g., duration, sensation, or oral habits). For example: "January 12, 2007: a soft, red papillary lesion located on the buccal mucosa opposite the maxillary left first premolar; measuring 5 mm in an anterior-posterior direction and 6 mm in a superior-inferior direction."

Documenting Measurements. It is best to use anatomic references rather than "length" or "width" to document your measurements on the chart (e.g., as the anterior-posterior measurement and the superior-inferior measurement).

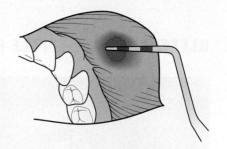

Determining the Height of a Raised Lesion. Place the probe tip on normal tissue alongside of the deviation. Imagine a line at the highest part of the deviation, and record this measurement as the height.

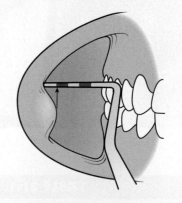

Determining the Depth of a Sunken Lesion. Carefully place the probe tip in the deepest part. Imagine a line running from edge to edge of the deviation. The depth is the distance from this imaginary line to the base of the deviation.

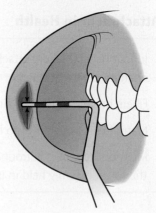

TOOTH MOBILITY

Mobility is the loosening of a tooth in its socket. Mobility may result from loss of bone support to the tooth. Most periodontal charts include boxes for documenting tooth mobility.

1. Horizontal tooth mobility is the ability to move the tooth in a facial-lingual direction in its socket. Horizontal tooth mobility is assessed by putting the handles of two dental instruments on either side of the tooth and applying alternating moderate pressure in the facial-lingual direction against the tooth—first with one, then with the other instrument handle.
2. Vertical tooth mobility, the ability to depress the tooth in its socket, is assessed using the end of an instrument handle to exert pressure against the occlusal or incisal surface of the tooth.
3. There are many mobility-rating scales for recording tooth mobility on a periodontal chart. One useful rating scale is indicated in Table 21-2.

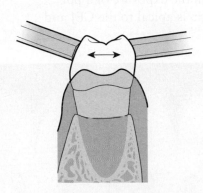

Assessing Horizontal Tooth Mobility. Using the ends of two handles, apply alternating pressure, first from the facial and then from the lingual aspects of the tooth.

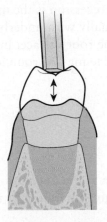

Assessing Vertical Tooth Mobility. Use the end of an instrument handle to exert pressure against the occlusal surface or incisal edge of the tooth.

TABLE 21-2.	Mobility Scale
Classification	**Description**
Class 1	Slight mobility, up to 1 mm of horizontal displacement in a facial-lingual direction
Class 2	Moderate mobility, greater than 1 mm of horizontal displacement in a facial-lingual direction
Class 3	Severe mobility, greater than 1 mm of displacement in a facial-lingual direction combined with vertical displacement (tooth depressible in the socket)

LEVEL OF THE GINGIVAL MARGIN

The level of the gingival margin can change over time in response to trauma, medications, or disease. Three possible relationships exist between the gingival margin and the cemento-enamel junction (CEJ) of the tooth.

1. **Gingival margin is at the CEJ.** This is the natural position of the gingival margin.
2. **Gingival margin significantly covers the CEJ.**
   a. In this instance, the gingiva covers a significant portion of the tooth crown.
   b. The position of the gingival margin may be coronal to the CEJ owing to (1) swelling (edema), (2) an overgrowth of the gingival tissues caused by certain medications that a patient takes to treat a medical condition, and/or (3) an increase in the fibrous connective tissue of the gingiva caused by a long-standing inflammation of the tissue.
3. **Gingival margin is significantly apical to the CEJ.**
   a. When the gingival margin is significantly apical to the CEJ, a portion of the root surface is exposed in the mouth. This relationship is known as gingival recession.
   b. Gingival recession is the movement of the gingival margin from its normal position—usually with underlying loss of bone—resulting in the exposure of a portion of the root surface. In recession, the gingival margin is apical to the CEJ and the papillae may be rounded or blunted.

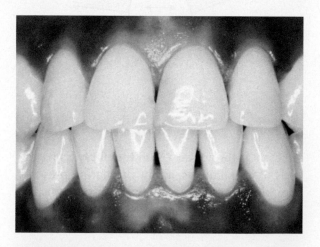

Gingival Margin at the Cemento-Enamel Junction (CEJ). The gingival margin is at the CEJ in this photograph.

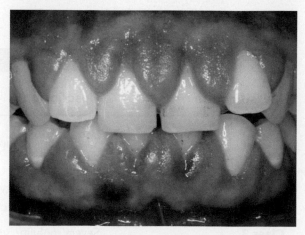

Gingival Margin Significantly Covers the Cemento-Enamel Junction (CEJ). The gingival margin is significantly coronal to the CEJ in this photograph.

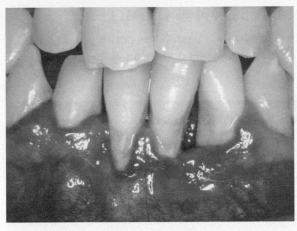

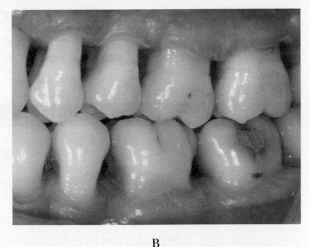

A   B

Gingival Margin Significantly Apical to (CEJ). This relationship, known as recession, leads to exposure of the root surface. **A.** Gingival recession on the facial aspect of three teeth. **B.** Gingival recession on the facial aspect of the posterior teeth.

TECHNIQUE TO DETERMINE THE GINGIVAL MARGIN LEVEL

When tissue swelling or recession is present, a periodontal probe is used to measure the distance that the gingival margin is apical or coronal to the CEJ.

1. For gingival recession. If gingival recession is present, the distance between the CEJ and the gingival margin is measured using a calibrated periodontal probe. This distance is recorded as the gingival margin level.
2. When the gingival margin covers the CEJ. If the gingival margin covers the CEJ, the distance between the margin and the CEJ is estimated using the following technique:
    a. Position the tip of the probe at a 45-degree angle to the tooth.
    b. Slowly move the probe beneath the gingival margin until the junction between the enamel and cementum is detected.
    c. Measure the distance between the gingival margin and the CEJ. This distance is recorded as the gingival margin level.

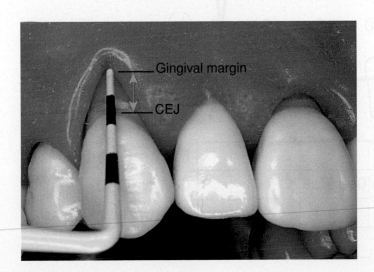

Gingival margin

CEJ

Measuring Tissue Recession. The extent of gingival recession is measured in millimeters from the gingival margin to the cemento-enamel junction (CEJ).

DOCUMENTING GINGIVAL MARGIN LEVEL ON A CHART

Gingival margin level measurements are recorded on a periodontal chart. Most periodontal charts include rows of boxes that are used to record the gingival margin level on the facial and lingual aspects of the teeth.

Box 21-1. Recording the Gingival Margin Level

Customarily, the following notations indicate the gingival margin level on a periodontal chart:

- A zero (**0**) indicates that the gingiva is at the cemento-enamel junction (CEJ; normal level of gingival margin)
- A negative (**−**) number indicates that the gingiva significantly covers the CEJ
- A positive (**+**) number indicates gingival recession

Sample Periodontal Chart With Gingival Margin Levels

On the sample periodontal chart shown below, the gingival margin level is charted in the row of boxes labeled "GM to CEJ"—gingival margin to cemento-enamel junction. In addition, the level of the gingival margin may be drawn across the teeth on a periodontal chart. In this example chart, the level of the gingival margin is significantly coronal to the CEJ on teeth 22, 23, and 24. The gingival margin level is normal for teeth 20 and 21. Recession is present on teeth 18 and 19.

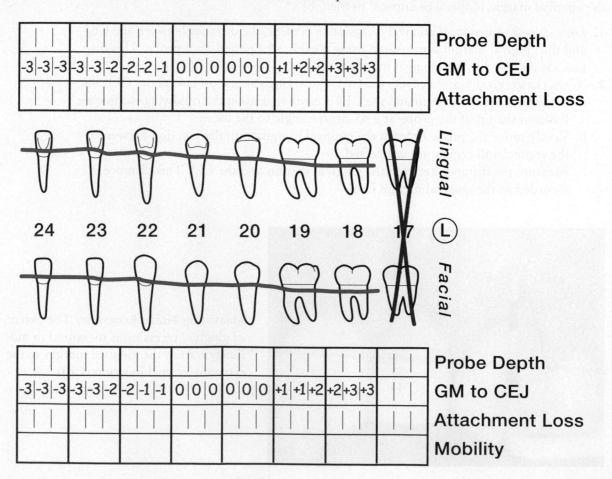

Section 3
Assessments That Require Calculations

Information collected during the periodontal assessment is used to make certain calculations that provide valuable information about the health of the periodontal tissues. The most common calculations are the clinical attachment level and width of the attached gingiva.

CLINICAL ATTACHMENT LEVEL

The clinical attachment level (CAL) refers to the estimated position of the structures that support the tooth as measured with a periodontal probe. The CAL provides an estimate of a tooth's stability and the loss of bone support.

1. Two terms are commonly used in conjunction with the periodontal support system: clinical attachment level and clinical attachment loss. Both of these terms may be abbreviated as CAL and can be used synonymously.
2. Clinical attachment loss (CAL) is the extent of periodontal support that has been destroyed around a tooth.
3. As an example of the use of these two terms, a clinician might report that the "*clinical attachment levels* were calculated for the facial surface of tooth 32 and there is 6 mm of *clinical attachment loss.*"

Box 21-2. Rationale for Computing CAL

- *Probing depths* are not reliable indicators of the extent of bone support because these measurements are made from the gingival margin. The position of gingival margin changes with tissue swelling, overgrowth, and recession.

- *Clinical attachment levels* (CALs) are calculated from measurements made from a fixed point that does not change—the cemento-enamel junction (CEJ). Because the bone level in health is approximately 2 mm apical to the CEJ, clinical attachment levels provide a reliable indication of the extent of bone support for a tooth.

CALCULATING CLINICAL ATTACHMENT LEVEL

A competent clinician must understand the procedure for determining the CAL for the three possible relationships of the gingival margin to the CEJ.

1. The gingival margin may be apical to the CEJ, cover the CEJ, or be at the CEJ.
2. Two measurements are used to calculate the clinical attachment level: (a) the probing depth and (b) the level of the gingival margin (distance from CEJ to gingival margin). Note that both of these measurements are routinely taken and documented on a periodontal chart.

Calculating CAL in the Presence of Gingival Recession. When recession is present, the CAL is calculated by ADDING the probing depth to the gingival margin level.

For example:

Probing depth measurement:	4 mm
Gingival margin level:	+2 mm
Clinical attachment loss:	6 mm

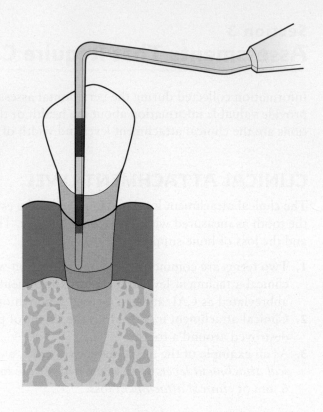

Calculating CAL When the Gingival Margin Covers the CEJ. When the gingival margin is coronal to the CEJ, the CAL is calculated by SUBTRACTING the gingival margin level from the probing depth.

For example:

Probing depth measurement:	9 mm
Gingival margin level:	–3 mm
Clinical attachment loss:	6 mm

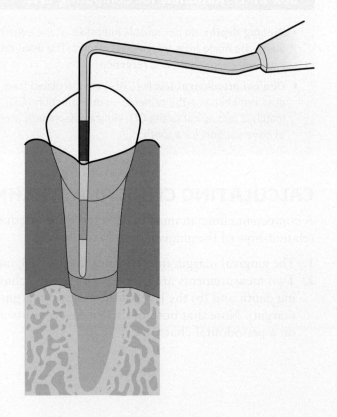

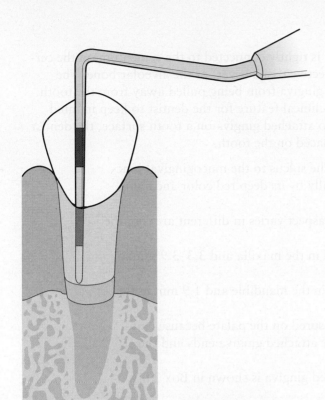

Calculating CAL When the Gingival Margin is at the CEJ. When the gingival margin is at the CEJ, no calculations are needed because the probing depth and the clinical attachment level are equal.

For example:
Probing depth measurement:	6 mm
Gingival margin level:	0 mm
Clinical attachment loss:	6 mm

DOCUMENTING CLINICAL ATTACHMENT LEVELS

On this sample periodontal chart, all three possible relationships of the gingival margin to the CEJ are demonstrated. On tooth 28, the gingival margin is at the level of the CEJ. On teeth 25 to 27, the gingival margin covers the CEJ. On teeth 29 and 31, the gingival margin is apical to (below) the CEJ.

Lingual

		32		31			30			29			28			27			26			25	
Probe Depth				4	3	3				3	2	3	3	3	4	4	5	5	5	5	6	6	6	6
GM to CEJ				+5	+4	+3				+2	+2	+1	0	0	0	-1	-2	-2	-2	-2	-3	-3	-4	-4
Attachment Loss				9	7	6				5	4	4	3	3	4	3	3	3	3	3	3	3	2	2

(R)   32   31   30   29   28   27   26   25

Facial

		32		31			30			29			28			27			26			25	
Probe Depth				3	3	2				2	1	2	2	2	3	3	4	4	4	4	5	5	5	5
GM to CEJ				+4	+4	+3				+2	+2	+1	0	0	0	-1	-2	-2	-2	-2	-2	-2	-2	-2
Attachment Loss				7	7	5				4	3	3	2	2	3	2	2	2	2	2	3	3	3	3
Mobility																								

WIDTH OF ATTACHED GINGIVA

The attached gingiva is the part of the gingiva that is tightly connected to the cementum on the cervical-third of the root and to the periosteum (connective tissue cover) of the alveolar bone. The function of the attached gingiva is to keep the free gingiva from being pulled away from the tooth. The width of the attached gingiva is an important clinical feature for the dentist to keep in mind when planning restorative procedures. If there is no attached gingiva on a tooth surface, the dentist is limited in the types of restorations that can be placed on the tooth.

1. The attached gingiva extends from the base of the sulcus to the mucogingival junction. The alveolar mucosa can be detected visually by its deep red color and shiny appearance.
2. The width of the attached gingiva on the facial aspect varies in different areas of the mouth.
   a. It is widest in the anterior teeth (3.5–4.5 mm in the maxilla and 3.3–3.9 mm in the mandible).
   b. It is narrowest in premolar regions (1.8 mm in the mandible and 1.9 mm in the maxilla).
   c. The width of the attached gingiva is not measured on the palate because clinically it is not possible to determine where the attached gingiva ends and the palatal mucosa begins.
3. The formula for calculating the width of attached gingiva is shown in Box 21-3.

Box 21-3. Width of the Attached Gingiva

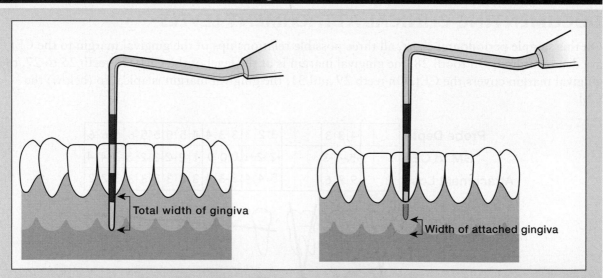

Formula: Calculate the width of the attached gingiva by subtracting the probing depth from the total width of the gingiva.

STEP 1: Measure the total width of the gingiva from the gingival margin to the mucogingival junction.

STEP 2: Measure the probing depth (from the gingival margin to the base of the pocket).

STEP 3: Calculate the width of the attached gingiva by subtracting the probing depth from the total width of the gingiva.

Section 4
Assessment With Furcation Probes

FURCATION INVOLVEMENT

A furcation is the place on a multirooted tooth where the root trunk divides into separate roots. The furcation is termed a bifurcation on a two-rooted tooth and a trifurcation on a three-rooted tooth.

1. The furcation area is the space—apical to the root trunk—between two or more roots.
2. In health, the furcation area cannot be probed because it is filled with alveolar bone and periodontal ligament fibers.
3. Furcation involvement is a loss of alveolar bone and periodontal ligament fibers in the space between the roots of a multirooted tooth.
   a. Furcation involvement results when periodontal infection invades the area between and around the roots.
   b. Furcation involvement frequently signals a need for periodontal surgery after completion of periodontal debridement. Therefore, detection and documentation of furcation involvement is a critical component of the comprehensive periodontal assessment.

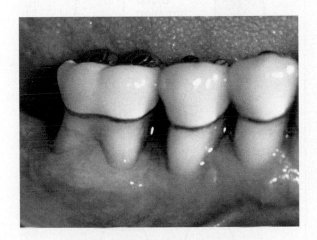

Clinically Visible Furcation. The furcation of this mandibular first molar is visible in the mouth because of bone loss and tissue recession.

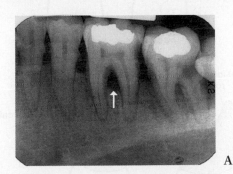

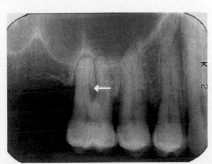

Radiographic Evidence of Furcation Involvement. A, This radiograph shows furcation involvement on the mandibular first molar. **B,** This radiograph shows furcation involvement on a maxillary first molar. (Courtesy of Dr. Robert P. Langlais.)

REVIEW OF ROOT FURCATION MORPHOLOGY

The ability to mentally visualize root furcation morphology is important for effective assessment and instrumentation of periodontal patients.

Box 21-4. Root Furcation Morphology

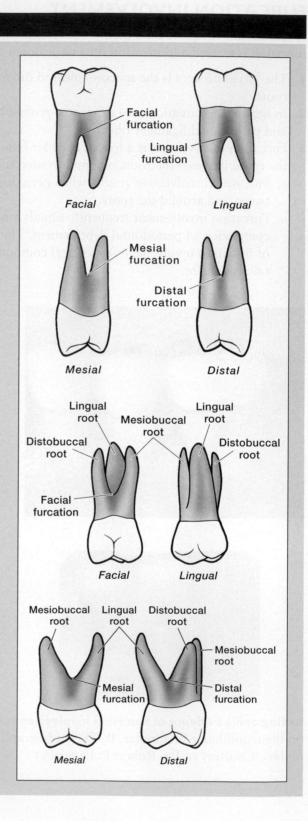

Mandibular molars usually are bifurcated with *mesial and distal roots.*

Maxillary first premolars can be bifurcated with *buccal and palatal roots.* When bifurcated, the roots of a maxillary first premolar separate many millimeters apical to the cemento-enamel junction.

Maxillary molar teeth usually are trifurcated with *mesiobuccal, distobuccal, and palatal* (lingual) *roots.*

On the mesial surface of a maxillary molar, the furcation is located more toward the lingual surface.

On the distal surface of a maxillary molar, the furcation is located near the center of the tooth.

DESIGN CHARACTERISTICS OF FURCATION PROBES

A furcation probe is a type of periodontal probe used to evaluate the bone support in the furcation areas of bifurcated and trifurcated teeth.

1. Furcation probes have curved, blunt-tipped working-ends that allow easy access to the furcation areas.
2. Examples of furcation probes are the Nabers 1N and 2N.

Furcation Probes. Probe **B** has black bands from 3 to 6 mm and from 9 to 12 mm. Furcation probes with millimeter markings often are used in research studies.

Other furcation probes, such as probe **A**, do not have millimeter markings.

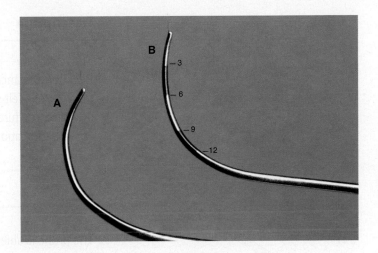

WORKING-END SELECTION

The correct working-end of the probe has been selected if the lower (terminal) shank is positioned parallel to the tooth surface being examined. The incorrect working-end has been selected if the lower shank is perpendicular to the long axis of the tooth surface being examined.

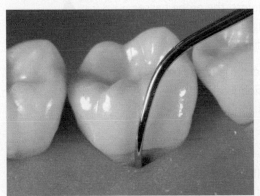
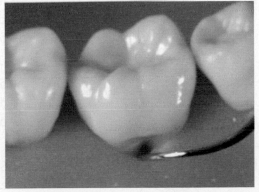

Working-End Selection for Furcation Probe. A, The correct end of a furcation probe has been selected if the lower shank is positioned parallel to the long axis of the tooth surface being examined. **B,** The incorrect working-end has been selected if the lower shank is perpendicular to the tooth surface being examined.

FOUR CLASSIFICATIONS OF FURCATION INVOLVEMENT

Furcation involvement should be recorded on a periodontal chart using a scale that quantifies the *severity (or extent) of the furcation invasion.* Table 21-3 shows a common furcation-rating scale and charting symbols.

TABLE 21-3. Charting Symbols for Furcation Classifications		
Class	**Description**	**Symbol**
I	The concavity—just above the furcation entrance—on the root trunk can be felt with the probe tip; however, the furcation probe cannot enter the furcation area.	∧
II	The probe is able to partially enter the furcation—extending approximately one third of the width of the tooth—but it is not able to pass completely through the furcation.	△
III	In *mandibular molars,* the probe passes completely through the furcation between the mesial and distal roots. In *maxillary molars,* the probe passes between the mesiobuccal and distobuccal roots and touches the palatal root.	▲
IV	Same as a class III furcation involvement except that the entrance to the furcation is visible clinically owing to tissue recession.	◆

DOCUMENTING FURCATION INVOLVEMENT

On this sample periodontal chart, all four classes of furcation involvement are represented. Tooth 2 has a class IV furcation involvement on the facial aspect. Tooth 3 has a class I furcation involvement on the facial aspect between the mesiobuccal and distobuccal roots. On the lingual aspect, tooth 2 has a class III furcation involvement between the distobuccal and palatal roots and a class II furcation involvement between the mesiobuccal and palatal roots.

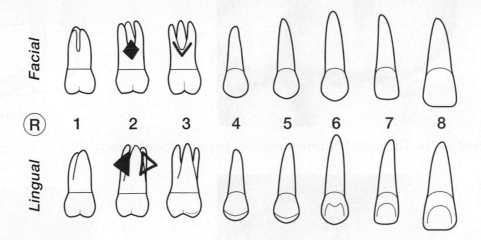

TECHNIQUE PRACTICE WITH FURCATION PROBES

Directions:

1. Use a skull, periodontal typodont or mount an acrylic mandibular molar, maxillary first premolar, and maxillary first molar in modeling clay or plaster. Mount the teeth so that the furcation areas are exposed.
2. Position the probe at the gingival line at a location near where the furcation is suspected.
3. Direct the probe beneath the gingival margin. At the base of the pocket, rotate the probe tip toward the tooth to fit the tip into the entrance of the furcation.

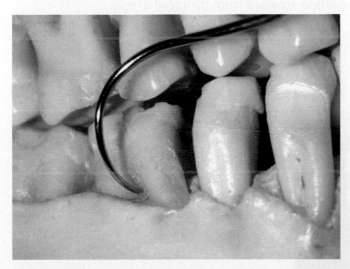

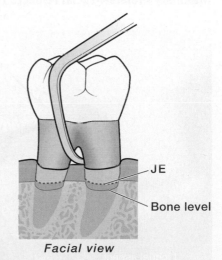

Facial view

Mandibular Molars. The facial furcation is accessed from the facial. The lingual furcation of a mandibular molar is accessed from lingual.

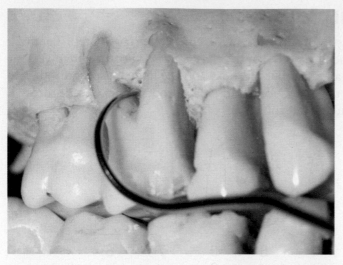

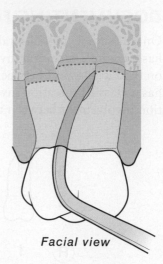

Facial view

Maxillary First Molar. The mesial furcation accessed from the facial aspect.

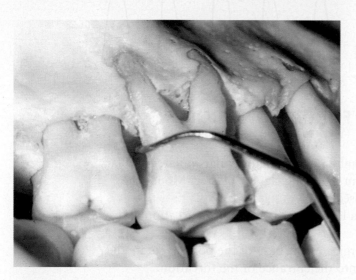

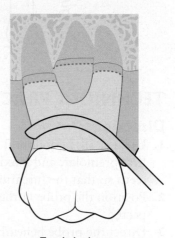

Facial view

Maxillary Molars—Facial Aspect. The distal furcation accessed from the facial aspect.

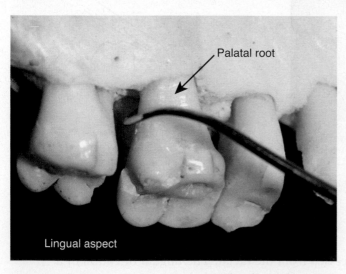

Palatal root

Lingual aspect

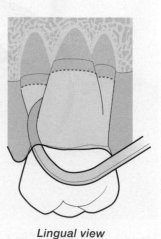

Lingual view

Maxillary Molars—Lingual Aspect. The distal furcation accessed from the lingual aspect.

Section 5
Skill Application

PRACTICAL FOCUS
Periodontal Assessment Case: Mr. Temple

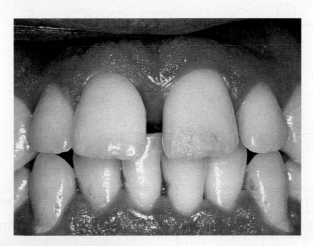

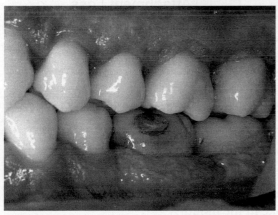

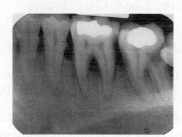

Mr. Temple: Assessment Data
1. Generalized bleeding upon probing.
2. Deposits
   a. Moderate supragingival plaque on all teeth. Light subgingival plaque on all surfaces with moderate subgingival plaque on the proximal surfaces on all teeth.
   b. Supragingival calculus deposits—light calculus on lingual surfaces of mandibular anteriors.
   c. Subgingival calculus deposits—small-sized deposits on all teeth; medium-sized deposits on all proximal surfaces.

Mr. Temple: Periodontal Chart

4	3	5	5	4	6	6	6	6	6	5	6	6	6	6	8	9	8	8	7	7			Probe Depth
0	0	0	0	0	0	0	0	0	0	0	0	0	0	0	0	0	0	0	0	0			GM to CEJ
																							Attachment Loss

Teeth (Lingual): 24 23 22 21 20 19 18 17 (L)

Teeth (Facial): 24 23 22 21 20 19 18 17

4	3	4	4	4	5	4	2	4	5	4	5	5	5	6	7	8	7	7	6	7			Probe Depth
0	0	0	0	0	0	+1	+3	+1	0	0	0	0	0	0	0	0	0	0	0	0			GM to CEJ
																							Attachment Loss
													2		1								Mobility

Mr. Temple: Case Questions

1. Use the information recorded on Mr. Temple's chart to calculate the attachment loss on the facial and lingual aspects for teeth 18 to 24.

2. Describe the characteristics of the class I mobility on tooth 18. Describe the characteristics of class II mobility on tooth 19.

3. Describe the characteristics of the furcation involvement on teeth 18 and 19 (i.e., What does this level of furcation involvement look like in the mouth?)

4. Do the assessment data indicate healthy sulci or periodontal pockets in this quadrant? Explain which data you used to determine the presence of sulci or pockets.

5. If the gingival margin level information had NOT been documented on this chart, would the probing depth measurements *alone* be an accurate indicator of the level of bone support present? Why?

6. Based on the assessment information, which type of explorer would you select to explore the teeth in this quadrant? Which instruments would you select for calculus removal in this quadrant: sickle scalers, universal curets, area-specific curets? Explain your rationale for instrument selection.

Periodontal Assessment Case: Mrs. Blanchard

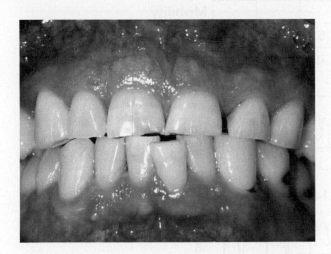

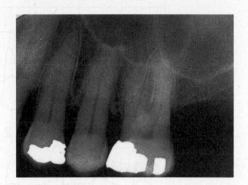

Mrs. Blanchard: Assessment Data

1. Generalized bleeding upon probing.
2. Deposits
   a. Light supragingival plaque on all teeth. Light subgingival plaque on all surfaces.
   b. Supragingival calculus deposits—light calculus on lingual surfaces of mandibular anteriors and facial surfaces of maxillary molar.
   c. Subgingival calculus deposits—small-sized deposits on all teeth.

Mrs. Blanchard: Periodontal Chart

																								Mobility
3	2	3	2	1	3	3	2	4	5	5	3	4	3	5	4	5	6							**Probe Depth**
+4	+5	+4	+5	+6	+5	+4	+5	+4	+3	+4	+3	+2	+2	+1	+1	+1	+1							**GM to CEJ**
																								Attachment Loss

Facial

9   10   11   12   13   14   15   16   (L)

Lingual

4	3	4	3	3	4	4	3	5	6	5	4	5	4	5	5	6	7							**Probe Depth**
+4	+5	+4	+5	+6	+5	+4	+5	+4	+3	+4	+3	+2	+2	+1	+1	+1	+1							**GM to CEJ**
																								Attachment Loss

Mrs. Blanchard: Case Questions

1. Use the information recorded on Mrs. Blanchard's chart to calculate the attachment loss on the facial and lingual aspects for teeth 9 to 14.

2. When assessing tooth 14 for mobility, up to 1 mm of horizontal movement in a facial-lingual direction was evident. Determine the classification of mobility for tooth 14, and enter it on the chart.

3. What class furcation involvement is present on the facial aspect of tooth 14? No furcation involvement is present between the mesiobuccal root and the palatal root. In addition, there is no furcation involvement between the distobuccal root and the palatal root. How would you explain this finding?

4. Do the assessment data indicate healthy sulci or periodontal pockets in this quadrant? Explain which data you used to determine the presence of sulci or pockets.

5. If the gingival margin level information had NOT been documented on this chart, would the probing depth measurements *alone* be an accurate indicator of the level of bone support present? Why?

6. Based on the assessment information, which type of explorer would you select to explore the teeth in this quadrant? Which instruments would you select for calculus removal in this quadrant: sickle scalers, universal curets, area-specific curets? Explain your rationale for instrument selection.

SKILL EVALUATION MODULE 21	ADVANCED PROBING TECHNIQUES

Student: _____

Evaluator: _____

Date: _____

Anterior Area 1 = _____

Posterior Area 2 = _____

PART 1—ASSESSMENT TECHNIQUE ON STUDENT PARTNER

EVALUATOR: Indicate **S** or **U**. Each **S** equals 1 point, each **U** equals 0 points.

	Area 1	Area 2
CRITERIA:	E	E
Position:		
Demonstrates correct principles of positioning for the clinician, patient, equipment, and area		
Dental Mirror:		
Uses the mirror correctly for retraction and/or indirect vision		
Infection Control and Communication:		
Maintains infection control throughout the assessment procedure		
Explains assessment procedure to the patient		
Intraoral Fulcrum and Grasp:		
Fulcrums on same arch, near tooth being instrumented		
Probing Technique:		
Positions probe parallel to the tooth surface		
Keeps tip in contact with the tooth surface and uses small walking strokes within the sulcus to cover the entire circumference of each tooth		
Tilts probe and extends tip beneath contact area to assess interproximal area		
Attached Gingiva:		
Measures the amount of attached gingiva on one tooth in each area		
OPTIONAL GRADE PERCENTAGE CALCULATION		
Part 1: Total points (18 possible points)		
Part 2: Total points (24 possible points)		
Part 3: Total points (8 possible points)		
Calculate Total S's for Parts 1, 2, and 3.		
Grand Total of S's _____ divided by Total Points Possible **(50)** equals the Percentage Grade _____		

Continue with evaluation PARTS 2 and 3 on the following page.

Student: _____

PART 2—PROBING DEPTH MEASUREMENTS ON STUDENT PARTNER

Evaluator calls out a tooth number in each quadrant to be probed on student partner (six readings per tooth).

S = student probing depth reading is within 1 mm of the evaluator's finding for the tooth.

U = student probing depth reading is not within 1 mm of the evaluator's finding for the tooth

QUADRANT	ASPECT	TOOTH #	STUDENT READINGS			EVALUATOR READINGS		
1	Facial	#						
	Lingual							
2	Facial	#						
	Lingual							
3	Facial	#						
	Lingual							
4	Facial	#						
	Lingual							

OPTIONAL GRADE PERCENTAGE CALCULATION—Part 2

Total number of readings within 1 mm of evaluator's measurement _____. (24 possible points)

EVALUATOR—Transfer total number of points to page 1 of Assessment Evaluation Form.

PART 3A—FURCATIONS ASSESSMENT ON PERIODONTAL TYPODONT

On a periodontal typodont, uses furcation probe to assess a mandibular first molar (2 possible points) and a maxillary first molar (3 possible points).

PART 3B—CALCULATING ATTACHMENT LOSS

Calculate the clinical attachment loss. S = correct calculation. U = incorrect calculation.

Tooth A	Tooth B	Tooth C
Probing Depth = 2 mm	Probing Depth = 3 mm	Probing Depth = 6 mm
GM to CEJ = +5 mm	GM to CEJ = +4 mm	GM to CEJ = −3 mm
Attachment Loss =	Attachment Loss =	Attachment Loss =

OPTIONAL GRADE PERCENTAGE CALCULATION—Part 3

Total number of S evaluations for technique with furcation probe _____. (5 possible points)

Total number of correct CAL calculations _____. (3 possible points)

EVALUATOR—Transfer total number of points to page 1 of the Assessment Evaluation Form.

Instruments for Advanced Root Debridement

Module Overview

Periodontitis causes alveolar bone loss that exposes the tooth roots to dental plaque biofilm. Treatment of periodontally involved patients requires specialized instruments with longer shank lengths and miniature working-ends for instrumentation of root concavities and furcation areas. This module presents a variety of periodontal instruments that have been developed to increase treatment effectiveness on root surfaces within deep periodontal pockets. The technique practice at the end of the module provides step-by-step instructions for debridement of multirooted teeth.

Module Outline

Key Terms

Root concavity	Miniature working-end	Endoscope
Extended shank	Magnification loupes	Dental endoscope

Learning Objectives

1. Describe characteristics of root morphology that make root instrumentation challenging.

2. Identify instruments that are appropriate for root instrumentation.

3. Compare and contrast standard curets, extended shank curets, and miniature curets.

4. Given any instrument, identify where and how it may be used on the dentition.

5. Demonstrate the use of an explorer on extracted or acrylic teeth including exploration of root concavities and the furcations of multirooted teeth.

6. Demonstrate the use of an extended shank or miniature curet on a periodontal typodont (or acrylic teeth).

Section 1
Root Surface Anatomy

ROOT CONCAVITIES AND FURCATIONS

Instrumentation for a patient with periodontal involvement requires advanced instrumentation skills because of the concavities found on the roots of most teeth and the furcation areas exposed on some posterior teeth. In health, most of the tooth root is surrounded by alveolar bone. In disease, bone support is lost, which exposes the root to dental plaque biofilm and requires instrumentation of these surfaces.

Effective debridement of the root surfaces requires the clinician to have a complete knowledge of root morphology. Most instrumentation on roots is performed on surfaces that are hidden beneath the gingival margin. A clear mental picture of root anatomy and a keen tactile sense are necessary for subgingival instrumentation to be successful.

1. A root concavity is a linear developmental depression in the root surface. Root concavities commonly occur on:
   a. Proximal surfaces of anterior and posterior teeth
   b. Facial and lingual surfaces of molar teeth
2. In health, root concavities are covered with alveolar bone and help to secure the tooth in the bone.
3. In periodontitis, bone loss exposes the root concavities.
   a. If the gingival margin has receded, these concavities can be seen in the mouth.
   b. If the gingival margin is near the cemento-enamel junction (CEJ), the root concavities remain hidden beneath the tissue in a periodontal pocket.
4. It is difficult for a patient to successfully remove plaque from root surface concavities. Likewise, instrumentation of these areas by a clinician requires skill and an attention to root anatomy.

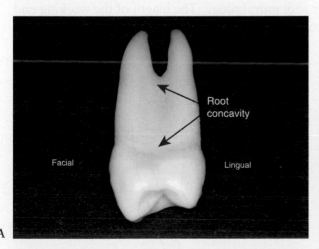 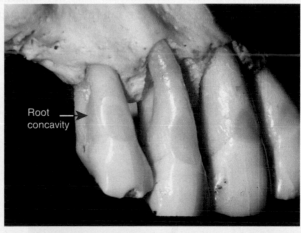

Concavity on the Mesial Surface of a Maxillary Premolar Tooth. A, Maxillary right first premolar showing the linear mesial concavity commonly found on this tooth. **B,** This photograph shows the distal root concavity on a maxillary first premolar that was exposed during a periodontal surgical procedure.

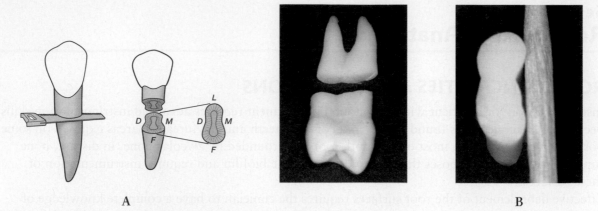

A   **B**

Plaque Removal From Root Concavities. A, A tooth is cut to expose the cross section of the root. **B,** The root of the maxillary first premolar in cross section. A toothpick will not remove plaque from the root concavity because the toothpick spans the depression and does not enter it.

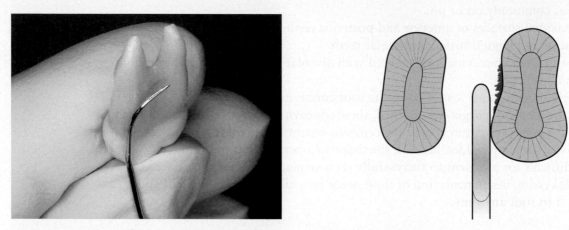

Incorrect Technique Causes the Working-End to Span the Concavity. A problem can occur during instrumentation when the clinician does not consider root morphology. The length of the working-end will span the depression, leaving the concavity untouched.

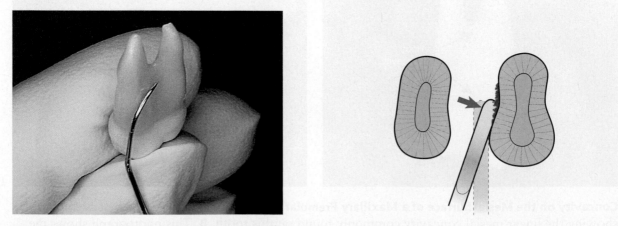

Correct Technique for Adaptation to the Concavity. Correct instrumentation technique involves rolling the handle to direct the leading-third of the working-end into the root concavity. Note that the middle- and heel-thirds of the working-end are rotated toward the adjacent tooth.

REVIEW OF ROOT MORPHOLOGY

TABLE 22-1.   Root Concavities and Furcations

Teeth   Characteristics

Mandibular Anteriors

Single-rooted teeth with deep, linear concavities on the mesial and distal surfaces

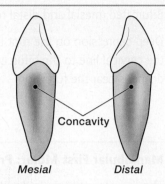

Maxillary Anteriors

Single-rooted teeth that may have proximal root concavities

Lateral incisors may have a palatal groove on the cingulum that extends onto the cervical-third of the lingual surface.

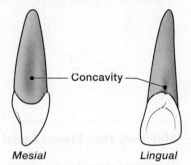

Premolars

The mandibular premolars and the maxillary second premolars are single-rooted teeth that may have deep linear concavities on the mesial and distal surfaces.

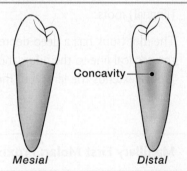

Maxillary First Premolar

The root of this tooth may be bifurcated and has a deep linear mesial concavity. The distal concavity is less pronounced.

When bifurcated, the roots of a maxillary first premolar separate many millimeters apical to the cemento-enamel junction.

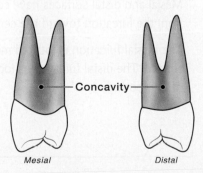

TABLE 22-1. Root Concavities and Furcations (continued)

Teeth	Characteristics

Mandibular First Molar: Facial and Lingual Aspects

Bifurcated, mesial and distal roots.

Deep depression on the root trunk that extends from the cervical line to the bifurcation. This depression deepens near the furcation.

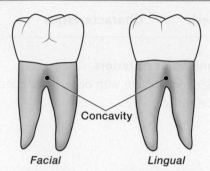

Mandibular First Molar: Proximal Aspects

The mesial root has a wide, shallow concavity.

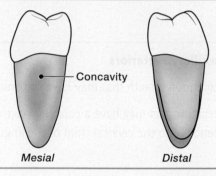

Maxillary First Molar: Facial and Lingual Aspects

Trifurcated mesiobuccal, distobuccal, and palatal (lingual) roots.

The root trunk has a deep depression that extends from the cervical line to the bifurcation. A longitudinal groove extends the length of the palatal root.

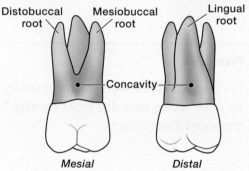

Maxillary First Molar: Proximal Aspects

Mesial and distal surfaces have concavities extending from the furcation toward the cervical line.

The mesial furcation is located more toward the lingual surface. The distal furcation is located near the center of the tooth.

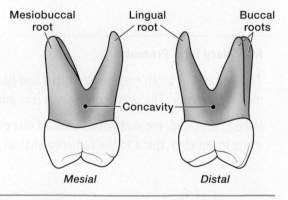

Section 2
Technique Practice: Exploration of Root Concavities and Furcations

Directions: For this technique practice, you will need the following items:

1. An appropriate explorer for root exploration, such as an 11/12-type explorer with an extended shank
2. The following acrylic or extracted teeth:
   - Maxillary first premolar
   - Maxillary first molar
   - Mandibular first molar

Note to Course Instructor: A source of acrylic teeth with anatomically correct roots is Kilgore International, Inc. (800) 892-9999 or online at http://www.kilgoreinternational.com.

MAXILLARY FIRST PREMOLAR: PROXIMAL CONCAVITY

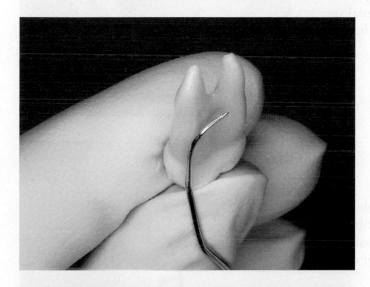

1. **Adaptation to Proximal Concavity—Incorrect.** First, span the concavity using incorrect adaptation and explore the root surface. To experience working in a periodontal pocket, close your eyes as you explore. Notice how the explorer seems to slip across the surface of the root.

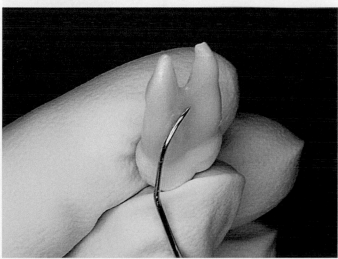

2. **Adaptation to Proximal Concavity—Correct.** Roll the handle slightly to direct the tip-third of the explorer into the concavity. Close your eyes and feel the difference as the tip explores the concavity, rather than just spanning the depression. This is the sensation that you should feel when working within a deep periodontal pocket.

3. **Explore the Mesial Surface From the Facial Aspect.** It is important to explore the mesial surface from both the facial and lingual aspects. First, practice exploring the mesial surface from the facial aspect as pictured here.

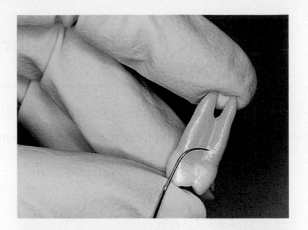

4. **Explore the Mesial Surface From the Lingual Aspect.** Next, practice exploring the mesial surface from the lingual aspect as pictured here.

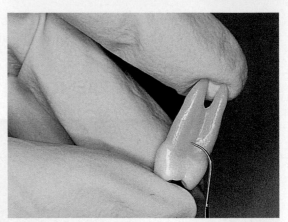

5. **Basic Working-End Position.** As you explore the concavity, note how difficult it is to completely adapt the explorer tip to the concavity using the basic instrumentation technique used for exploring tooth crowns.

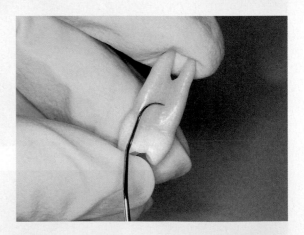

6. **Advanced Working-End Position.** Proximal root concavities can be more effectively explored by positioning the working-end in a tip-up position. Use horizontal strokes to explore the concavity.

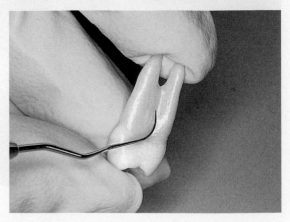

MANDIBULAR FIRST MOLAR: CONCAVITIES AND FURCATION

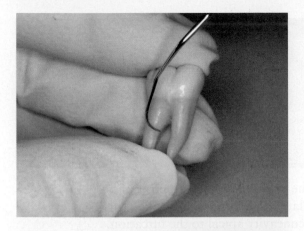

1. **Furcation—Mesial Portion of Distal Root.** Use the leading-third of the tip to explore the mesial portion of the distal root.

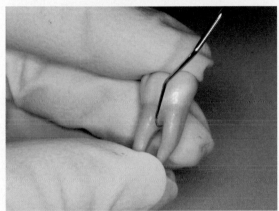

2. **Furcation—Roof.** Use the explorer tip to explore the roof of the furcation.

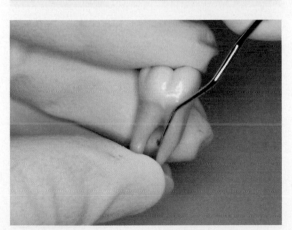

3. **Furcation—Distal Portion of Mesial Root.** Explore the distal portion of the mesial root.

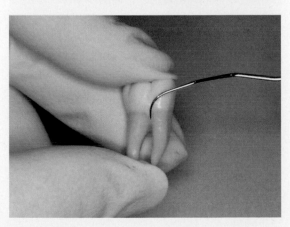

4. **Facial Depression.** Most mandibular molars have a deep depression on the root trunk that extends from the cervical line to the bifurcation. A tip-down position of the explorer is most effective for exploring this depression. As you explore, note that the depression deepens near the furcation.

MAXILLARY FIRST MOLAR: CONCAVITIES AND FURCATION

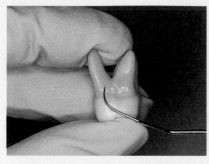
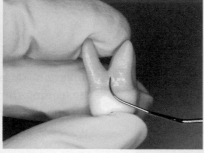
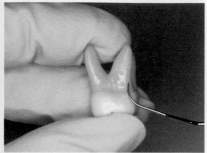

1. **Concavity—Advanced Technique.** Practice using the explorer in a tip-up position to explore the distal surface of the maxillary first molar with a horizontal stroke. This is the most effective approach for adapting to the concavity apical to the furcation.

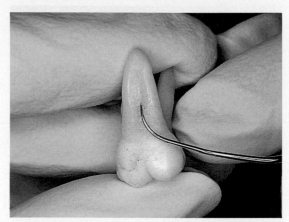

2. **Palatal Root Depression.** A tip-up approach with horizontal strokes is most effective when exploring the narrow linear depression on the palatal (lingual) root of a maxillary molar.

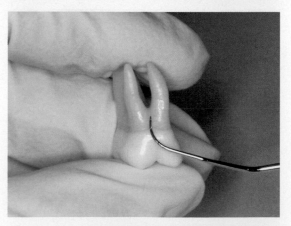

3. **Facial Depression.** Most maxillary molars have a deep depression on the root trunk that extends from the cervical line to the bifurcation. Use a tip-up position and horizontal strokes to explore this area of the molar.

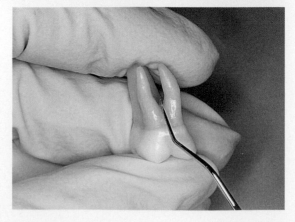

4. **Furcation—Roof.** Use the explorer tip to explore the roof of the furcation.

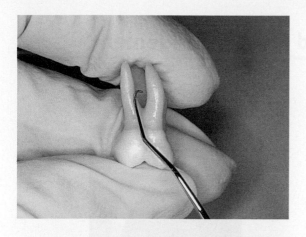

5. **Furcation—Mesial Portion of Distal Root.** Use the leading-third of the tip to explore the mesial portion of the distal root.

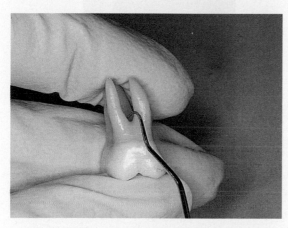

6. **Furcation—Distal Portion of Mesial Root.** Explore the distal portion of the mesial root.

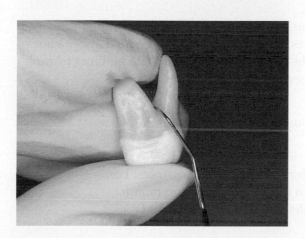

7. **Furcation—Mesial Surface.** The mesial furcation between the mesiobuccal and palatal roots is located more toward the lingual surface. Therefore, the mesial furcation is explored more easily from the lingual aspect.

The distal furcation is located near the center of the tooth and may be explored from either the facial or the lingual approach.

Section 3
Universal Curets for Advanced Root Debridement

LANGER MINIATURE CURETS

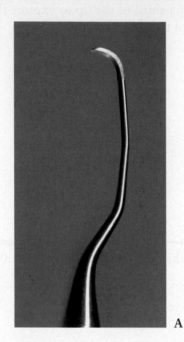
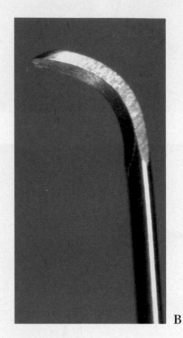

A

B

Miniature Langer Curet. A, A posterior Langer curet with a miniature working-end. **B,** Close up of the working-end on a Langer miniature curet.

Langer curets with extended shanks and miniature working-ends are universal curets that have been modified to increase their effectiveness on root surfaces. Examples are the Hu-Friedy Langer Mini Five miniature curets. The Langer curet can be thought of as a hybrid design that combines features of a universal curet with features typical of an area-specific curet.

1. Design characteristics of a Langer universal curet:
   a. Working-end with a face that is at a 90-degree angle to the lower shank.
   b. Two parallel working, cutting edges.
2. Langer curets differ from other universal curets in three important respects:
   a. Each curet is limited to use only on certain teeth and certain tooth surfaces. For this reason, several Langer curets are required to instrument the entire mouth.
   b. A Langer curet has a long complex functional shank design like that of a Gracey curet.
   c. A set of three Langer curets—the Langer 5/6, 1/2, 3/4—is needed to instrument the entire dentition. The Langer 17/18—which facilitates access to the posterior teeth—may be used on molar teeth.
3. Langer curets are available in several designs. *For root surface debridement, Langer miniature curets are recommended.*
   a. Standard Langer—designed for instrumenting pockets 4 mm or less in depth.
   b. Rigid Langer—provides increased strength for removal of tenacious deposits.
   c. Extended shank Langer—designed for instrumenting pockets greater than 4 mm in depth.
   d. Miniature working-end Langer—designed for access into deep narrow pockets.

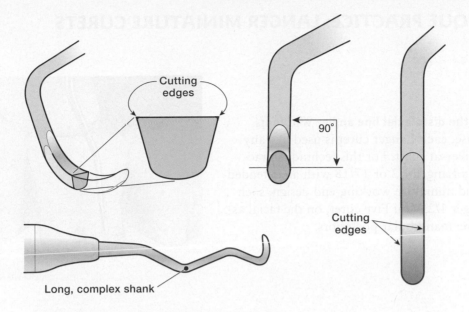

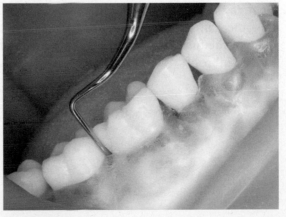

TABLE 22-2.	Langer Curet Application
Curet	**Area of Use**
Langer 5/6	Anterior teeth
Langer 1/2	Mandibular posterior teeth
Langer 3/4	Maxillary posterior teeth
Langer 17/18	Posterior teeth

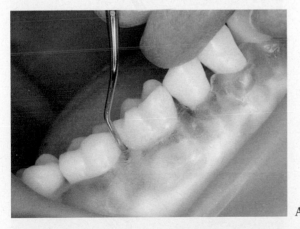

Comparison of Langer 1/2 and 17/18. A, Adaptation of the Langer 1/2 can be difficult when the patient is unable to open widely. **B,** The modified shank design of the Langer 17/18 makes it easier to position the lower shank parallel to the mesial surface of molar teeth.

TECHNIQUE PRACTICE: LANGER MINIATURE CURETS

1. **Begin at the distofacial line angle.** Within its area of use, each Langer curet is used like any other universal curet. For this technique practice, use a Langer 1/2 or 17/18 with an extended shank and miniature working-end design, such as a Langer 1/2 Mini Five curet, on the facial aspect of the mandibular posteriors.

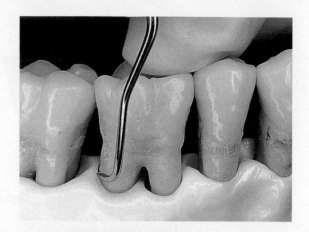

2. **Debride the mesial portion of the distal root.** Instrument the furcation area and the mesial portion of the distal root.

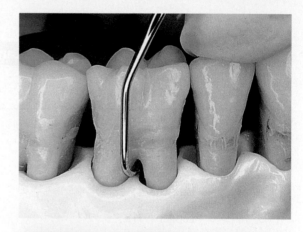

3. **Debride the distal portion of the mesial root.** Use the other cutting edge on this working-end to debride the furcation and the distal portion of the mesial root.

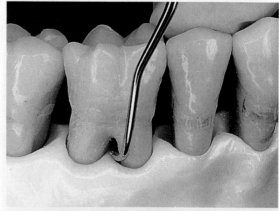

4. **Instrument the mesial surface.** Complete the mesial surface of the first molar.

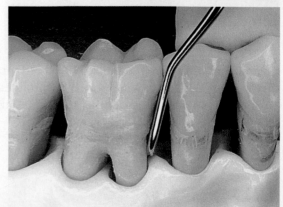

Section 4
Modified Gracey Curets for Advanced Root Debridement

INTRODUCTION TO MODIFIED GRACEY CURET DESIGNS

Standard area-specific curets are designed for instrumenting root surfaces in periodontal pockets of 4 mm or less in depth. To increase treatment effectiveness on root surfaces in periodontal pockets greater than 4 mm in depth, modified Gracey curet designs were developed.

1. An extended shank Gracey curet has a *lower shank that is 3 mm longer* than the lower shank of a standard area-specific curet.
2. A miniature Gracey curet has a *shorter, thinner working-end* and a *lower shank that is 3 mm longer* than that of a standard Gracey curet.

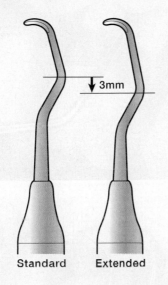

Standard   Extended

Comparison of Standard and Extended Shank Gracey Curets.
The instrument on the left has a standard shank.

The instrument on the right has a lower shank that is 3 mm longer. The overall shank length for the instrument on the right, however, is the same as that of a standard Gracey curet.

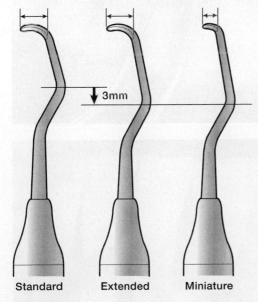

Standard   Extended   Miniature

Comparison of Standard, Extended Shank, and Miniature Gracey Curets.
The extended shank Gracey curet has a lower shank that is 3 mm longer than that of the standard curet.

The miniature Gracey curet has a longer lower shank and a working-end that is half the length of a standard or extended curet.

Application of Curets with Standard and Extended Shanks.
The curet on the right with a standard shank is used to instrument root surfaces in periodontal pockets that are 4 mm or less in depth.

The curet on the left with an extended shank is used to instrument root surfaces in periodontal pockets greater than 4 mm in depth.

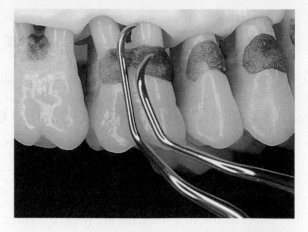

Gracey Extended Shank Design. This modified Gracey curet has a longer lower shank that provides improved access to the root surfaces.

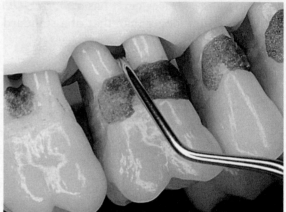

Comparison of Extended Shank and Miniature Gracey Curets.
The instrument on the left is a modified Gracey curet with an extended shank.

The instrument on the right is a miniature Gracey curet with a working-end that is 50 percent shorter than that of a standard Gracey curet.

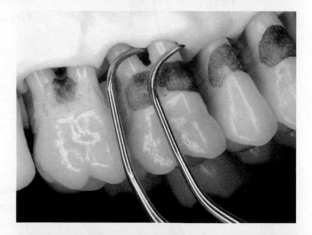

Miniature Curet on Anterior Root Surface.
The miniature Gracey curet works well on the narrow roots of the anterior teeth.

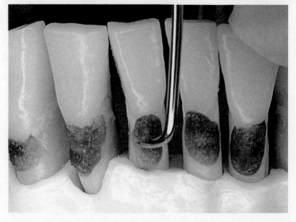

APPLICATION OF GRACEY CURETS AND MODIFIED GRACEY DESIGNS

Area-specific curets with extended shanks and miniature working-ends are modifications of the standard Gracey series. These curets can be applied to the same tooth surfaces as the original Gracey series. There are no 17/18 curets in either the extended shank or miniature curet designs because the standard Gracey 17/18 has a longer shank length and a shorter, slightly thinned working-end.

TABLE 22-3.	Curet Application
Curets	**Areas of Application**
Curets 1, 2, 3, 4	Anterior teeth: all tooth surfaces
Curets 5 and 6	Anterior teeth: all tooth surfaces
	Premolar teeth: all tooth surfaces
	Molar teeth: facial, lingual, mesial surfaces
Curets 7, 8, 9, 10	Anterior teeth: all surfaces
	Premolar teeth: all surfaces
	Posterior teeth: facial and lingual surfaces
Curets 11 and 12	Anterior teeth: mesial and distal surfaces
	Posterior teeth: mesial surfaces
	Posterior teeth: facial, lingual, mesial surfaces
Curets 13 and 14	Anterior teeth: mesial and distal surfaces
	Posterior teeth: distal surfaces
Curets 15 and 16	Posterior teeth: facial, lingual, mesial surfaces
Curets 17 and 18	Posterior teeth: distal surfaces

MODIFIED GRACEY CURETS WITH EXTENDED SHANKS

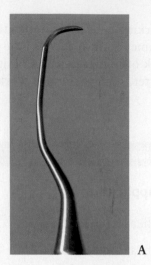 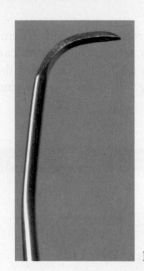

Modified Gracey Curets with Extended Shank Length. A, A modified Gracey curet with a longer, extended shank. **B,** Close up of the working-end of Gracey curet with an extended shank length.

Modified Gracey curets with extended shanks are designed to debride root surfaces within deep pockets more than 4 mm in depth.

1. Examples of extended shank Gracey curets include the Hu-Friedy Manufacturing Company's After Five curets and the American Eagle Instruments' Gracey +3 Deep Pocket curets.
2. The design characteristics of the After Five and Gracey +3 Deep Pocket curets differ from those of standard Gracey curets in two important respects:
   a. **Longer Lower Shank.** The extended lower shank is 3 mm longer than the lower shank of a standard Gracey curet.
   b. **Thinner Working-End.** The working-end is 10 percent thinner than that of a standard Gracey curet. The thinner working-end facilitates insertion beneath the gingival margin and reduces tissue distention away from the root surface.

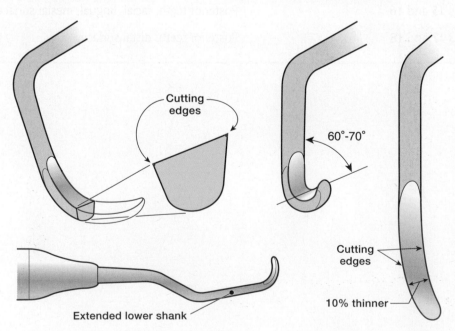

MODIFIED GRACEY CURETS WITH MINIATURE WORKING-ENDS

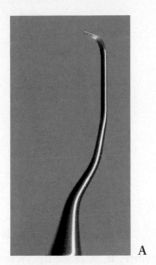 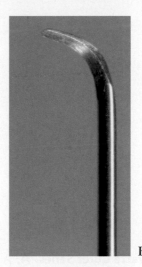

A   B

Miniature Gracey Curet. A, A modified Gracey curet with a smaller working-end. **B,** Close up of a miniature Gracey curet.

Miniature Gracey curets are designed for use in narrow deep pockets more than 4 mm in depth to debride root branches, midlines of anterior roots, root concavities, and furcation areas. The design characteristics of the Hu-Friedy Mini Five and American Eagle Instruments' Gracey +3 Access curets differ from those of standard Gracey curets in three important respects:

1. **Longer Lower Shank.** The extended lower shank is 3 mm longer than the lower shank of a standard Gracey curet. The longer lower shank permits access to root surfaces within periodontal pockets greater than 4 mm in depth.
2. **Thinner Working-End.** The working end is 10 percent thinner than that of a standard Gracey curet. The thinner working-end facilitates insertion beneath the gingival margin and reduces tissue distention away from the root surface.
3. **Shorter Working-End.** The miniature working-end is half the length of a standard Gracey curet.

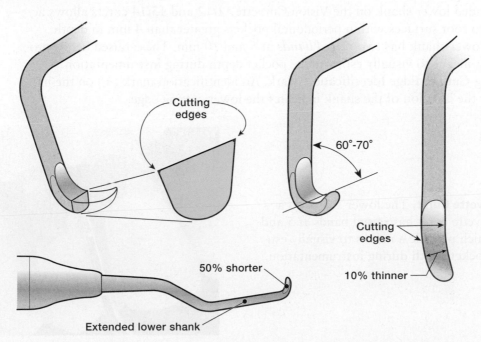

Cutting edges

60°-70°

Cutting edges

50% shorter

10% thinner

Extended lower shank

VISION CURVETTE MINIATURE CURETS

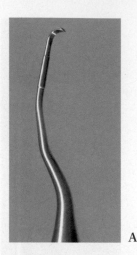

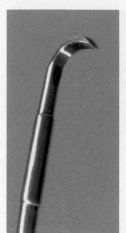

A   B

The Vision Curvette Curet Series. A, A miniature Vision Curvette. **B,** A close up view of the working-end of a Vision Curvette.

Hu-Friedy Manufacturing Company's Vision Curvette curets are another design modification of the original Gracey curet designs. The design characteristics of Vision Curvette area-specific curets differ from those of standard Gracey curets in several respects:

1. **Working-End Length.** The Vision Curvette working-end is shortened to half the length of a standard Gracey curet.
   a. The shorter working-end allows the entire length of the working-end to be adapted to the root surface.
   b. The miniature working-end provides improved access to root concavities, furcation areas of posterior teeth, and midlines of anterior teeth.
2. **Working-End Curvature.** The working-end is more curved than that of a standard Gracey curet. This working-end design facilitates adaptation to curved root surfaces.
3. **Shank Design.**
   a. Extended lower shank on the Vision Curvette 11/12 and 13/14 curets allows access to root surfaces within periodontal pockets greater than 4 mm in depth.
   b. The lower shank has two *raised bands* at 5 and 10 mm. These raised bands provide a means to visually estimate the pocket depth during instrumentation.
4. **Working-Cutting Edge Identification Mark.** An identification mark (+) on the handle near the junction of the shank indicates the lower cutting edge.

Vision Curvette Curet. The lower shank on a Vision Curvette curet has raised bands at 5 and 10 mm, which provide a means to visually estimate the pocket depth during instrumentation.

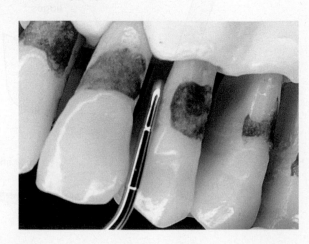

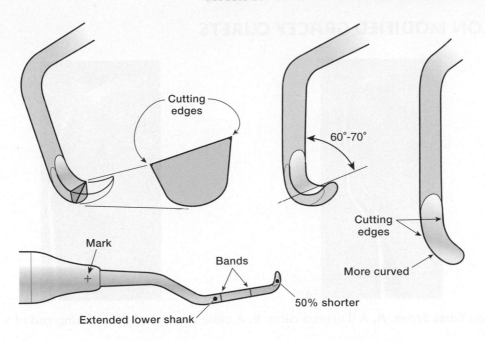

TABLE 22-4.   Vision Curvette Curet Application

Curet	Area of Use
Vision Curvette Sub-Zero	Anterior teeth
Vision Curvette 1/2	Anterior and premolar teeth
Vision Curvette 11/12	Mesial, facial, and lingual surfaces of molars
Vision Curvette 13/14	Distal surfaces of molar teeth

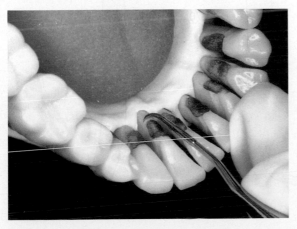
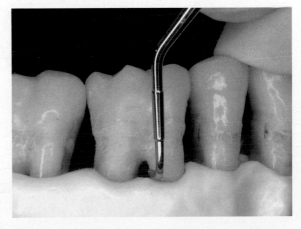

Vision Curvette Working-End. The shorter working-end of a Vision Curvette curet facilitates adaptation to narrow anterior root surfaces and the furcation areas of molar teeth.

TURGEON MODIFIED GRACEY CURETS

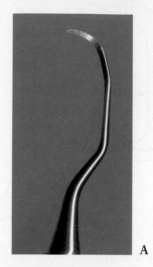
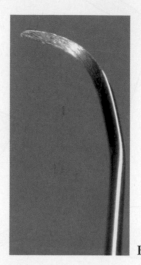

A

B

The Turgeon Curet Series. A, A Turgeon curet. **B,** A close up view of the working-end of a Turgeon curet.

The Turgeon curets are another design modification of the original Gracey curet designs. The design characteristics of Turgeon area-specific curets differ from those of standard Gracey curets in several respects:

1. The working-end of a Turgeon curet is narrower in size than that of a standard Gracey curet. The narrower working-end is easier to insert.
2. The cross section has been modified as shown in the illustration below. Some clinicians find this design easier to sharpen than the traditional Gracey curets.

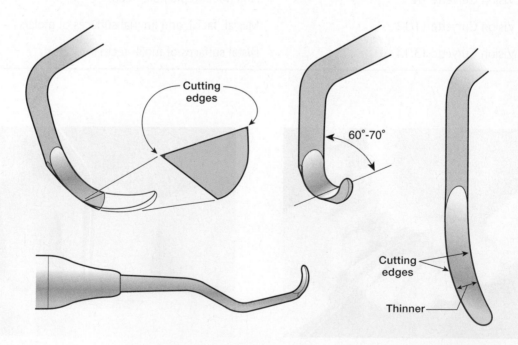

Section 5
Specialized Root Instruments

QUÉTIN FURCATION CURETS

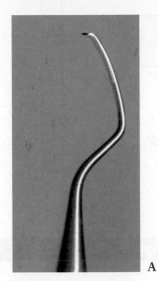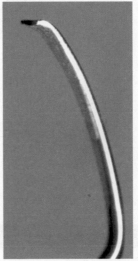

A
B

Quétin Furcation Curet. A, A Quétin curet. **B,** A close up view of the working-end of a Quétin curet.

The Quétin furcation curets are specialized instruments used to debride furcation areas and root concavities.

1. **Working-End Design.**
   a. Each miniature working-end has a single, straight cutting edge.
   b. The corners of the cutting edges and the back of the working-end are rounded to minimize the potential for gouging the tooth surface.
2. **Working-End Size.** Each working-end is available in either 0.9-mm or 1.3-mm size.

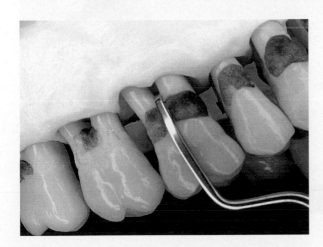

Quétin Curet in Furcation. The Quétin 1 curet used on the furcation roof of a maxillary first molar.

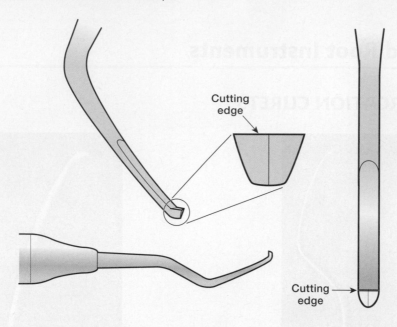

Cutting edge

Cutting edge

TABLE 22-5.	Quétin Curet Application
Curet	**Area of Use**
Quétin 1	Facial and lingual surfaces of posterior teeth
Quétin 2	Mesial and distal surfaces of posterior teeth
Quétin 3	Facial and lingual surfaces of anterior teeth

Quétin Curet in the Mesial Furcation. The Quétin 2 curet used in the mesial furcation of a maxillary first molar. The mesial furcation is accessed from the lingual aspect of the molar.

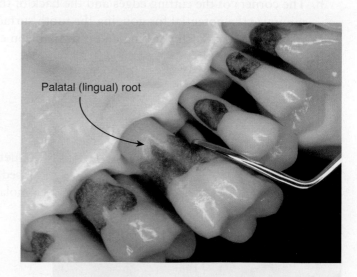

Palatal (lingual) root

O'HEHIR DEBRIDEMENT CURETS

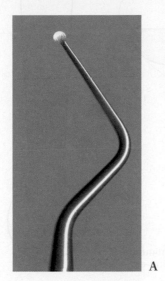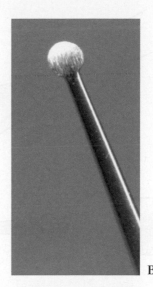

A   B

The O'Hehir Curets. A, An O'Hehir curet. **B,** A close up view of the working-end of an O'Hehir curet.

The O'Hehir Debridement curets are a new type of area-specific curet designed to remove light residual calculus deposits and bacterial contaminants from the entire root surface. These instruments are used with gentle stroke pressure with either push or pull strokes.

1. **Shape of Working-End.** The working-end of an O'Hehir curet is a tiny circular disk.
2. **Cutting Edge.**
   a. The entire circumference of the working-end is a cutting edge. This design allows the instrument to be used with a push or pull stroke in any direction—vertical, horizontal, or oblique.
   b. The working-end curves into the tooth for easy adaptation in furcations, developmental grooves, and line angles.
3. **Shank Design.** These curets have extended lower shanks for easy access into deep periodontal pockets.

TABLE 22-6.	O'Hehir Debridement Curet Application
Curet	**Area of Use**
O'Hehir 1/2	Facial and lingual surfaces of posterior teeth
O'Hehir 3/4	Mesial and distal surfaces of posterior teeth
O'Hehir 5/6	Anterior teeth
O'Hehir 7/8	Anterior teeth with deep pockets

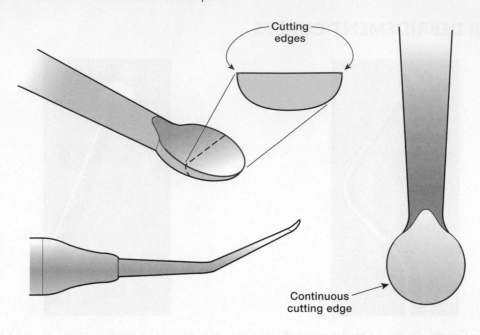

Cutting edges

Continuous cutting edge

TECHNIQUE PRACTICE: FURCATION AND DEBRIDEMENT CURETS

Directions: Practice the use of specialized furcation and debridement instruments using one of the following sets: Quétin furcation series, DeMarco furcation series, or O'Hehir debridement series. If these instruments are not available, read the technique practice to learn about these specialized instruments.

1. **Facial Instrument.** Use the facial instrument from the Quétin furcation series, DeMarco furcation series, or O'Hehir debridement series on the facial surface of the mandibular first molar.

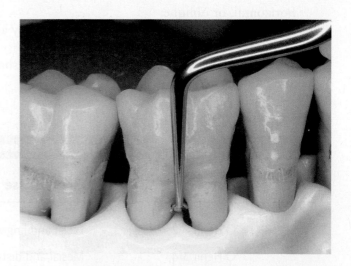

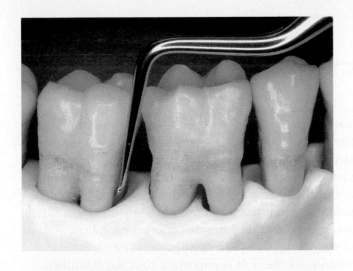

2. **Mesial Instrument.** Adapt the mesial instrument to the mesial surface of the mandibular second molar. How well does the mesial instrument adapt to the linear concavities on the proximal root surfaces?

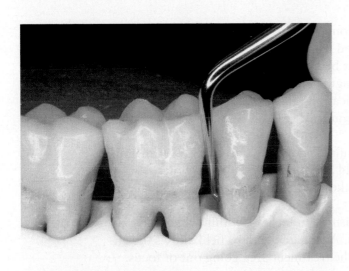

3. **Distal Instrument.** Apply the distal instrument to the distal root concavity on the mandibular second premolar.

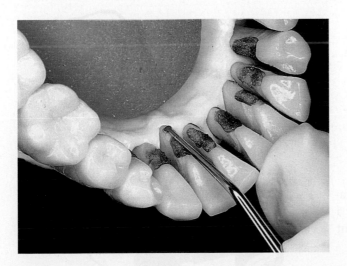

4. **Access to the Lingual Surfaces of the Mandibular Anteriors.** If you have the O'Hehir instruments, adapt the O'Hehir 7/8 curet to the lingual surfaces of the mandibular anterior teeth. This instrument features a 15-mm long shank, which provides access to the base of even the deepest periodontal pocket.

Section 6
Technological Advances

MAGNIFICATION LOUPES

Magnification through surgical telescopes—known as **magnification loupes**—can be a technological aid during periodontal instrumentation. Clinicians using appropriate magnification loupes report decreased eyestrain and an improved visual sharpness. Magnification may reduce the tendency to lean forward in an attempt to obtain a better view of the treatment area and therefore reduces musculoskeletal strain to the clinician's neck, back, and shoulder muscles. For these reasons, some dental and dental hygiene programs have begun including magnification loops in their instrument kits.[1] As with most equipment, how the loupes are used determines whether this equipment is beneficial in reducing musculoskeletal strain. A poorly fitted or incorrectly used magnification system is more likely to exacerbate musculoskeletal problems than solve them. It is important that the magnification system be properly fitted to the clinician.

1. Factors in selecting appropriate magnification.[2]
   a. **Working distance**—the distance measured from the eyes to the viewed object.
   b. **Field of view**—the total size of the object being viewed through the loupes.
      1) The most popular magnification strengths for periodontal debridement are 2.0X, 2.5X, and 2.6X. These magnifications allow the clinician to view the entire mouth at one time. Higher magnification levels result in a smaller field of view.
      2) The lowest level of magnification required should be selected. Lower magnification levels increase the depth of field and minimize the blind-zone.
      3) Too great a level of magnification makes it difficult to keep the treatment area steady in the field of vision.
   c. **Depth of field**—the distance range—measured in inches—within which the object being viewed remains in sharp focus. Adequate depth of field allows the clinician to move his or her head without the treatment area going out of focus.

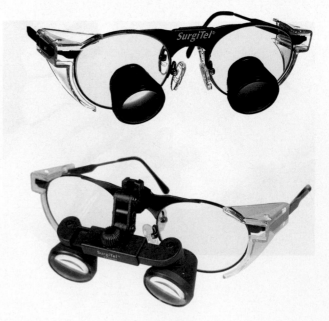

Through-the-Lens Style. Through-the-lens style compound-lens loupes provide low to medium magnification. (Courtesy of SurgiTel/General Scientific Corporation.)

Flip-Up Style. The flip-up style of the magnification system allows the clinician to adjust from a magnified view to a nonmagnified view without removing the eyewear. (Courtesy of SurgiTel/General Scientific Corporation.)

d. Angle of declination—the angle between (1) the line of sight made with the eyes in neutral position and (2) the actual line of sight made with the eyes inclined downward to view the treatment area. Declination angles among clinicians range from 15 to 44 degrees. Each clinician, however, has a unique optimal declination angle determined by the individual's most balanced seated position.
   1) If the declination angle of the loupes is too small, the clinician will have to tip the chin toward the chest to view the treatment area through the loupes.
   2) If the declination angle is too great, the clinician will have to tilt the head backward to view the treatment area through the loupes.
e. Blind zone—an area of vision between the unmagnified peripheral field of vision and the magnified center of the field of vision.
   1) The blind zone presents the most difficulty when an instrument is being moved into or out of the magnified field of view. Injury to the patient or the clinician is a possibility as the instrument is moved through the blind spot. Most clinicians simply move the loupes aside until a stable fulcrum has been established with the instrument.
   2) The lowest magnification should be selected to minimize the size of the blind zone.

2. Types of magnification equipment available.
   a. Single-Lens Loupes.
      1) Low magnification.
      2) Limited depth of field and working distance.
      3) Preset declination angle.
      4) This type can distort the shape and color of objects.
   b. Compound-Lens Loupes.
      1) Low to medium magnification.
      2) Greater depth of field.
      3) Adjustable declination angle.
      4) Available with achromatic lenses that produce a color-correct image.
   c. Prism Telescopic Loupes.
      1) Best magnification.
      2) Widest depth of field.
      3) Adjustable declination angle and wider fields of view.
3. Design Styles.
   a. Through-the-lens styles have the magnification telescopes mounted directly to the eyewear or headband.
   b. Flip-up styles have the magnification telescopes attached to the eyeglasses by a hinged bracket. The bracket allows the clinician to obtain nonmagnified vision by rotating the telescopes above the eyewear or headband.

TABLE 22-7. Magnification Systems

Advantages of Magnification	Disadvantages of Magnification
• Improved vision and decreased eyestrain	• Equipment cost
• Decreased fatigue of neck, back, and shoulder muscles	• Two weeks to two months needed to become proficient in using magnification
• Improved eye protection	• Cross-contamination potential if loupes are adjusted during treatment

SUBGINGIVAL ENDOSCOPE TECHNOLOGY

An endoscope is an illuminated optic instrument used to view the interior of a body cavity or organ. This flexible optic instrument has been used for many years in medicine to diagnose gastric ulcers, locate the source of gastrointestinal bleeding, examine the esophagus and stomach, and detect abnormalities of the lower colon. Recently, a dental endoscope has been introduced for subgingival use in the diagnosis and treatment of periodontal disease.[3]

1. The dental endoscope consists of a fiber optic camera covered with a disposable sterile sheath.
    a. The endoscope fits into modified periodontal instruments that are inserted into the periodontal pocket to provide the clinician with direct vision of subgingival root conditions.
    b. The sheath delivers water irrigation that flushes the pocket while the endoscope is in use.
    c. The modified periodontal instruments that can be attached to the endoscope for subgingival use include explorers, curets, and ultrasonic instruments.
2. The endoscope is attached to a flat screen monitor that provides a clear picture of subgingival conditions. It enables the clinician to see subgingival calculus deposits and caries. With the dental endoscope, clinicians can actually see subgingival deposits instead of only detecting deposits with an explorer.
3. The dental endoscope is not recommended for routine subgingival instrumentation because this process would be too time-consuming.
    a. Instead, the endoscopic examination is recommended for pockets 4 mm or more in depth that continue to bleed at a reevaluation appointment conducted 4 to 6 weeks after completion of periodontal debridement procedures.
    b. The dental endoscope allows the clinician to see the root surface and into furcations to locate any remaining calculus deposits.

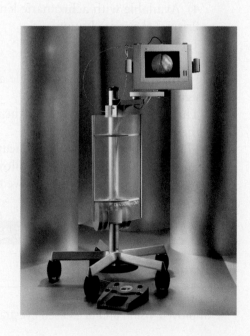

The Perioscopy System. The dental subgingival endoscope from DentalView, Inc., is called the Perioscopy System. The Perioscopy System consists of a fiber optic camera covered with a disposable sterile sheath that is fitted into modified periodontal instruments. The endoscope is attached to a color monitor that provides a clear picture of actual subgingival conditions. (Courtesy of DentalView, Inc., Irvine, CA.)

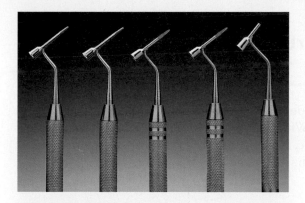

Modified Instruments. Shown here are the modified periodontal explorers that are used with the Perioscopy System. (Courtesy of DentalView, Inc., Irvine, CA.)

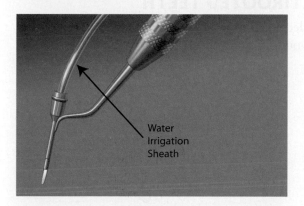

Water Irrigation Sheath

Modified Periodontal Instruments. Modified periodontal instruments attached to the endoscope are inserted into the periodontal pocket. An endoscopic sheath delivers water irrigation that flushes the pocket while the modified instrument is in use. (Courtesy of DentalView, Inc., Irvine, CA.)

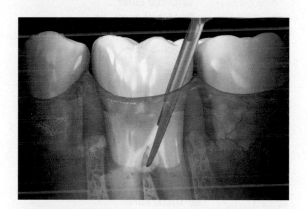

Modified Tip in Pocket. The modified periodontal instruments of the Perioscopy system are about the size of a periodontal probe and are easily inserted into a periodontal pocket. (Courtesy of DentalView, Inc., Irvine, CA.)

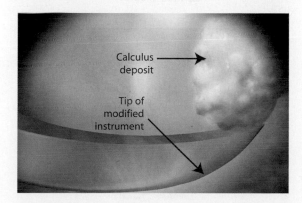

Calculus deposit

Tip of modified instrument

Tooth Surface Through Endoscope. Real-time images of the actual subgingival conditions are displayed on a color monitor. (Courtesy of DentalView, Inc., Irvine, CA.)

Section 7
Technique Practice: Basic Instrumentation of Multirooted Teeth

Periodontal debridement is complicated when furcation areas, root concavities, and multiple roots have been exposed because of loss of alveolar bone. With multirooted teeth, the best approach is to instrument each root as a separate tooth. For example, imagine that the two roots of a mandibular molar tooth are the single roots of two premolar teeth.

STEP-BY-STEP TECHNIQUE ON MULTIROOTED TEETH

Directions: Miniature area-specific curets with extended shanks are recommended for this technique practice. Practice instrumentation on a periodontal typodont or an acrylic tooth model.

1. **Begin with the root trunk.** Debride the root trunk using the distal curet on the distal surface and the mesial curet on the facial and mesial surfaces.

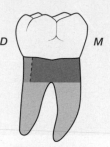

☐ Distal curet
■ Mesial curet

2. **Instrument the root branches.** Treat each root branch as if it were the root of a single rooted tooth.

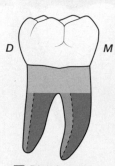

☐ Distal curet
■ Mesial curet

3. **Distal portion of distal root.** Use the *distal* curet to instrument the distal portion of the distal root, beginning at the line angle.

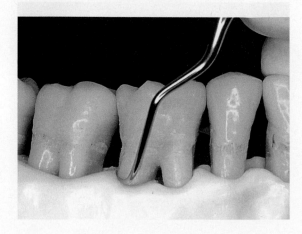

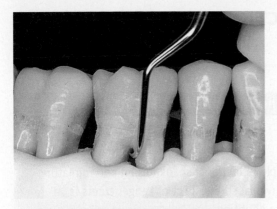

4. **Distal portion of mesial root.** Using the *distal* curet, instrument the distal portion of the mesial root.

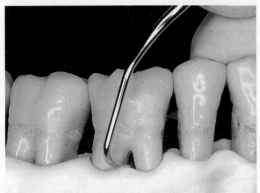

5. **Mesial portion of distal root.** Beginning at the line angle, use the *mesial* curet to debride the mesial portion of the distal root.

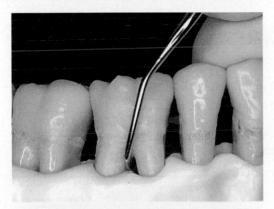

6. **Furcation.** Instrument the mesial side of the furcation using the *mesial* curet.

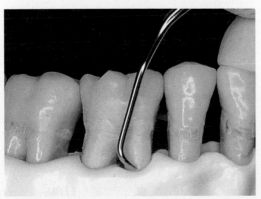

7. **Mesial portion of mesial root.** Use the *mesial* curet to debride the mesial portion of the mesial root and the mesial surface of the root.

NOTE TO COURSE INSTRUCTOR: Advanced techniques for instrumentation of root surfaces are covered in Module 23, Advanced Techniques for Root Surface Debridement.

SUMMARY SHEET: INSTRUMENT SELECTION FOR ADVANCED ROOT DEBRIDEMENT

TABLE 22-8. Instruments for Advanced Root Debridement	
Instrument	**Design Characteristics**
Langer Mini 5	Universal curet with long complex functional shank design and miniature working-ends. Unlike other universal curets, a set of Langer curets is needed to instrument the entire dentition.
Turgeon	Area-specific curets with a modified cross sectional design. Modified working-end shape provides a cutting edge that is easier to sharpen. Narrower working-end is easier to insert.
After Five Gracey +3 Deep Pocket	Extended lower shank and thinner working-end. Slim working-end is easier to insert but is not as strong. Extended shank allows access to surfaces 5 mm or more apical to cemento-enamel junction.
Mini Five Gracey +3 Access	Thin miniature working-end and extended lower shank. Tiny working-end aids in access to root concavities, furcation areas, and midline regions of anterior roots. Thin working-end is limited to use on light deposits.
Vision Curvette Quétin Furcation	Shorter, more curved working-ends facilitate access to root concavities, furcation areas, and midlines of anterior teeth.
DeMarco Furcation	Specialized instruments for use in furcations and concavities. Single cutting edge with rounded corners and a rounded back.
O'Hehir Debridement	Disc-shaped working-end with a continuous cutting edge; used for root surface debridement and deplaquing.

REFERENCES

1. Sunell, S. and L. Maschak, Positioning for clinical dental hygiene care. Preventing back, neck and shoulder pain. Probe, 1996. 30(6): 216–219.

2. Chang, B.J., Ergonomic benefits of surgical telescope systems: selection guidelines. J Calif Dent Assoc, 2002. 30(2): 161–169.

3. Stambaugh, R.V., et al., Endoscopic visualization of the submarginal gingiva dental sulcus and tooth root surfaces. J Periodontol, 2002. 73(4): 374–382:

Section 8
Skill Application

PRACTICAL FOCUS
Periodontal Assessment Case: Mrs. Jefferson

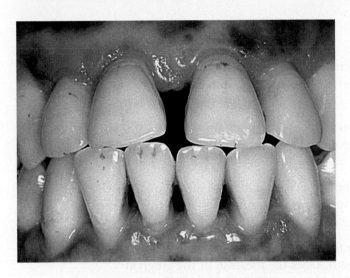

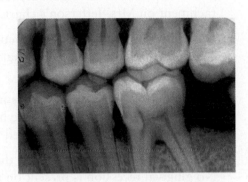

Mrs. Jefferson: Periodontal Chart

3	3	3	3	2	3	3	2	3	5	6	6	6	6	6	7	6	6							Probe Depth
+1	+1	+1	+2	+2	+2	+2	+4	+2	+1	0	0	0	0	0	0	0	0							GM to CEJ
																								Attachment Loss

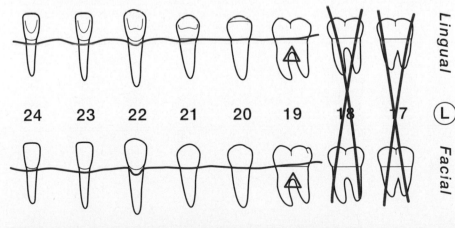

Lingual

24   23   22   21   20   19   18   17   Ⓛ

Facial

3	2	3	2	2	2	2	1	3	4	5	5	5	5	5	6	5	5							Probe Depth
+1	+1	+1	+2	+2	+2	+2	+4	+2	+1	0	0	0	0	0	0	0	0							GM to CEJ
																								Attachment Loss
																								Mobility

Mrs. Jefferson: Assessment Data

1. Generalized bleeding upon probing.
2. Deposits
   a. Moderate supragingival plaque on all teeth.
   b. Supragingival calculus deposits—light calculus on lingual surfaces of the mandibular anteriors and molar teeth.
   c. Subgingival calculus deposits—small-sized deposits on all teeth; medium-sized deposits on all proximal surfaces.

Mrs. Jefferson: Case Questions

1. Use the information recorded on Mrs. Jefferson's chart to calculate the attachment loss on the facial and lingual aspects for teeth 19 through 24. Enter the loss of attachment on Mrs. Jefferson's chart.

2. Is mobility or furcation involvement present in the quadrant charted above? If so, which teeth are involved, and what is the extent of the mobility and/or furcation involvement?

3. Does the assessment data indicate normal bone levels or bone loss in this quadrant? Does the assessment data indicate healthy sulci or periodontal pockets in this quadrant? Explain which data you used to make these determinations.

4. The gingival margin is located at the cemento-enamel junction for teeth 19 and 20. No gingival recession is present on these teeth. Does the location of the gingival margin make the instrumentation of these teeth more difficult or less difficult?

5. Do you expect to instrument any root concavities or furcation areas while debriding the teeth in this quadrant? If so, indicate which teeth will probably have root concavities and/or furcation areas to be instrumented.

6. Based on the assessment information, select explorer(s), probe(s), and calculus removal instruments that would be appropriate for instrumentation of this quadrant. List the instruments you would select and explain your rationale for instrument selection.

Student: _____

Evaluator: _____

Date: _____

EQUIPMENT FOR THIS SKILL EVALUATION: An assortment of instruments including (1) some of which are limited to supragingival use, (2) some that are appropriate for subgingival instrumentation up to 4 mm in depth, and (3) some that are appropriate for subgingival instrumentation at depths greater than 4 mm. If instruments are not available, a variety of pictures from this textbook can be used. For demonstration of exploring technique, use a periodontal typodont or acrylic tooth models.

DIRECTIONS FOR STUDENT: Use **Column S.** Evaluate your skill level as: **S** (satisfactory) or **U** (unsatisfactory).

DIRECTIONS FOR EVALUATOR: Use **Column E.** Indicate: **S** (satisfactory) or **U** (unsatisfactory). Each **S** equals 1 point, each **U** equals 0 points.

CRITERIA:	S	E
Instrument Selection:		
Correctly divides the instruments provided into the three categories described under EQUIPMENT above		
Instrument Design of Two Instruments From Category 3:		
Instrument 1 correctly describes the design characteristics that make this instrument appropriate for subgingival instrumentation at depths greater than 4 mm		
Instrument 2—correctly describes the design characteristics that make this instrument appropriate for subgingival instrumentation at depths greater than 4 mm		
Exploring Technique for Root Surfaces: Premolar Tooth		
Demonstrates and explains correct technique for exploration of the mesial root concavity		
Demonstrates and explains technique for exploration of the mesial root surface from both aspects		
Demonstrates and explains technique for using horizontal strokes to assess the mesial root concavity		
Exploring Technique for Root Surfaces: Mandibular First Molar		
Demonstrates and explains correct technique for exploration of the mesial portion of the distal root		
Demonstrates and explains correct technique for exploration of the roof of the furcation		
Demonstrates and explains correct technique for exploration of the distal portion of the mesial root		
Exploring Technique for Root Surfaces: Maxillary First Molar		
Demonstrates and explains correct technique for using horizontal strokes on the distal root surface		
Demonstrates and explains correct technique for exploring the linear depression on the palatal root		
Demonstrates and explains correct technique for exploration of the mesial furcation		
OPTIONAL GRADE PERCENTAGE CALCULATION Total **S**'s in each E column.		

Sum of **S**'s _____ divided by Total Points Possible (**12**) equals the Percentage Grade _____

SKILL EVALUATION MODULE 22   INSTRUMENTS FOR ADVANCED ROOT DEBRIDEMENT

Student: _____

EVALUATOR COMMENTS

_____
_____
_____
_____
_____
_____
_____
_____
_____
_____
_____
_____
_____
_____
_____
_____
_____

Box for sketches pertaining to written comments.

Advanced Techniques for Root Surface Debridement

Module Overview

This module explains advanced instrumentation techniques for root surface debridement. Treating root surfaces located within deep periodontal pockets is challenging, especially on posterior teeth. Advanced fulcruming techniques can facilitate access and adaptation to these root surfaces. Instrumentation of root surfaces within deep periodontal pockets is further complicated by root surface anatomy, including root concavities, fissures, and furcation areas. This module presents advanced fulcruming techniques and strategies for debridement of root surfaces.

Module Outline

Key Terms

Fulcrum	Modified intraoral fulcrum	Basic extraoral fulcrum
Intraoral fulcrum	Cross arch fulcrumOpposite	Finger assist fulcrum
Extraoral fulcrum	arch fulcrum	
Advanced fulcrum	Finger-on-finger fulcrum	

Learning Objectives

1. Select instruments that are appropriate for root instrumentation.

2. Demonstrate each of the following fulcrums in an appropriate sextant of the dentition for the fulcrum: modified intraoral, cross arch, opposite arch, finger-on-finger, extraoral, and finger assist.

3. Select the correct working-end of an area-specific curet for use in a toe-down or toe-up position on the mesial and distal tooth surfaces.

4. Demonstrate horizontal strokes in a proximal root concavity, and explain the rationale for using horizontal strokes in concavities.

5. Demonstrate horizontal strokes in the concavity located between the cemento-enamel junction and the furcation area of multirooted teeth, and explain the rationale for using horizontal strokes in this area.

6. Demonstrate horizontal strokes at the distofacial and distolingual line angles, and explain the rational for using horizontal strokes at line angles.

7. Demonstrate instrumentation of the furcation area on a mandibular first molar.

8. Demonstrate instrumentation of the furcations on a maxillary first molar from the facial aspect. Instrument only those furcations that are best accessed from the facial aspect.

9. Demonstrate instrumentation of the furcations on a maxillary first molar from the lingual aspect. Instrument only those furcations that are best accessed from the lingual aspect.

10. Demonstrate an opposite arch fulcrum with a finger assist on the proximal surfaces of a maxillary first molar.

Section 1
Fulcruming Techniques

INTRODUCTION TO FULCRUMING TECHNIQUES

A fulcrum is a finger rest used to stabilize the clinician's hand during periodontal debridement. There are three categories of fulcrums.

1. An intraoral fulcrum is stabilization of the clinician's dominant hand by placing the pad of the ring finger on a tooth near to the tooth being instrumented.
2. An extraoral fulcrum is stabilization of the clinician's hand outside the patient's mouth, usually on the chin or cheek. An extraoral fulcrum is useful in gaining access to root surfaces within deep periodontal pockets.
3. An advanced fulcrum is a variation of an intraoral or extraoral finger rest used to gain access to root surfaces within deep periodontal pockets.

STANDARD INTRAORAL FULCRUM

Fulcruming the ring finger on a tooth provides stability while working in a patient's mouth with sharp instruments. A standard intraoral fulcrum provides the best stability for the clinician's hand, decreases the likelihood of injury to the patient or clinician, and provides the best leverage and strength during instrumentation.

TABLE 23-1. The Standard Intraoral Fulcrum	
Technique	Tip of ring finger rests on a stable tooth surface
Location	On the same arch as the treatment area, near the tooth being instrumented
Advantages	• Provides the most stable, secure support for the hand
	• Provides leverage and power for instrumentation
	• Provides excellent tactile transfer to the fingers
	• Allows hand and instrument to work together effectively
	• Permits precise stroke control
	• Allows forceful stroke pressure with the least amount of stress to the hand and fingers
	• Decreases the likelihood of injury to the patient if he or she moves unexpectedly during instrumentation
Disadvantages	• May be difficult to obtain parallelism of the lower shank to the tooth surface for access to deep pockets
	• May not be practical for use in edentulous areas

ADVANCED FULCRUMING TECHNIQUES

There are times when it is difficult to obtain parallelism with the lower shank or to adapt the cutting edge when using a standard intraoral fulcrum. In instances in which a standard intraoral fulcrum doesn't seem to work well, an advanced fulcruming technique can improve access to the tooth surface. For example, when working within a deep periodontal pocket, sometimes it is difficult to position the lower shank parallel to the root surface being treated. This is especially true for the maxillary molars. In such instances, advanced fulcruming techniques are useful in obtaining parallelism.

1. Advanced fulcruming techniques require greater clinician skill and are helpful when working in areas of limited access, such as a narrow deep pocket.
2. Advanced fulcrums should be used selectively in areas of limited access and/or to maintain neutral body position.
3. Advanced fulcruming techniques are not intended to replace the intraoral fulcrum because it places the least amount of strain on the clinician's muscles. An advanced fulcrum should be used if an intraoral fulcrum is not effective or possible.
4. Before attempting advanced fulcruming techniques, the clinician should have mastered the fundamentals of neutral position and standard fulcruming technique.
   a. Bad habits with fundamental techniques cannot be corrected by the use of advanced fulcrums.
   b. A clinician with poor fundamental techniques will compound his or her problems by attempting to use advanced fulcrums. Unorthodox methods of instrumentation may serve as a quick fix for achieving an end product, but usually at the expense of the clinician's musculoskeletal system.
   c. Before attempting advanced fulcruming techniques, the student should self-evaluate his or her skill level with a standard intraoral fulcrum and request a critique from an instructor.

TABLE 23-2. Benefits and Drawbacks of Advanced Fulcruming Techniques	
Advantages	**Disadvantages**
• Easier access to maxillary second and third molars	• Require a greater degree of muscle coordination and instrumentation skill to achieve calculus removal
• Easier access to deep pockets on molar teeth	• Greater risk for instrument stick
• Improved parallelism of the lower shank to molar teeth	• Reduce tactile information to the fingers
• Facilitate neutral wrist position for molar teeth	• May cause more muscle strain
	• Not well tolerated by patients with limited opening or temporomandibular joint problems

SUMMARY SHEET: ADVANCED FULCRUMING TECHNIQUES

	TABLE 23-3. Advanced Fulcruming Techniques	
Type		**Description**
Modified Intraoral		Intraoral fulcrum with an altered point of contact between the middle and ring fingers in the grasp
Cross Arch		Intraoral fulcrum in which the finger rest is established on opposite side of arch from the treatment area
Opposite Arch		Intraoral fulcrum in which the finger rest is established on opposite arch from the treatment area
Finger-on-Finger		Intraoral fulcrum in which a finger of the nondominant hand serves as the resting point for the dominant hand
Basic Extraoral		Extraoral fulcrum in which the dominant hand rests against the patient's chin or cheek
Finger Assist		A finger of the nondominant hand is used to concentrate lateral pressure against the tooth surface and help control the instrument stroke

MODIFIED INTRAORAL FULCRUM

The modified intraoral fulcrum is achieved by combining an altered modified pen grasp with a standard intraoral fulcrum. This technique is particularly useful when instrumenting the maxillary teeth. It involves altering the point of contact between the middle and ring fingers in the grasp. In a standard modified pen grasp, the middle and ring fingers contact one another near the tips of the fingers. For the modified intraoral fulcrum, the middle and ring fingers contact one another near the middle knuckle region of the fingers. The modified intraoral fulcrum should not be confused with a split fulcrum. In a split fulcrum, there is no contact between the middle and ring fingers.

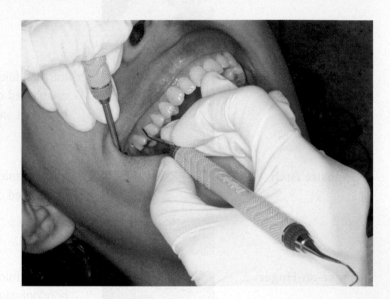

The Modified Intraoral Fulcrum. This photograph shows a right-handed clinician demonstrating a modified intraoral fulcrum. The clinician rests the ring finger of her right hand on the maxillary centrals. This fulcrum provides stable support for the clinician's hand while improving access to the difficult to reach proximal root surfaces of the maxillary molars.

CROSS ARCH FULCRUM

The cross arch fulcrum is accomplished by resting the ring finger on a tooth on the opposite side of the arch from the teeth being instrumented (e.g., resting on the left side of the mandible to instrument a mandibular right molar).

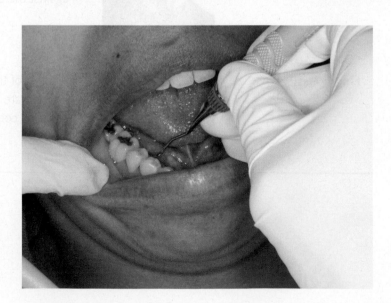

Cross Arch Fulcrum. This photograph shows a cross arch fulcrum demonstrated by a right-handed clinician. The clinician fulcrums on the mandibular left premolars while instrumenting the lingual aspect of the mandibular right posteriors.

OPPOSITE ARCH FULCRUM

The opposite arch fulcrum is an advanced fulcrum used to improve access to deep pockets and to facilitate parallelism to proximal root surfaces. It is accomplished by resting the ring finger on the arch opposite the treatment area (e.g., resting on the mandibular arch to instrument maxillary teeth).

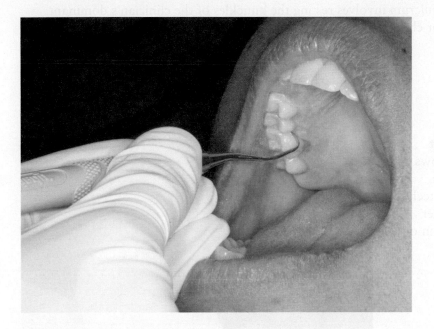

Opposite Arch Fulcrum. In this example, an opposite arch fulcrum rests on the mandibular anterior teeth.

FINGER-ON-FINGER FULCRUM

The finger-on-finger fulcrum is accomplished by resting the ring finger of the dominant hand on the index finger of the **nondominant** hand. This technique allows the clinician to fulcrum in line with the long axis of the tooth to improve parallelism of the lower shank to the tooth surface. The nondominant index finger provides a stable rest for the clinician's dominant hand and provides improved access to deep periodontal pockets.

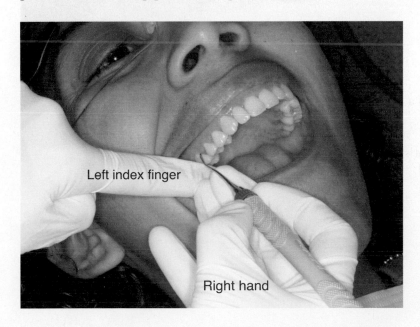

Left index finger

Right hand

Finger-on-Finger Fulcrum. This photograph shows a finger-on-finger fulcrum used by a right-handed clinician. The fulcrum finger of the right hand rests on the index finger of the clinician's left hand.

BASIC EXTRAORAL FULCRUMS

The basic extraoral fulcrum involves resting the fingers or palm of the hand against the patient's chin or cheeks.

Knuckle-Rest Technique

One technique for an extraoral fulcrum involves resting the knuckles of the clinician's dominant hand against the patient's chin or cheek.

Extraoral Fulcrum—Knuckle-Rest Technique. This photograph shows a basic extraoral fulcrum using the knuckle-rest technique. For this technique, the clinician rests his or her knuckles against the patient's chin or cheek.

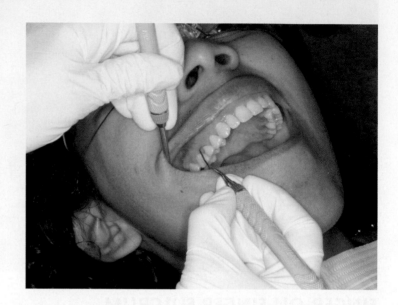

Chin-Cup Technique

Another technique for an extraoral fulcrum involves the clinician cupping the patient's chin in the palm of his or her dominant hand.

Extraoral Fulcrum—Chin-Cup Technique This photograph shows a basic extraoral fulcrum using the chin-cup technique. For this technique, the clinician cups the patient's chin in the palm of his or her hand.

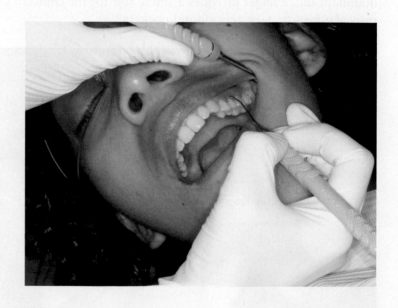

FINGER ASSIST FULCRUM

A finger assist fulcrum is accomplished by using the index finger of the nondominant hand *against the shank* of a periodontal instrument to assist in the instrumentation stroke. The finger of the non-dominant hand is placed against the instrument shank to (1) concentrate lateral pressure against the tooth surface and (2) help control the working-end throughout the instrumentation stroke. The finger assist fulcrum can be combined with a basic intraoral fulcrum; however, most commonly a finger assist fulcrum is used with an extraoral fulcrum or an opposite arch fulcrum. The combination of a finger assist fulcrum with another advanced fulcruming technique, such as an opposite arch fulcrum, is an extremely effective technique for removing calculus deposits from root surfaces located within deep periodontal pockets.

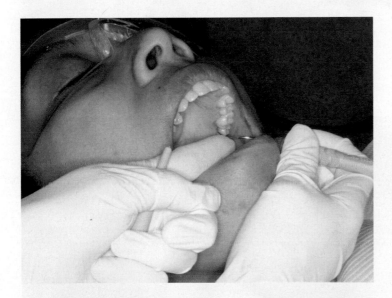

Finger Assist Fulcrum—Example 1. This photograph shows a right-handed clinician applying a finger assist fulcrum behind the instrument shank. Here, the clinician is debriding the distal surface of the maxillary first molar.

The clinician is using an extraoral arch fulcrum.

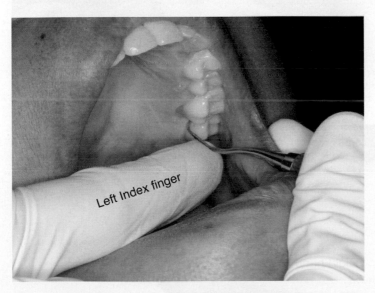

Left Index finger

Example 1—close-up view. This photograph is a closer view of the finger assist fulcrum pictured above. The clinician is using the index finger of the left hand to apply pressure behind the shank, thus *concentrating lateral pressure with the cutting edge forward against the distal surface* of the first molar.

Finger Assist Fulcrum—Example 2.
This photograph shows a finger assist fulcrum demonstrated by a right-handed clinician on the lingual aspect of the maxillary left posteriors. The clinician uses the index finger of the left hand to apply pressure against the instrument shank.

The clinician is using an opposite arch fulcrum on the mandibular arch.

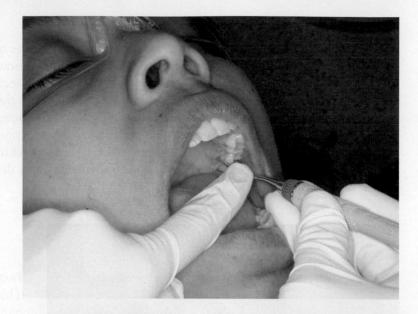

Example 2—close-up view. This photograph is a closer view of the finger assist fulcrum pictured above. The clinician uses the index finger of the left hand to apply pressure against the shank, thus *concentrating lateral pressure with the cutting edge against the mesial surface* of the first molar.

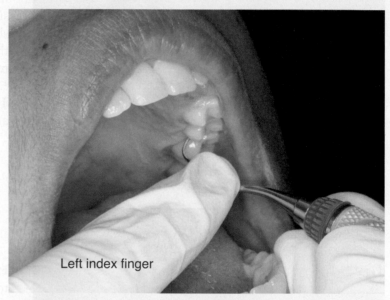

Left index finger

Finger Assist Fulcrum—Example 3.
This photograph shows a finger assist fulcrum on the mandibular anteriors. The right-handed clinician—seated behind the patient—positions the left index finger on the shank to stabilize a short horizontal stroke. The finger assist fulcrum helps the clinician to control the horizontal strokes by concentrating pressure precisely on the cutting edge.

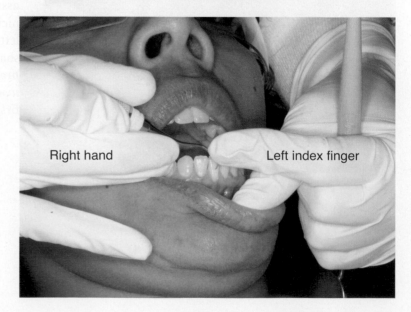

Right hand

Left index finger

Section 2
Anatomical Features That Complicate Instrumentation

ROOT CONCAVITIES AND DEPRESSIONS

Root surface morphology can greatly complicate instrumentation, especially when the roots are hidden from view within deep periodontal pockets. These anatomical features include root concavities and depressions and, occasionally, root fissures. The Technique Practice, located in Section 3 of this module, explains how to use horizontal strokes to remove calculus from root concavities and depressions.

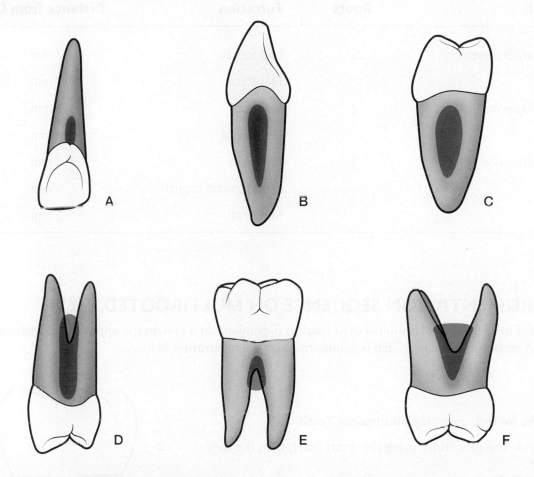

Root Concavities, Depressions, and Fissures. Examples of root surface morphology (shaded areas) that can hinder debridement:

A. *Palatal groove* on mandibular lateral incisor that extends onto the cervical third of the root surface.

B. *Deep, linear root concavities* on the proximal surfaces of mandibular canine.

C. *Wide, shallow root concavity* on the mesial surface of mandibular molar.

D. *Deep, linear, proximal root concavities* and *furcation* on maxillary first premolar.

E. *Deep depression on root trunk* and *furcation* on mandibular molar.

F. *Proximal concavities* extending from the *furcation* to cemento-enamel junction on maxillary molar.

ROOT FURCATIONS

Instrumentation is complicated on molar teeth when furcation areas are exposed because of bone loss. Furcation exposure can be encountered in pockets as shallow as 4 mm in depth. Gher and Vernino[1] demonstrated that furcations could be located at as little as 3 mm from the cemento-enamel junction (Table 23-1).

TABLE 23-4.	**Location of Furcations**		
Tooth	**Roots**	**Furcation**	**Distance from CEJ**
Maxillary first premolar	2	Mid-mesial	7 mm
		Mid-distal	7 mm
Mandibular molar	2	Mid-facial	3 mm
		Mid-lingual	4 mm
Maxillary molar	3	Mid-facial	4 mm
		Mesial toward lingual	3 mm
		Mid-distal	5 mm

INSTRUMENTATION SEQUENCE ON MULTIROOTED TEETH

Successful debridement of a multirooted tooth is dependent on a systematic approach to instrumentation. A recommended approach is summarized on the illustration below.

Sequence for Instrumenting Multirooted Teeth

1. Debride the root trunk using the distal curet, then the mesial curet.
2. Treat each root as a separate tooth. Use the distal curet on the distal portion of each root.
3. Use the mesial curet on the mesial portions of each root.
4. Treat the roof of the furcation and the concavity coronal to the furcation entrance with the mesial curet.
   a. Use the toe of the curet against the roof of the furcation.
   b. Position the curet in a toe-down position, and use horizontal strokes in the concavity.

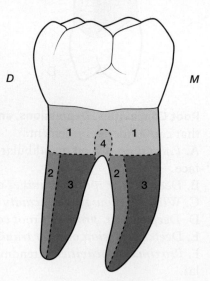

Section 3
Technique Practice: Horizontal Strokes

Working-end selection requires some thought when using an area-specific curet in a toe-down or toe-up position for horizontal strokes. Because area-specific curets have only one working-cutting edge per working-end, it is necessary to use the other working-end when making horizontal strokes on mesial and distal surfaces.

DIRECTIONS:

1. For this technique practice, you need (1) a periodontal typodont or an acrylic mandibular molar, (2) Gracey 11/12 and 13/14 standard, miniature, or extended shank curets, (3) a container of brightly colored nail polish, and (4) a bottle of nail polish remover.
2. On each working-end, paint the *lower cutting edge and its lateral surface* with nail polish.
3. Follow steps 4 through 6 to practice selecting the correct working-end for horizontal strokes with an area-specific curet.

HORIZONTAL STROKES ON MESIAL AND DISTAL SURFACES

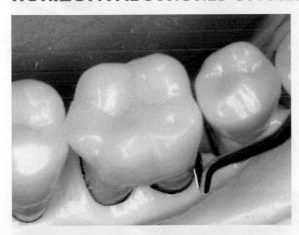

4. **Vertical Strokes on Mesial Surface.** Adapt the Gracey 11 curet to the *mesial surface of a mandibular right molar.* Note that the lower cutting edge with the nail polish is adapted against the mesial surface. The Gracey 11 is the correct working-end for making vertical strokes across the mesial surface.

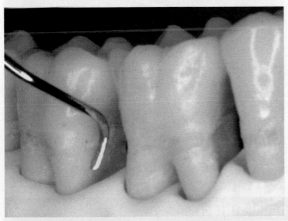

5. **Horizontal Strokes on Mesial Surface.** Next, position the Gracey 11 in a toe-down position and adapt it to the mesial surface. Note that the lower cutting edge colored with the nail polish is not adapted to the mesial surface.

The correct working-end is the Gracey 12 when making horizontal strokes on the proximal surface of the mandibular right molar from the facial aspect.

Box 23-1. Horizontal Strokes on Proximal Surfaces

Switch working-ends to make horizontal strokes on either the distal or mesial surface of a tooth. For distal surfaces, if the G13 is used for vertical strokes, use the G14 for horizontal strokes. For mesial surfaces, if the G11 is used for vertical strokes, use the G12 for horizontal strokes.

6. **Horizontal Strokes on Distal Surface.** Select the correct working-end of a G13/14 curet for use on the distal surface when making vertical strokes.

   Now position the same curet in a toe-down position on the distal surface. Again, the lower cutting edge is not adapted to the distal surface. The opposite working-end is the correct one to use with horizontal strokes on the distal surface.

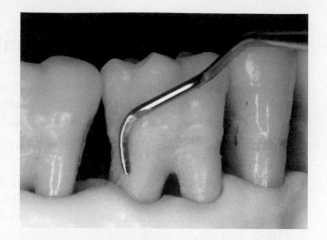

HORIZONTAL STROKES ON FACIAL AND LINGUAL SURFACES

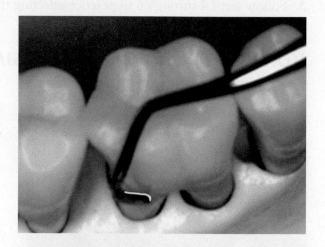

7. **Oblique Strokes on Facial Surface.** Select the correct working-end of a G11/12 curet for use on the facial surface. Note that the lower cutting edge with the nail polish is adapted against the facial surface.

8. **Horizontal Strokes on Facial Surface.** Reposition the same working-end in a toe-down position for horizontal strokes. The same working-end is used for both oblique and horizontal strokes on the facial surface of the molar.

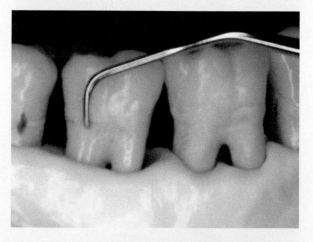

Box 23-2. Horizontal Strokes on Facial and Lingual Surfaces

There is no need to switch working-ends to make horizontal strokes on either the facial or lingual surface of a tooth.

Section 4
Technique Practice: Maxillary Arch

DIRECTIONS: Miniature area-specific curets with extended shanks such as the Hu-Friedy Mini Five are recommended for this technique practice. This technique practice is best accomplished on a periodontal typodont.

MAXILLARY RIGHT POSTERIORS, FACIAL ASPECT—DISTAL SURFACES

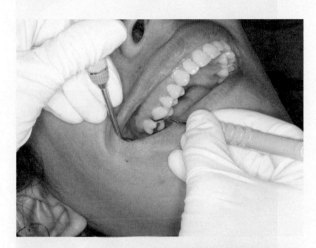

Technique Summary for Distal Surfaces of Facial Aspect
1. Extraoral fulcrum using knuckle-rest technique
2. Thumb provides lateral pressure forward against distal surfaces
3. Vertical and oblique strokes

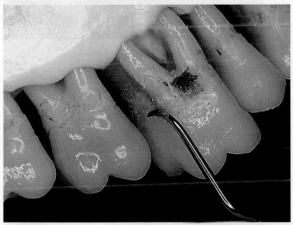

4. **Distal Concavity of First Molar.** Use the distal curet. Rotate the handle slightly to adapt the toe-third of the cutting edge to the distal concavity.

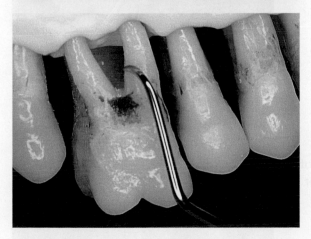

5. **Distal Portion of the Mesial Root.** Use the distal curet on the distal portion of the mesial root.

MAXILLARY RIGHT POSTERIORS, FACIAL ASPECT—MESIAL SURFACES

Technique Summary for Mesial Surfaces of Facial Aspect

1. Extraoral fulcrum using knuckle-rest technique
2. Index finger provides lateral pressure back against mesial surfaces
3. Vertical and oblique strokes

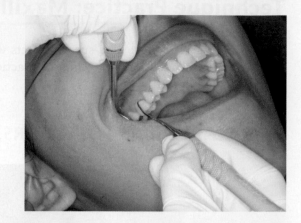

4. **Mesial Portion of the Distal Root.** Use the mesial curet on the mesial portion of the distal root.

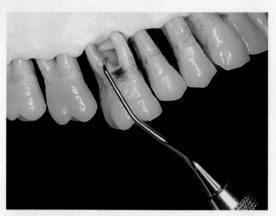

5. **Mesial Portion of the Distal Root—close-up view.** The mesial curet is used to debride the mesial portion of the distal root and the roof of the furcation.

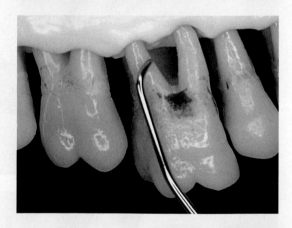

6. **Mesial Surface of the First Premolar.** The maxillary first premolar has the deepest concavity in the entire dentition. Use the mesial curet to debride the mesial concavity. Rotate the toe-third of the cutting edge toward the root surface to adapt to the concavity.

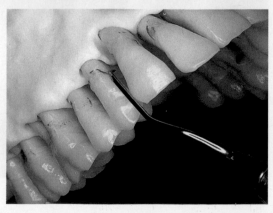

CURET TOE-UP, HORIZONTAL STROKES—DISTAL CONCAVITIES

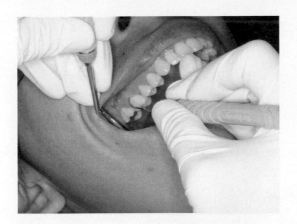

Technique Summary for Distal Concavities
1. Modified intraoral fulcrum
2. Working-end in the toe-up position with Gracey miniature 7 or 13 curet
3. Thumb provides lateral pressure forward against distal concavity
4. Short horizontal strokes

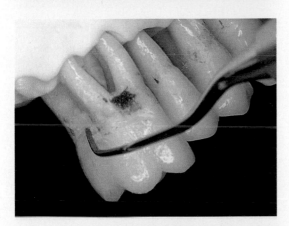

5. **Distal Concavity of First Molar.** Use a distal curet in the distal concavity; the Gracey miniature 7/8 works well in this area. Use the opposite working-end from the one that you used to make vertical strokes on the distal.

   Use the curet in a toe-up position, adapt the lower cutting edge, and make a series of horizontal strokes. This technique facilitates calculus removal from the concavity.

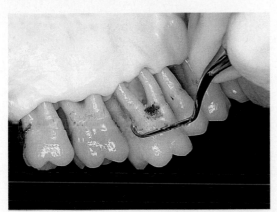

6. **Distal Concavity and Distofacial Line Angle.** After making a series of horizontal strokes in the distal concavity, make a series of short horizontal strokes around the distofacial line angle.

   The line angle is one of the most common places where calculus deposits are missed. Making horizontal strokes around the line angle is the best technique to avoid missing deposits in this area.

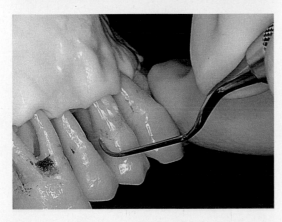

7. **Distal Concavity of First Premolar.** Use the distal curet in a toe-up position to make a series of short controlled horizontal strokes in the distal concavity.

CURET TOE-UP, HORIZONTAL STROKES—MESIAL CONCAVITIES

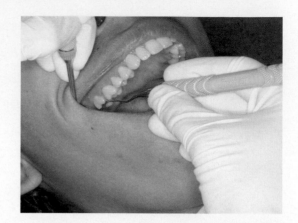

Technique Summary for Facial and Mesial Concavities
1. Extraoral fulcrum
2. Working-end in the toe-up position
3. Thumb provides lateral pressure on the facial concavity; index finger provides lateral pressure on the mesial root concavity.
4. Short horizontal strokes

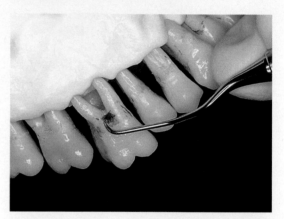

5. **Facial Concavity.** A common area for missed calculus deposits is the broad concavity that extends from the furcation to the cemento-enamel junction on molar teeth. Use the Gracey miniature 12 curet in a toe-up position to make short horizontal strokes in the depression.

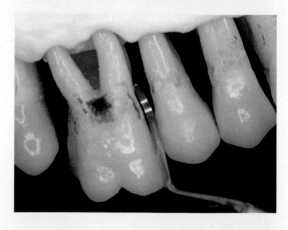

6. **Mesial Concavity of Molar.** Use the Gracey miniature 11 curet in a toe-up position to make horizontal strokes in the concavity. This is the opposite working-end from the one you would use to make vertical strokes on the mesial surface.

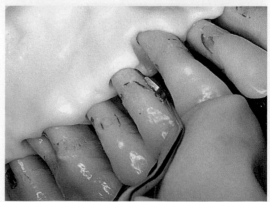

7. **Mesial Concavity of Premolar.** Use the Gracey miniature 11 curet in a toe-up position to make horizontal strokes in the concavity.

MAXILLARY LEFT POSTERIORS, LINGUAL ASPECT—DISTAL SURFACES

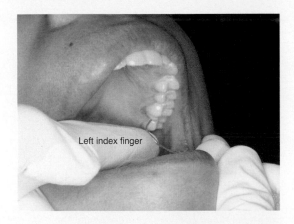

Left index finger

Technique Summary for Distal Surfaces
1. Extraoral fulcrum with a finger assist
2. Index finger of nondominant hand provides lateral pressure forward against distal surface
3. Vertical strokes

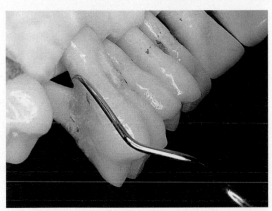

4. **Distal Concavity.** Use a distal curet to debride the distal concavity with vertical strokes. It is important to rotate the toe-third of the curet to adapt to the concavity.

   Use the index finger of your nondominant hand to apply pressure behind the shank, thus *concentrating pressure with the cutting edge forward against the distal surface* of the first molar.

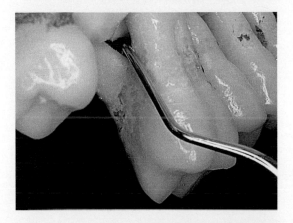

5. **Distal Furcation.** The distal furcation entrance is located near the midline of the tooth and therefore can be instrumented from both the facial and lingual aspects.

   Use the distal curet to instrument the distal furcation.

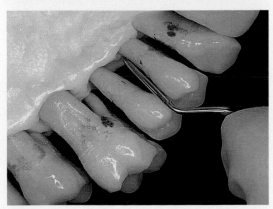

6. **Distal Surface of Premolar.** Use the distal curet on the distal surface. Use the index finger of your nondominant hand to apply pressure behind the shank, thus *concentrating pressure with the cutting edge forward against the distal surface* of the premolar.

MAXILLARY LEFT POSTERIORS, LINGUAL ASPECT—MESIAL SURFACES

Technique Summary for Mesial Surfaces
1. Extraoral fulcrum with a finger assist
2. Index finger of nondominant hand provides lateral pressure back against mesial surface
3. Vertical strokes

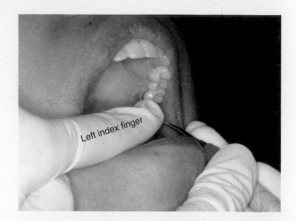

4. **Lingual Surface of Palatal Root.** The palatal root commonly has a deep depression. Use the mesial curet to make a series of small overlapping vertical and oblique strokes. Use the index finger of your nondominant hand to apply pressure against the shank, thus *concentrating pressure with the cutting edge against the lingual surface* of the first molar.

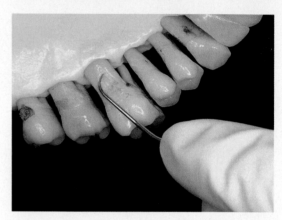

5. **Mesial Furcation.** The entrance to the mesial furcation is located toward the lingual aspect, rather than at the midline of the mesial surface. Because of its location, the entrance is best accessed from the lingual aspect using a mesial curet.

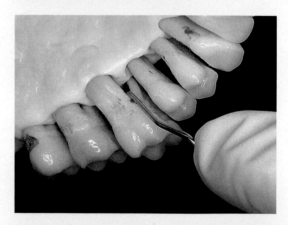

6. **Mesial Furcation—close-up view.** Use the mesial curet to instrument the furcation.

Use the index finger of your nondominant hand to apply pressure against the shank, thus *concentrating pressure with the cutting edge back against the mesial surface* of the first molar.

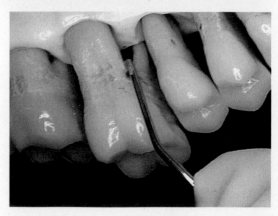

CURET TOE-UP, HORIZONTAL STROKES—DISTAL CONCAVITIES

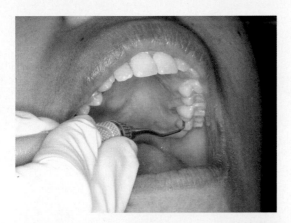

Technique Summary for Distal Concavities
1. Cross arch fulcrum
2. Working-end in the toe-up position
3. Index finger provides lateral pressure forward against distal surface; thumb provides lateral pressure on the lingual surface
4. Short horizontal strokes

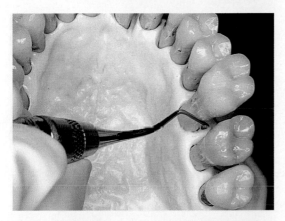

5. **Distal Concavity of Molar.** The linear concavities often are difficult to debride using vertical strokes.

   Use the miniature curet in a toe-up position (toward the palate) with horizontal strokes to debride the concavity. This is the opposite working-end from the one you would use to make vertical strokes on the distal surface.

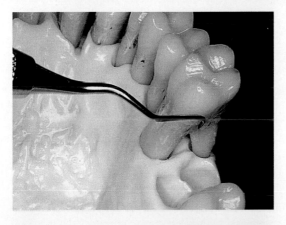

6. **Distal Concavity—close-up view.** Use the distal curet in a toe-up position. Make a series of controlled horizontal strokes.

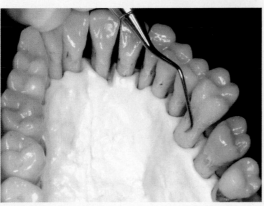

7. **Palatal Root Depression.** The palatal root has a narrow root depression that is difficult to instrument using vertical strokes.

   Use the miniature curet in a toe-up position with a series of short horizontal strokes. Begin making strokes at the base of the pocket, then move coronally slightly, and repeat the process.

MAXILLARY ANTERIORS, FACIAL ASPECT

Technique Summary for Facial Aspect
1. Standard intraoral
2. Working-end in the toe-up position
3. Thumb provides lateral pressure against the facial surface
4. Short horizontal strokes

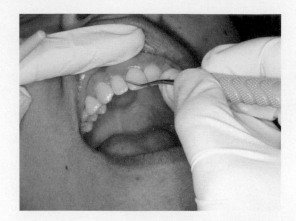

5. **Mesial Surface.** Use an anterior curet in a toe-up position on the mesial surface of the maxillary right central. Make short horizontal stokes across the distal surface and around the line angle of the tooth.

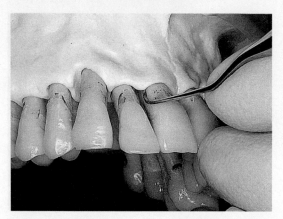

6. **Facial Surface.** The roots of anterior teeth are narrow, and it can be difficult to use vertical strokes when working within a deep pocket. Instead, use the curet in a toe-up position, and make a series of horizontal strokes on the root surface.

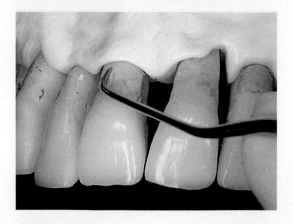

MAXILLARY ANTERIORS, LINGUAL ASPECT

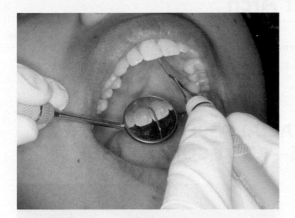

Technique Summary for Lingual Aspect Using Vertical Strokes
1. Opposite arch fulcrum with a finger assist
2. Thumb provides lateral pressure against the lingual surface
3. Vertical strokes

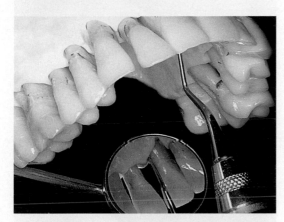

4. **Lingual and Mesial Surfaces.** Use an opposite arch fulcrum with an anterior curet. Note that the root tapers toward the lingual.

   Use the index finger of your nondominant hand to apply pressure against the shank.

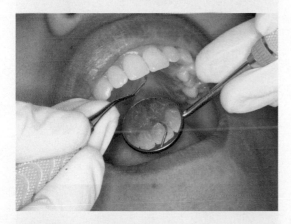

Technique Summary for Lingual Aspect Using Horizontal Strokes
1. Standard intraoral fulcrum
2. Working-end in a toe-up position
3. Index finger provides pressure against lingual surface
4. Short horizontal strokes

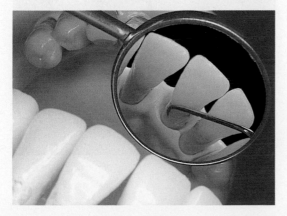

5. **Lingual Aspect.** The root of the maxillary central tapers toward the lingual, making the root very narrow on the lingual surface. Use an anterior curet in a toe-up position to make short horizontal strokes.

Section 5
Technique Practice: Mandibular Arch

DIRECTIONS: Miniature area-specific curets with extended shanks such as the Hu-Friedy Mini Five are recommended for this technique practice. This technique practice is best accomplished on a and periodontal typodont.

MANDIBULAR RIGHT POSTERIORS, FACIAL ASPECT AND CURET TOE-DOWN, HORIZONTAL STROKES—ROOT CONCAVITIES

Furcation—Facial Aspect

1. Standard intraoral fulcrum
2. Working-end in a toe-down position
3. Thumb lateral provides pressure
4. Short horizontal strokes

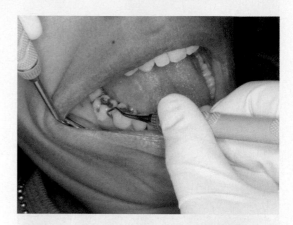

5. **Distal Root Concavity.** Use a distal curet in a toe-down position. Make a series of short, horizontal strokes.

   After instrumenting the concavity, make a series of short horizontal strokes around the distofacial line angle.

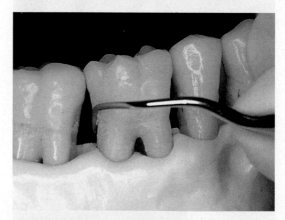

6. **Distal Concavity of Premolar.** Use a distal curet in a toe-down position with horizontal strokes to debride the distal root concavity of the first premolar.

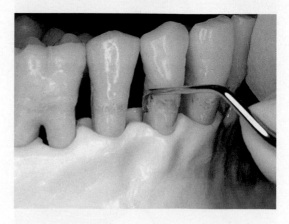

MANDIBULAR ANTERIORS

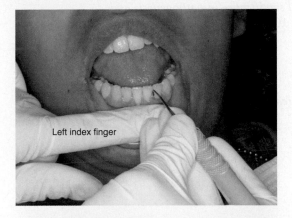

Left index finger

Facial Aspect—Mesial Surface
1. Finger-on-finger fulcrum
2. Working-end in a toe-down position
3. Thumb lateral provides pressure
4. Short horizontal strokes

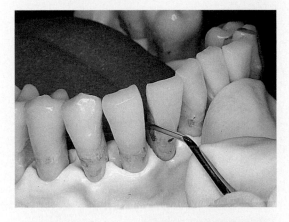

5. **Mesial Concavity.** Use an anterior curet in a toe-down position. Make a series of short horizontal strokes in the mesial root concavity.

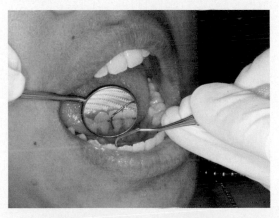

Lingual Aspect—Lingual Surface
1. Standard intraoral fulcrum
2. Working-end in a toe-down position
3. Thumb lateral provides pressure
4. Short horizontal strokes

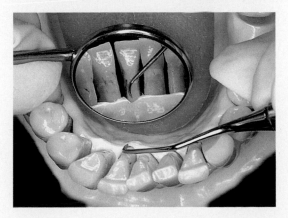

5. **Lingual Aspect.** The lingual root surfaces of the mandibular anteriors are very narrow. It is often difficult to make vertical strokes on these surfaces because the curet is wider than the pocket.

Use the curet in a toe-down position. Begin at the base of the pocket, and make a series of very short horizontal strokes across the lingual surface. Work your way up the root surface.

REFERENCE

1. Gher, M.E. and A.R. Vernino. *Root morphology—clinical significance in pathogenesis and treatment of periodontal disease.* J Am Dent Assoc, 1980. **101**(4): 627–633.

SUGGESTED READING

Bower, R. C. *Furcation morphology relative to periodontal treatment. Furcation root surface anatomy.* J Periodontol, 1979. **50**(7): 366–374.

Section 6
Skill Application

PRACTICAL FOCUS

Complete the following chart.

Tooth	Anatomical Considerations for Instrumentation	Instrumentation Techniques
Example: Mandibular second molar	1. *Mesial and distal root concavity* 2. *Facial concavity above furcation* 3. *Bifurcation*	1. *Curet toe-down, horizontal strokes* 2. *Curet toe-down, horizontal strokes* 3. *Debride each root as a separate tooth: distal curet for distal portions of each root; mesial curet for mesial portions of roots and for roof of the concavity*
Mandibular central incisor		
Maxillary canine		

Tooth	Anatomical Considerations for Instrumentation	Instrumentation Techniques
Maxillary first premolar		
Mandibular first premolar		
Mandibular first molar		
Maxillary first molar		

Student: _____

Evaluator: _____

Date: _____

DIRECTIONS FOR STUDENT: Use **Column S.** Evaluate your skill level as: **S** (satisfactory) or **U** (unsatisfactory).

DIRECTIONS FOR EVALUATOR: Use **Column E.** Indicate: **S** (satisfactory) or **U** (unsatisfactory). Each **S** equals 1 point, each **U** equals 0 points.

CRITERIA:	S	E
Right-Handed Clinicians—Maxillary Left Posteriors, Lingual Aspect:		
Left-Handed Clinicians—Maxillary Right Posteriors, Lingual Aspect:		
Selects an appropriate curet and demonstrates an opposite arch fulcrum with a finger assist for the distal surface of the first molar		
Selects an appropriate curet and demonstrates an opposite arch fulcrum with a finger assist for the mesial surface of the first molar		
Selects an appropriate curet and demonstrates instrumentation of the distal furcation on the first molar tooth (on typodont or tooth model)		
Selects an appropriate curet and demonstrates instrumentation of the mesial furcation on the first molar tooth. States whether the mesial furcation should be accessed from the facial or lingual aspect and explains the rationale		
Right-Handed Clinicians—Maxillary Right Posteriors, Facial Aspect:		
Left-Handed Clinicians—Maxillary Left Posteriors, Facial Aspect:		
Selects an appropriate curet and demonstrates a modified fulcrum for this sextant		
Selects an appropriate curet and demonstrates instrumentation of the broad facial concavity adjacent to the furcation area		
Selects an appropriate curet and demonstrates the toe-up technique for the instrumentation of the mesial concavity on the first premolar		
Right-Handed Clinicians—Maxillary Left Posteriors, Lingual Aspect:		
Left-Handed Clinicians—Maxillary Right Posteriors, Lingual Aspect:		
Selects an appropriate curet and demonstrates a cross arch fulcrum for this sextant		
Selects an appropriate curet and demonstrates the toe-up technique for the instrumentation of the distal root concavity on the first molar		
Selects an appropriate curet and demonstrates the toe-up technique for the instrumentation of the palatal root depression		
Mandibular Anteriors, Facial Aspect, Surfaces Toward:		
Selects an appropriate curet and, using a basic intraoral fulcrum, demonstrates the use of the curet in a toe-down technique on the central incisor, surface toward		
OPTIONAL GRADE PERCENTAGE CALCULATION Total **S**'s in each E column.		

Sum of **S**'s _____ divided by Total Points Possible (**11**) equals the Percentage Grade _____

| SKILL EVALUATION MODULE 23 | ADVANCED TECHNIQUES FOR ROOT SURFACE DEBRIDEMENT |

Student: _____

EVALUATOR COMMENTS

_____

_____

_____

_____

_____

_____

_____

_____

_____

_____

_____

_____

_____

_____

_____

_____

_____

_____

_____

Box for sketches pertaining to written comments.

Ultrasonic and Sonic Instrumentation

Module Overview

Electronically powered instrumentation uses rapid energy vibrations of a powered instrument tip to fracture calculus from the tooth surface and clean the environment of the periodontal pocket. This module presents principles of electronically powered instrumentation with sonic, magnetostrictive ultrasonic, and piezoelectric devices.

Module Outline

Key Terms

Electronically powered
    instrumentation
Slim-diameter
    instrument tips
Water-cooled
    instrument tip
Deplaquing
Fluid lavage

Cavitation
Acoustic turbulence
Frequency
Stroke
Resonant frequency
Automatically tuned
    ultrasonic devices

Manually tuned
    ultrasonic devices
Sonic devices
Piezoelectric ultrasonic
    devices
Magnetostrictive
    ultrasonic devices
Active tip area

Pre-procedural rinse
Tapping motions
Sweeping motions
Oblique "curet"
    technique
Vertical "probe"
    technique
Overhang removal

Learning Objectives

1. Discuss the role of electronically powered instrumentation in periodontal debridement.

2. Discuss the history and technological advances of electronically powered instrumentation.

3. Compare and contrast the advantages and limitations of electronically powered instrumentation.

4. Discuss the use of electronically powered instrumentation in the dental hygiene treatment plan to facilitate and enhance periodontal debridement.

5. Compare and contrast sonic and ultrasonic devices.

6. Compare and contrast automatically and manually tuned ultrasonic devices.

7. Compare and contrast standard and slim instrument tip design.

8. Identify pretreatment considerations before the initiation of electronically powered instrumentation.

9. Discuss medical and dental contraindications for electronically powered instrumentation.

10. Discuss criteria for the selection of instrument tips.

11. Explain proper infection control for electronically powered instrumentation.

12. Prepare an electronically powered device for use.

13. Select appropriate instrument tips for the patient case.

14. Demonstrate correct technique for use of an ultrasonic device, including treatment room and patient preparation, patient/clinician positioning, armamentarium selection/set-up, cord management, grasp, fulcrum, tip activation, tip insertion, stroke, and fluid evacuation.

15. Demonstrate the correct amount of stroke pressure and different strokes used with an electronically powered instrument.

16. Properly maintain electronically powered instruments.

Section I
Introduction to Electronically Powered Instrumentation

HISTORY OF ELECTRONICALLY POWERED DEVICES

Electronically powered instrumentation uses rapid energy vibrations of a powered instrument tip to fracture calculus from the tooth surface and clean the environment of the periodontal pocket. Ultrasonic and sonic devices are electronically powered instruments for the removal of calculus deposits and plaque biofilms. These electronically powered devices were developed with the goal of making calculus removal easier and faster with less patient discomfort and clinician fatigue. Initially introduced in the late 1950s, electronically powered instruments were bulky and limited to removing heavy supragingival calculus deposits. In the late 1980s, slim-diameter instrument tips were developed that are smaller in size than curets. Slim-diameter instrument tips are used to disrupt plaque biofilms and remove calculus deposits from deep periodontal pockets and furcation areas. Modern electronically powered devices have an indispensable role in periodontal debridement.

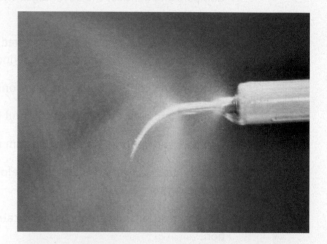

Water-Cooled Instrument Tips. Electronically powered devices use water-cooled instrument tips. Water constantly exists near the point of the instrument tip. (Courtesy of Odonto-Wave.)

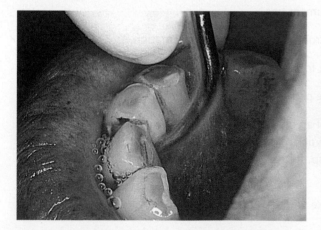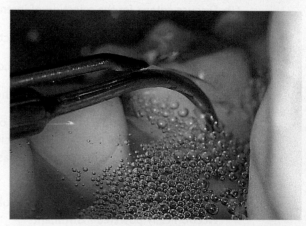

Powered Instrumentation. Rapid energy vibrations of the powered instrument tip fracture calculus from the tooth surface and clean the environment of the periodontal pocket. (Photographs courtesy of Dave Selander, Parkell USA.)

TABLE 24-1.	A Timeline for Electronically Powered Devices
Date	**Event**
Late 1950s	The first electronically powered debridement devices are developed.
1960s & 1970s	Electronically powered devices are used to remove heavy calculus deposits. Bulky instrument tip design limited use to supragingival instrumentation or where tissue allowed easy subgingival insertion. The Gracey curet is the primary instrument for use within periodontal pockets.
Late 1980s	Slim-diameter instrument tips are developed for electronically powered devices. Slim-diameter tips are significantly smaller than the working-end of a standard Gracey curet.
1990s	Research studies established that bacterial products are easily removed from the root surfaces, leading to a new approach to instrumentation and the conservation of cementum.
Today	Modern electronically powered slim-diameter instrument tips have been shown to be as effective as hand instruments for removing subgingival calculus deposits, plaque biofilms, and bacterial products from periodontally involved teeth.

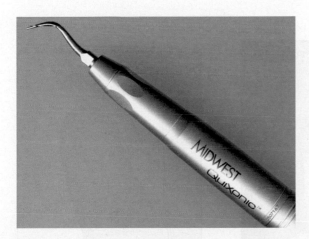

A. **Sonic Device**

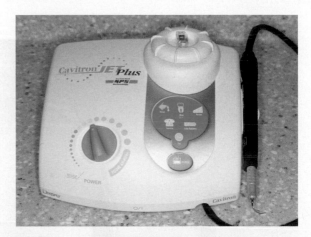

B. **Ultrasonic Device**

There are two types of electronically powered devices: sonic and ultrasonic. Sonic handpieces attach to the dental unit's compressed air line. Ultrasonic devices have an electric generator and do not need to be connected to the dental unit. The two types of ultrasonic devices are the (A) magnetostrictive and (B) piezoelectric ultrasonic units.

EFFECTIVENESS OF ELECTRONICALLY POWERED INSTRUMENTATION

The 1996 World Workshop in Periodontics review of nonsurgical periodontal instrumentation states that the best instrumentation results are probably achieved by the combined use of electronically powered devices and hand-activated instrumentation. Research investigations indicate that electronically powered devices are not only as effective as hand instrumentation but also have some advantages over hand instrumentation.

1. **Removal of Calculus.** Powered instrumentation has been shown to be as effective as hand instrumentation.[1–10]
2. **Removal of Plaque.** Powered instruments are especially effective in deplaquing—the disruption or removal of the subgingival plaque biofilm from root surfaces and the pocket space.[11, 12]
3. **Access to Furcations.** Slim-diameter instrument tips are more effective in treating Class II and III furcations when used by experienced clinicians.[6, 13–15]
4. **Conservation of Cementum.** Used with proper technique, electronically powered instruments used on low or medium power settings seem to do less damage to the root surface than hand instruments.[18, 19]
5. **Pocket Penetration.** Slim-diameter instrument tips penetrate deeper into periodontal pockets than hand instruments.[18, 21–28]
6. **Irrigation (Lavage).** A constant stream of water exits near the point of the electronically powered instrument tip. This water stream within the periodontal pocket is termed the fluid lavage. Water irrigation of the pocket washes toxic products and free-floating bacteria from the pocket and provides better vision during instrumentation by removing blood from the treatment site.[30–33]

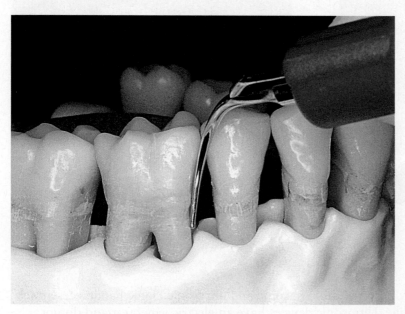
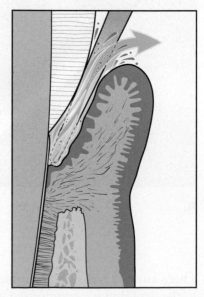

A

B

Pocket Penetration of Tip and Fluid Lavage. A, Slim-diameter instrument tips penetrate deeper into periodontal pockets and reach the base of the pocket better than hand instruments. **B,** Research has shown that the water lavage reaches a depth that is equal to the depth reached by the powered instrument tip.

7. **Bactericidal Effect.** The fluid stream flowing through the powered instrument tip produces two effects that are unique to powered instruments: cavitation and acoustic turbulence. These actions are capable of disrupting bacterial cell walls and may also dislodge plaque biofilms *slightly beyond the reach* of the powered instrument tip.[6, 7, 34, 35]
   a. Just the act of holding an activated ultrasonic tip in the periodontal pocket is destructive to the bacteria. This ability to "destroy from a distance" might be likened to an opera singer's ability to break a glass by singing a certain note.
   b. **Cavitation** is the formation of tiny bubbles in the fluid; when these tiny bubbles collapse, they produce shock waves that destroy bacteria by tearing the bacterial cell walls.
   c. **Acoustic turbulence** is swirling effect produced within the confined space of a periodontal pocket by the continuous stream of fluid flowing over the vibrating instrument tip. This intense swirling effect disrupts the plaque biofilm.
8. **Shorter Instrumentation Time.** Several studies have shown that instrumentation time may be reduced when using powered instruments as compared with hand instruments.[18, 29]

LIMITATIONS OF ELECTRONICALLY POWERED INSTRUMENTATION

1. **Aerosol Production.** Powered instruments have been shown to generate high levels of contaminated aerosols.[36–40]
   a. Dental aerosols are airborne particles dispersed into the surrounding environment by dental equipment such as high-speed handpieces and electronically powered instruments. Microorganisms in the dental aerosols have been shown to survive for up to 24 hours.
   b. Surface disinfection and barriers are particularly important when using electronically powered instruments.
   c. Laminar airflow systems that filter microorganisms from the air can significantly reduce the number of airborne organisms in the dental environment.
   d. The use of antimicrobial mouth rinses before treatment with an electronically powered instrument can reduce bacterial counts in aerosols by about 92 percent.[40]
2. **Effect on Cardiac Pacemakers.** Modern pacemakers are shielded against everyday electromagnetic interference, such as interference from microwave ovens.
   a. In the dental setting, *magnetostrictive* ultrasonic instruments and ultrasonic bath cleaners may interfere with certain styles of cardiac pacemakers.[4, 41–43] *Piezoelectric* ultrasonic devices do not generate a magnetic field and therefore do not interfere with the functioning of cardiac pacemakers.[41–43]
   b. In a recent position paper, the American Academy of Periodontology recommends that dental healthcare workers avoid exposing patients with cardiac pacemakers to magnetostrictive ultrasonic devices.[4]
3. **Reduced Tactile Sensitivity.** Clinicians experience less tactile sensitivity when using powered instruments than when using hand instruments.
4. **Infection Control.**
   1. Infection control can be compromised because some electronically powered devices have components that cannot be sterilized.
   2. When selecting an electronically powered device for purchase, consider whether the unit's handpiece and fluid reservoir bottles (if available) can be autoclaved.

Section 2
Mechanisms of Action

How efficiently an electronically powered instrument removes plaque biofilms and calculus deposits is determined by the instrument tip's vibration frequency, stroke length, stroke motion, and the surface of the instrument tip in contact with the tooth.

FREQUENCY

Electronically powered devices use an electric current to produce rapid vibrations of the instrument tip. Frequency refers to how many times the electronically powered instrument tip vibrates per second.

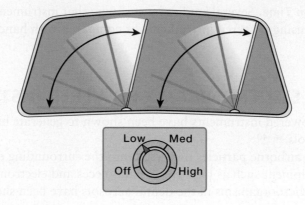

The frequency of an electronically powered instrument can be compared with the settings for the windshield wipers on a car.

1. When the wiper setting is on low, the wipers go back and forth only a few times per minute. Similarly, when the frequency of a powered instrument is low, the instrument tip vibrates fewer times per second.
2. When the wiper setting is on high, the windshield wipers go back and forth many times per minute. Correspondingly, when the frequency of a powered instrument is high, the instrument tip vibrates more times per second.

STROKE

Stroke refers to how far the instrument tip moves during one cycle. Another term for stroke is amplitude. Ultrasonic electronically powered devices have a *power knob* that is used to change the length of the stroke. Higher power delivers a longer, more forceful stroke; lower power delivers a shorter, less forceful stroke.

1. **Lower Power.** Using the example of a child on a swing, low power would be a gentle push against the child's back, causing the swing to move forward a short distance before returning to its starting position. Lower power causes the instrument tip to move a shorter distance.
2. **Higher Power.** Higher power causes the instrument tip to move a longer distance. This is similar to a forceful push against the child's back, causing the swing to travel a long distance before returning to its original position.

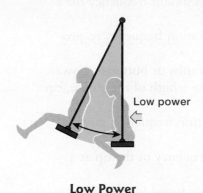

Low power

Low Power

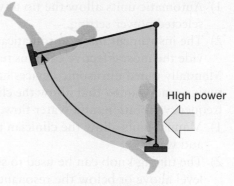

High power

High Power

CONTROLLING STROKE, FREQUENCY, AND WATER FLOW

Ultrasonic devices have controls that allow the clinician to adjust power and water flow. Some ultrasonic devices have a third control that allows the clinician to adjust the frequency.

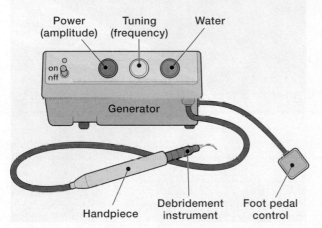

Power (amplitude)   Tuning (frequency)   Water

on off

Generator

Handpiece   Debridement instrument   Foot pedal control

Manually Tuned Ultrasonic Device. Manual ultrasonic devices have three control knobs or buttons—power, tuning, and water—that allow the clinician to adjust the length of the stroke, tip frequency vibration, and water flow.

1. **Power Adjustment.** The power setting on the ultrasonic device determines the length of the stroke—the distance the instrument travels back and forth in one cycle. On ultrasonic devices, the stroke is adjusted by turning the power knob on the ultrasonic unit.
   a. The power levels may be designated as ranges of high, medium, and low or 1, 2, 3, depending on the unit.
   b. Higher power settings deliver a longer, more forceful stroke. Lower power settings deliver a shorter, less powerful stroke. Because the instrument tip strikes the tooth with more force at higher power settings, higher power proves more uncomfortable for the patient and is more likely to damage the tooth surface.
   c. Research investigations found no difference in the effectiveness of ultrasonic instruments when operated at high power levels or medium power levels.[29] Use of the high power setting is not recommended.

2. **Frequency Adjustment—Tuning.** Tuning on ultrasonic devices may be either manual or automatic. In addition to the frequency tuning of the ultrasonic generator, each magnetostrictive ultrasonic instrument tip has its own natural vibration level. This level at which a magnetostrictive instrument insert vibrates naturally is called its resonant frequency.
   a. **Automatically tuned ultrasonic devices** have two control knobs or buttons—power and water—that allow the clinician to adjust the length of the stroke and the water flow.

1) Automatic units allow the tip to vibrate at its own resonant frequency for a selected power setting.
2) The instrument insert automatically adjusts the vibration frequency to provide the most effective calculus removal.

b. **Manually tuned ultrasonic devices** have three control knobs or buttons—power, tuning, and water—that allow the clinician to adjust the length of the stroke, tip frequency vibration, and water flow.
1) Manual units allow the clinician to adjust the vibration frequency, power, and water.
2) The tuning knob can be used to set the vibration frequency of the tip at a level above or below the resonant frequency.
3) One problem with manual units is that an incorrectly tuned instrument is ineffective for calculus removal. With manual units, the effectiveness of the powered instrument for calculus removal depends on the experience of the clinician in tuning the tip frequency.

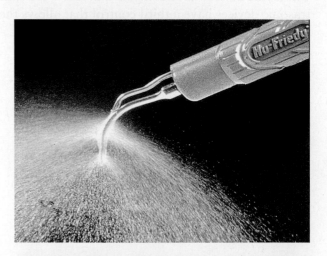

Tip Tuned for Calculus Removal. When tuned to provide the most effective calculus removal, the water should break into a fine mist—a halo of water—at the instrument tip. (Courtesy of Hu-Friedy Manufacturing Company, Inc.)

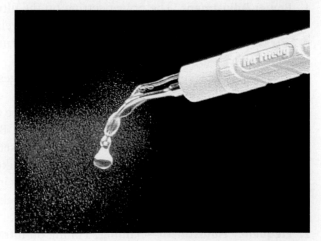

Tip Tuned for Deplaquing. When tuned for deplaquing, the water flow is adjusted so that the water halo is smaller and water drips from the instrument tip. (Courtesy of Hu-Friedy Manufacturing Company, Inc.)

WATER FLOW

Ultrasonic instrument tips must be cooled by fluid to prevent overheating of the vibrating instrument tip. Fluid, usually water, is used as a coolant. Fluid constantly flows thorough the ultrasonic handpiece and exits near the point of the instrument tip.

1. Most commonly, the electronically powered device is connected by a hose to a water outlet on the dental unit. In this case, water is the fluid used to cool the instrument tip.

2. Some ultrasonic devices have independent fluid reservoirs (bottles) that can be used to deliver distilled water or other fluid solutions to the instrument tip.

   a. Solutions commonly used for irrigation include distilled water, sterile saline, stannous fluoride, and chemotherapeutic agents (antimicrobials) such as chlorhexidine.

   b. The use of chemotherapeutic agents with ultrasonic instruments has been shown to enhance pocket depth reduction beyond that achieved by hand instrumentation or ultrasonic instrumentation with water.[30, 44, 45]

3. On ultrasonic devices, the clinician can adjust the volume and temperature of the water supplied to the instrument tip.

   a. Lower rates of water flow increase the heating of the handpiece and result in warmer water at the instrument tip. Too little water flow to the instrument tip can result in heat damage to the dental pulp.

   b. One of the most common mistakes made by beginning clinicians is using too little water. A warm handpiece is a sign of inadequate water flowing through the handpiece and instrument tip.

4. Water is provided to the instrument tip through either an external or internal fluid flow tube.

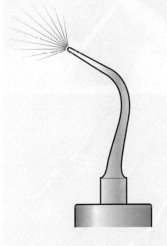

Water Adjustment for Tips with Internal Flow Tubes. For instrument tips with internal flow systems, the water flow should be adjusted so that the water breaks into a fine mist at the very end of the tip.

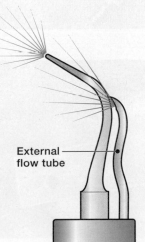

External flow tube

Water Adjustment for Tips with External Flow Tubes. For instrument tips with external flow tubes, the water flow should be adjusted so that the water breaks into a fine mist (1) near the end of the external flow tube and (2) at the very end of the tip.

Section 3
Features of Powered Devices

SONIC DEVICES

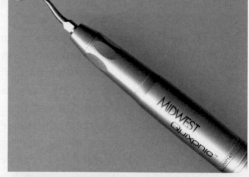

Sonic Device. Sonic electronically powered devices consist of a handpiece that attaches to the dental unit's high-speed handpiece tubing and interchangeable instrument tips.

Handpiece and Instrument Tips. Sonic instrument tips attach directly to the handpiece. Some devices have special wrenches to lock the instrument tip in the handpiece.

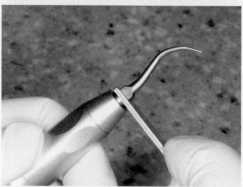

Instrument Tips. Example of slim-diameter sonic instrument tips for a sonic device.

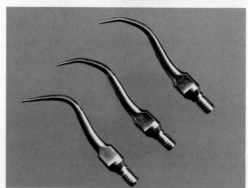

PIEZOELECTRIC ULTRASONIC DEVICES

Piezoelectric Ultrasonic Device. Piezoelectric ultrasonic devices are composed of a portable electronic generator, a handpiece, and instrument inserts.

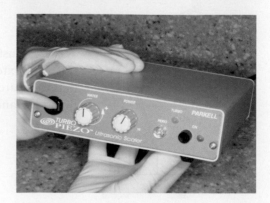

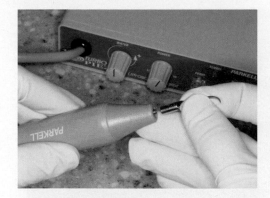

Piezoelectric Instrument Tips. Most piezoelectric devices have instrument tips that attach directly to the handpiece.

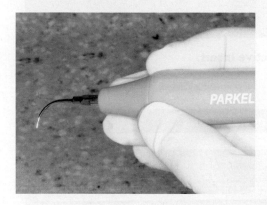

Piezoelectric Instrument Tip. This instrument tip is an example of a slim-diameter piezoelectric tip.

MAGNETOSTRICTIVE ULTRASONIC DEVICES

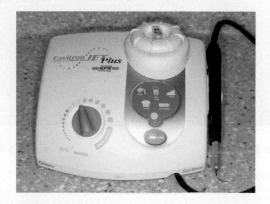

Magnetostrictive Ultrasonic Device. Magnetostrictive ultrasonic devices are composed of a portable unit that contains an electronic generator, a handpiece, and interchangeable instrument inserts.

Magnetostrictive Inserts. Most magnetostrictive devices have removable instrument inserts that fit into the handpiece. The components of a magnetostrictive insert are:

1. Metal stack—converts electrical power into mechanical vibrations
2. O-ring—a seal that keeps water flowing through the insert rather than flowing out the handpiece
3. Handle grip—portion of the insert grasped by the clinician during instrumentation.
4. Water outlet—provides water to the instrument tip
5. Working-end—portion of the instrument insert used for calculus removal and de-plaquing

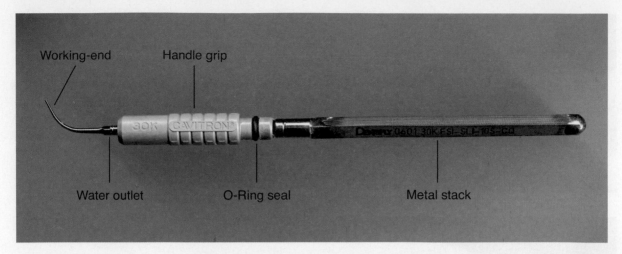

Components of a Magnetostrictive Insert.

TABLE 24-2. **Insert Frequency Options**

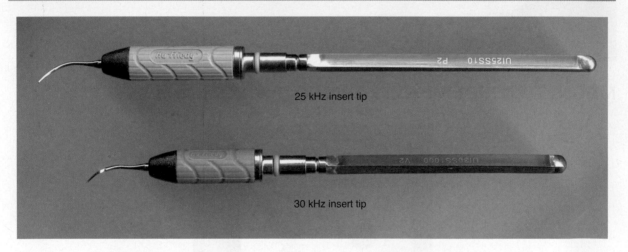

25 kHz insert tip

30 kHz insert tip

30 kHz Insert Tip	25 kHz Insert Tip
Work with 30 kHz devices only	Work with 25 kHz devices only
20,000 cycles per second	25,000 cycles per second
Shorter stroke length	Longer stroke length
About the same length as a hand instrument	Longer in length than a hand instrument

Section 4
Instrument Tips

A wide variety of instrument tip designs are available for the various sonic and ultrasonic devices. As mentioned previously, instrument tips from one device may not work with another manufacturer's handpiece. Sonic and piezoelectric devices usually have instrument tips that attach directly to the nosecone of the handpiece. Most magnetostrictive devices have instrument inserts. When you are purchasing an electronically powered device, one of the decisive factors should be the selection of instrument tips available for that device. The number of instrument tip designs offered for a particular device can vary from 3 to 75 tip designs. Some electronically powered devices do not offer slim-diameter instrument tips. It is important to select a device that offers both standard-diameter and slim-diameter instrument tips.

INSTRUMENT TIP SELECTION CRITERIA

Instrument tips vary in tip shape, diameter, length, and curvature. Factors to be considered when selecting an instrument tip for a particular task include:

1. The type of calculus deposits (small-, medium-, or large-sized deposits?)
2. The location of calculus deposits (deposits located (a) above the gingival margin, (b) 4 mm or less below the gingival margin, or (c) more than 4 mm below the gingival margin?)

TABLE 24-3. Instrument Tip Selection

Diameter		
	Standard-Diameter	**Slim-Diameter**
Characteristics	Standard-diameter	40 percent smaller in diameter
	Shorter shank lengths	Longer shank lengths
Use	Heavy deposit removal: mostly for supragingival use and for subgingival deposits easily accessed without undue tissue stretching	Light deposits and deplaquing
		Debridement of root concavities and furcations

TABLE 24-4. Common Instrument Tip Designs

Instrument	Description/Use
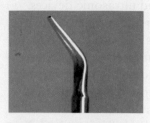	**Beavertail Tip:** Broad bulky tip, resembling a beaver's tail Supragingival: large-sized calculus ledges and stain; orthodontic cement
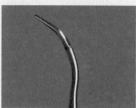	**Standard-Diameter Triple Bend Tip:** Standard-diameter tip with shank bends that facilitate access to proximal surfaces and around line angles Supragingival: small- to large-sized calculus deposits and stain
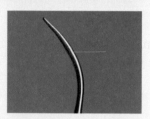	**Standard-Diameter Universal Tip:** Standard-diameter tip with curved shank and tapered tip Supragingival: small- to large-sized calculus deposits and stain Subgingival: deposits accessed without undue tissue stretching
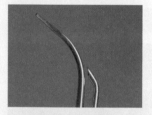	**Slim-Diameter Straight Tip:** Slim-diameter tip with extended shank and tapered tip; similar in design to a calibrated periodontal probe Subgingival: root surfaces located in periodontal pockets 4 mm or less in depth for calculus removal and deplaquing of root surfaces and concavities
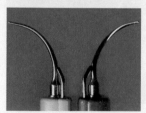	**Slim-Diameter Curved Tips (Right and Left):** Slim-diameter tip with extended shank and tapered tip; similar in design to a furcation probe; enhanced access to interproximal areas and root surfaces Subgingival: root surfaces located in pockets greater than 4 mm in depth for calculus removal and deplaquing of root surfaces, furcations, and concavities
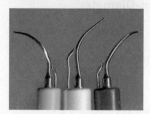	**Slim-Diameter Furcation Tips:** Slim-diameter tip with a ball end Subgingival: root surfaces located in periodontal pockets for deplaquing of furcation areas and root concavities

TABLE 24-5. Use of Straight and Curved Slim Tips

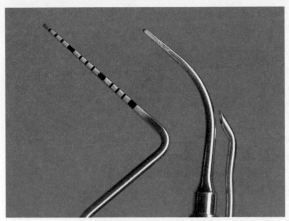

Slim-Diameter Straight Tips

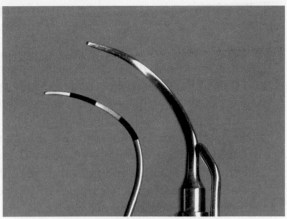

Slim-Diameter Curved Tips

Similar in design to a calibrated probe	Similar in design to a curved furcation probe
Designed for use on:	Designed for use on:
1. Anterior root surfaces	1. Posterior root surfaces located more than 4 mm apical to the CEJ
2. Posterior root surfaces that are 4 mm or less apical to (below) the cemento-enamel junction	2. Root concavities and furcations on posterior tooth

POWER SETTINGS FOR INSTRUMENTATION

The lowest effective power setting always should be used during electronically powered instrumentation. The high power setting should be avoided because studies have shown that this power setting is no more effective than the medium power setting. *Two criteria should be considered to determine the power setting for instrumentation: (1) the size of the calculus deposits and (2) the diameter of the instrument tip.*

TABLE 24-6. Instrument Selection

Instrumentation Task	Insert Diameter	Power Level
Large-sized calculus deposits	Standard-diameter	Medium
Medium-sized calculus deposits	Standard-diameter	Low to medium
	Slim-diameter	Low to medium
Small-sized calculus deposits	Slim-diameter	Low
Deplaquing	Slim-diameter	Low

ENERGY DISPERSION BY THE WORKING-END SURFACES

Electronically powered instrument tips disperse energy vibrations from each surface of the working-end. *By adapting the appropriate tip surface, the clinician can control energy dispersion and client sensitivity.*

1. **Energy Output.** Different amounts of energy are produced by the face, back, lateral surfaces, and point of an electronically powered instrument tip.
   a. **Point of the tip**—produces the greatest amount of energy vibrations.
   b. **Face of the tip** (concave surface)—produces the second greatest amount of energy vibrations.
   c. **Back of the tip** (convex surface)—produces less energy than the face or the point.
   d. **Lateral surfaces of the tip**—produce the least amount of energy vibrations.
2. **Adaptation.** Clinicians should follow manufacturer's recommendations for tip surface adaptation. In general, the following guidelines should be followed for all electronically powered instrumentation:
   a. **Point of the tip.** The point of the working-end should never be adapted to the tooth surface. The high energy output from the tip could damage the tooth.
   b. **Face of the tip.**
      1) The face should not be adapted to the tooth surface because of the high amount of energy it produces.
      2) The high energy output from the face could damage the tooth surface.
   c. **Back of the tip.**
      1) The backs of most ultrasonic and sonic instrument tips can be adapted to the tooth surface; follow the recommendations of the tip manufacturer.
      2) The back of magnetostrictive instrument tips (convex surface) is most effective in debriding root surfaces.
   d. **Lateral surfaces of the tip.** Adaptation of the lateral surfaces of the working-end is recommended with all sonic, piezoelectric, and magnetostrictive ultrasonic instruments.

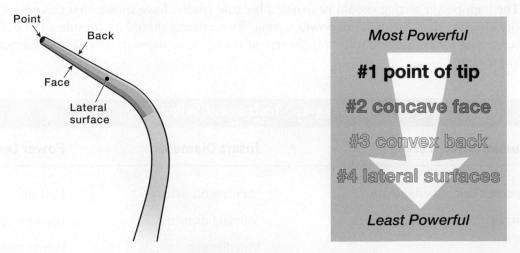

Energy Output of Working-End Surfaces.

ACTIVE TIP AREA

It is the vibration energy of a powered instrument tip that is responsible for calculus removal. The portion of the instrument tip that is capable of doing work is called the **active tip area.**

1. The active tip area ranges from approximately 2 to 4 mm of the length of the instrument tip.
2. *This means that the power to remove calculus is concentrated in the last 2 to 4 mm of the length of the tip.*
3. The higher the frequency of an electronic device, the shorter the active tip area.
   a. A 50 kHz device—active tip area is 2.3 mm long
   b. A 30 kHz device—active tip area is 4.2 mm long
   c. A 25 kHz device—active tip area is 4.3 mm long

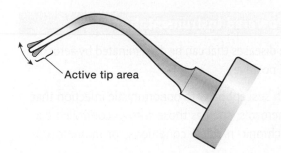
Active tip area

Active Tip Area. The power for calculus removal is concentrated in the active tip area (the last 2 to 4 mm of the tip).

INSTRUMENT TIP WEAR AND REPLACEMENT

The working-end of the powered instrument should be inspected regularly for signs of wear. With use, the instrument tip is worn down. As the instrument tip wears, effectiveness decreases. Some companies provide instrument tip wear guides that facilitate evaluation of instruments.

1. A rule of thumb is that 1 mm of wear results in approximately 25 percent loss of efficiency.
2. Approximately 50 percent loss of efficiency occurs at 2 mm of wear and the tip should be discarded at this point.

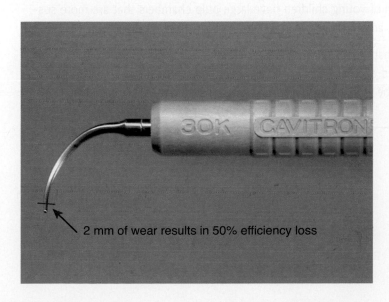
2 mm of wear results in 50% efficiency loss

Tip Wear. Instrument tips should be evaluated for tip wear. Tips should be discarded after 2 mm of wear.

Section 5
Treatment Preparation

CONTRAINDICATIONS FOR POWERED INSTRUMENTATION

Even with all the benefits of electronically powered instrumentation, it is important to remember that these instruments are not recommended for use with all patients. Before any treatment procedure, the patient's medical and dental history should be thoroughly reviewed. Electronically powered instrumentation is contraindicated for patients with certain medical and dental conditions.

TABLE 24-7.   **Contraindications for Powered Instrumentation**

1. **Communicable disease.** Individuals with communicable diseases that can be disseminated by aerosols (e.g., hepatitis, tuberculosis, respiratory infections, or HIV positive).

2. **High susceptibility to infection.** Individuals with a high susceptibility to opportunistic infection that can be transmitted by contaminated dental unit water or aerosols, such as those with uncontrolled diabetes or organ transplants, debilitated individuals with chronic medical conditions, or immunosuppressed individuals.

3. **Respiratory risk.** Individuals with respiratory disease or difficulty in breathing (e.g., those with a history of emphysema, cystic fibrosis, asthma). This patient would have a high risk of infection if he or she were to aspirate septic material or microorganisms from dental plaque into the lungs.

4. **Pacemaker.** The American Academy of Periodontology recommends that dental healthcare workers avoid exposing patients with cardiac pacemakers to magnetostrictive devices [4]. Piezoelectric ultrasonic devices do not interfere with pacemaker functioning.

5. **Difficulty in swallowing or prone to gagging.** Individuals with multiple sclerosis, amyotrophic lateral sclerosis, muscular dystrophy, or paralysis may experience difficulty in swallowing or be prone to gagging.

6. **Age.** Primary and newly erupted teeth of young children have large pulp chambers that are more susceptible to damage from the vibrations and heat produced by ultrasonic instrumentation.

7. **Oral conditions.** Avoid contact of instrument tip with hypersensitive teeth, porcelain crowns, composite resin restorations, demineralized enamel surfaces, or exposed dentinal surfaces. Not for use in those with titanium implants, unless the working-end of the powered instrument is covered with a specially designed plastic sleeve.

FLUSHING OF WATER TUBING

Scientific investigations have shown that dental unit waterlines may become significantly contaminated with microorganisms.[46, 47] This contaminated water is delivered to electronically powered instruments, dental handpieces, and air/water syringes. Although water from a municipal water source is safe for drinking, the presence of even small numbers of organisms can present problems for dental unit water quality. Potable drinking water is defined as less than 500 bacterial colony-forming units per milliliter (CFU/ml). Water recovered from dental units connected to municipal water supplies may contain millions of bacterial colony-forming units per milliliter.

Options to control water tubing contamination of electronically powered devices include a combination of:

1. **Self-contained reservoir.** Use an ultrasonic unit with a self-contained reservoir bottle that requires no waterline hook-up. The reservoir can be used to deliver distilled water or antimicrobial solution to the ultrasonic instrument tip.
2. **Point-of-use filter.** Install a filter in the dental unit waterline to physically reduce the numbers of microorganisms in the water flowing over the instrument tip. These filters are easily installed in existing dental unit waterlines.
3. **Flush the water tubing.** Flush the water tubing at the beginning of each day by stepping on the foot pedal to allow water to flow through the handpiece for at least 2 minutes at the start of the day and for a minimum of 30 seconds between patients. Flushing clears stagnant water from the tubing.

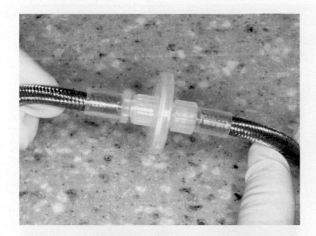

Point-of-Use Filter. Some ultrasonic devices have point-of-use filters preinstalled in the handpiece tubing that delivers water to the powered instrument.

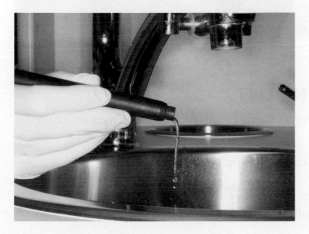

Flush Water Tubing. Flush the water tubing for a minimum of 2 minutes at the start of the day and for 30 seconds between patients.

PREPARING THE CLINICIAN AND PATIENT

As with any dental procedure, universal precautions must be used during ultrasonic instrumentation.

1. The clinician should wear a gown with a high neck and long sleeves, mask, protective eyewear or a face shield, and gloves.
2. Select a mask with a high bacterial filtration efficiency (BFE).[48] By definition, a mask with a high bacterial filtration efficiency effectively filters 98 percent of particles that are 3 microns or larger in size.
3. Because of the high level of aerosols generated by powered instrumentation, change masks every 20 minutes because a damp mask does not provide adequate protection.
4. Personal protective gear for the patient should include a plastic drape, towel or bib, and protective eyewear. The patient may prefer to cover his or her nose with a flat-style mask to limit inhalation of aerosols.
5. Administering a pre-procedural rinse to the patient is recommended to reduce the number of bacteria introduced into the patient's bloodstream and to control the release of aerosols into the surrounding environment. A 2-minute mouth rinse with either 0.12 percent chlorhexidine or an antiseptic mouth rinse such as Listerine Antiseptic before treatment is recommended for all patients.

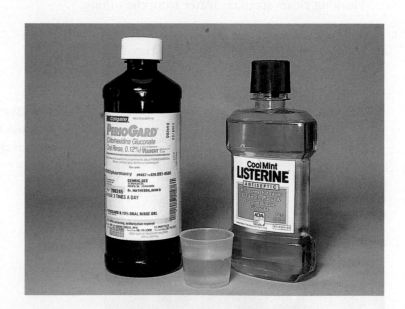

Pre-procedural Rinse. Administering a pre-procedural rinse is recommended to reduce the numbers of bacteria and other oral pathogens.

FLUID EVACUATION AND CONTAINMENT

Good fluid control is necessary to increase patient comfort and efficiency during instrumentation.

1. **Patient Positioning.**
   a. Position the patient in a supine position, and work with the head turned to the side and tipped slightly downward.
   b. Positioning the patient's head to the side causes the fluid generated by the instrument tip to pool in the corner of the mouth, where it can be suctioned or evacuated.

2. **Suction Devices.**
   a. A high-volume suction tip or a saliva ejector should be used for fluid control.
   b. A high-volume suction tip is recommended when working with an assistant; or, in some instances, the clinician can hold the suction tip rather than a mirror in the nondominant hand. It may be helpful to cut the suction tip in half for easier handling when working without an assistant.
   c. Another alternative when working alone is to ask the patient to hold a saliva ejector.
   d. Position the suction tip or saliva ejector in the corner of the mouth where fluid will pool.
   e. Deactivate the ultrasonic tip occasionally to keep excessive amounts of fluid from pooling in the corner of the mouth.
3. **Cupping Techniques.** It can be very frustrating for the patient to have his or her face and hair sprayed with the water from the instrument tip.
   a. Good water containment can be achieved through a combination of evacuation and use of the patient's lips and cheeks as fluid-deflecting barriers.
   b. When working on the mandibular anterior teeth, for example, pull the patient's lip up and out and away from the teeth to act as a barrier to deflect the water back into the mouth and as a cup to collect the water for evacuation.
   c. A similar technique is used for the posterior teeth, by holding the cheek away from the teeth to catch the water spray.

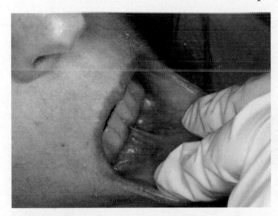
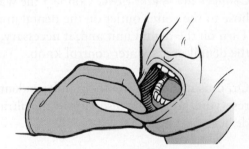

Fluid Control in Anterior Sextants. For anterior sextants, the lower and upper lips can be cupped to contain the water spray.

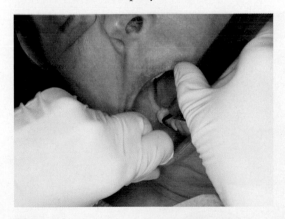
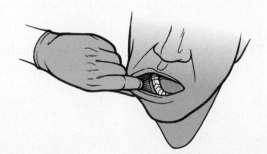

Fluid Control in Posterior Treatment Areas. For posterior treatment areas, hold the cheek between the thumb and index finger and pull out and up, or down, to form a cup.

TECHNIQUE PRACTICE: PREPARATION OF ULTRASONIC DEVICE

Certain steps should be followed when setting up an ultrasonic device. Follow the steps below to practice the recommended procedure for preparing an ultrasonic device for use. If your school does not have any ultrasonic equipment, read this section carefully to become familiar with the procedure.

1. **Put the Device in a Convenient Place.** The ultrasonic device should be located on a stable countertop or cart so that you have easy access to the device at the dental chair.

   Place barriers over the control knobs on the power generator.

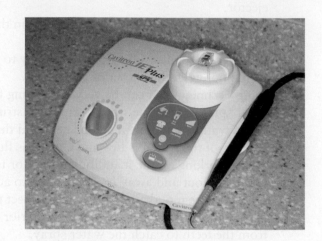

2. **Connect the Water Hose.** Connect the water hose to the water outlet on the dental unit. Turn on the dental unit and, if necessary, open the dental unit's water control knob.

   Or, if using a device with an independent fluid reservoir, attach the reservoir to the ultrasonic device.

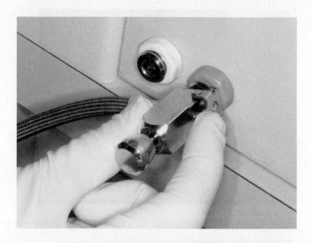

3. **Turn on the Unit.** Locate the power switch or button and turn on the ultrasonic unit.

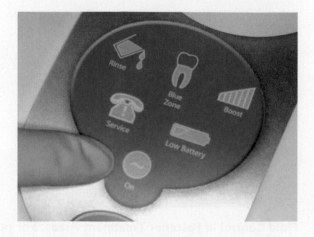

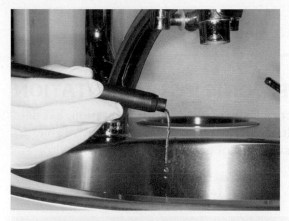

4. **Flush the Water Tubing.** Flush the handpiece tubing of stagnant water by holding the handpiece over a sink and stepping on the foot pedal to activate a steady stream of water.

   At the start of each day, flush the tubing for a minimum of 2 minutes. Between patients, flush the tubing for at least 30 seconds.

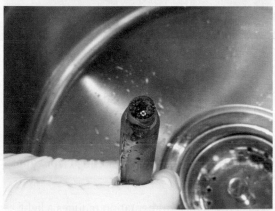

5. **Fill the Handpiece With Water.** Hold the handpiece upright and step on the foot pedal to fill the entire handpiece with water. While maintaining the handpiece in a vertical position, release the foot pedal. This step expels air bubbles from the handpiece that could cause overheating.

   Repeat this process whenever you change instrument inserts.

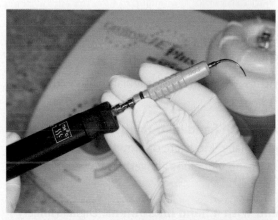

6. **Lubricate the O-ring and Seat the Insert.** Use your fingertips to lubricate the O-ring with water from the handpiece.

   Grasp the insert grip, keeping your hand and fingers away from the working-end of the insert. Grasping or pushing against the working-end can bend the instrument tip or cause injury to your hand. Gently twist the insert into the handpiece until it snaps into place.

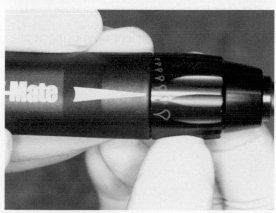

7. **Adjust the Water Spray.** The water spray is controlled by a knob on the unit or on the ultrasonic handpiece. Adjust the water flow to create a light mist at the working-end.

   The water spray should be adjusted each time that you change the power level during instrumentation.

Section 6
Instrumentation Technique

FUNDAMENTALS OF SONIC AND ULTRASONIC INSTRUMENTATION

Dr. Larry Burnett of Portland, Oregon, a master at electronically powered instrumentation, has developed what he refers to as his "secrets for effective ultrasonic subgingival debridement." Table 24-8 incorporates Dr. Burnett's secrets and provides a summary of principles for sonic and ultrasonic instrumentation.

TABLE 24-8. Ten Secrets for Successful Powered Instrumentation
1. **Insert Selection. Don't ask more of an instrument tip than it can deliver.** Use a standard-diameter tip for large- or medium-sized calculus deposits. Use a slim-diameter tip for small- to medium-sized deposits.
2. **Power Setting. Set the power setting lower than you think is necessary.** Use low to medium power settings for calculus removal and low power settings for deplaquing.
3. **Water Flow. Use more water than you think is necessary.** Ensure that the water flow is hitting the active portion of the tip. Adjust the water until a halo of water surrounds the tip or until a rapid drip is achieved.
4. **Grasp. Use a lighter grasp than you think is necessary.** Powered instrumentation requires a light, related grasp similar to that used when probing.
5. **Finger Rest. Use a more stable finger rest than you think is necessary.** Use a stable standard intraoral finger rest or one of the extraoral fulcrums described in Chapter 23.
6. **Angulation. Use less angulation than with a hand instrument.** The angulation should be as close to 0 degrees as possible and should never exceed 15 degrees.
7. **Lateral Pressure. Use much less lateral pressure than with hand instrumentation.** Touch the lateral surface lightly (gently) against the deposit or tooth surface. Moderate or firm pressure decreases the effectiveness of the instrument tip and can even stop the tip vibrations altogether! Powered instrumentation requires a light touch.
8. **Activation. Use more finger motion than you would with a hand instrument.** Digital (finger) activation is excellent for applying the light stroke pressure needed for powered instrumentation.
9. **Tip Motion. Never allow the instrument tip to be idle.** Keep the instrument tip moving at all times. Never continue to hold the tip on any one spot.
10. **Stroke Technique. Give each tooth adequate attention.** Cover every millimeter of the root surface with overlapping, horizontal, vertical, and oblique brushlike strokes.

HANDPIECE CORD MANAGEMENT

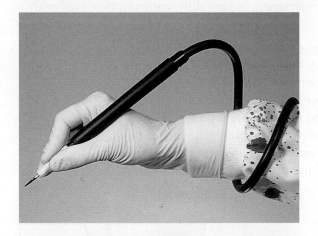

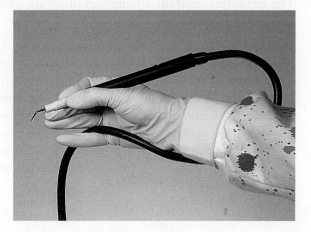

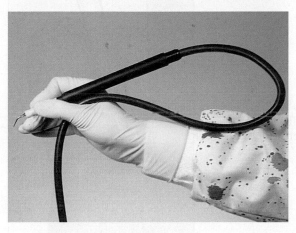

Management of Handpiece Cord. Some clinicians find that the cord tends to weigh down the end of the handpiece or causes the handpiece to twist during instrumentation. Several techniques are helpful in reducing the pull of the cord on the handpiece, such as wrapping the cord around the forearm, running it between the little and ring fingers, and resting it in the palm of the hand around the thumb.

STROKE DIRECTIONS

When the instrument tip is adapted to a tooth surface, it should be kept moving at all times using a combination of overlapping vertical, oblique, and horizontal strokes. Instrumentation strokes should be short and overlapping to cover every square millimeter of the root surface.

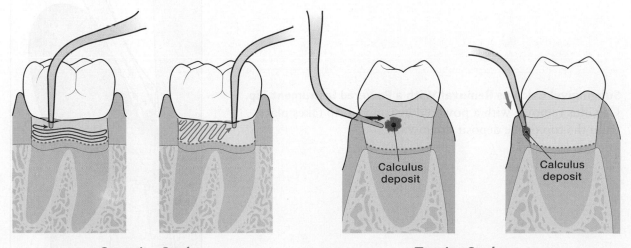

Sweeping Strokes   **Tapping Strokes**

APPROACH TO CALCULUS REMOVAL

The technique used for adaptation of an ultrasonic instrument is very different from that used with hand instruments.

1. Calculus Removal Technique with a Curet. A curet, such as a Gracey extended shank curet, must be *positioned apical to (below) the calculus deposit*—starting at the base of the pocket and working toward the cemento-enamel junction (CEJ). To be effective, a curet must be adapted at the proper angulation.

2. Calculus Removal with an Electronically Powered Instrument. A powered instrument tip works from the *top of the deposit downward*—starting near the CEJ and working toward the base of the pocket. There is no need to position the tip beneath the deposit. This is a great advantage when working in deep periodontal pockets.

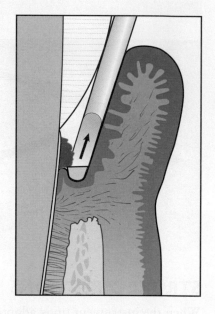

Subgingival Calculus Removal With a Curet. Calculus removal with a curet takes place from the base of the pocket upward toward the CEJ. Often it is difficult to position the curet under calculus deposits near the base of the pocket.

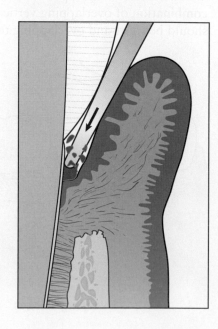

Subgingival Calculus Removal With a Powered Instrument Tip. Calculus removal with a powered instrument tip takes place from the top of the deposit downward.

REMOVING STUBBORN CALCULUS DEPOSITS

A common misconception among clinicians who are new to powered instrumentation is the belief that a single quick tap against a deposit will remove it. Powered instruments are very effective at removing calculus deposits, but they are not magic wands. Adequate time must be spent on a deposit to remove it. A calculus deposit does not vanish in a single tap; rather, tiny pieces fall away from the deposit as it is exposed to the instrument tip during a series of gentle strokes. Effective strategies for removing stubborn calculus deposits include:

1. **Proper Tip Selection.** As with hand instruments, the instrument tip is selected based on the size and location of the calculus deposit.
   a. **Standard-Diameter Tips.** Use standard-diameter tips to remove moderate to heavy deposits above the gingival margin and in shallow pockets.
   b. **Straight Slim-Diameter Tips.** Use straight slim-diameter tips to remove light to moderate calculus deposits on anterior teeth and on posterior root surfaces up to 4 mm below the CEJ.
   c. **Curved Slim-Diameter Tips.** Use curved right and left slim-diameter tips to remove light to moderate calculus deposits on posterior root surfaces greater than 4 mm below the CEJ.
2. **Attack the Deposit from All Directions.** Approach a deposit from a variety of directions. For example, interproximal deposits can be approached from both the facial and lingual aspects.
3. **Increase the Frequency.** If the electronically powered device can be manually tuned, use the tuning control knob to increase the frequency.
4. **Increase the Power.** If all the above strategies fail to remove the deposit, it is necessary to increase the power setting.

TIP ADAPTATION

The point of the working-end of an electronically powered instrument tip should never be adapted to the tooth surface. The high energy output from the point of the tip could damage the tooth surface.

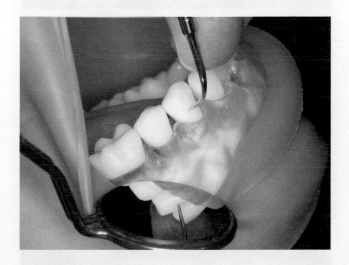

Incorrect Adaptation. Never adapt the point of the working-end to the tooth surface. Using the instrument tip in this manner can gouge cementum and dentin surfaces.

Powered instrument tips should be adapted with the either the *lateral surface or back parallel to the tooth surface being treated*. The working-end's face-to-tooth surface angulation should be as close to 0 degrees as possible and should never exceed 15 degrees.

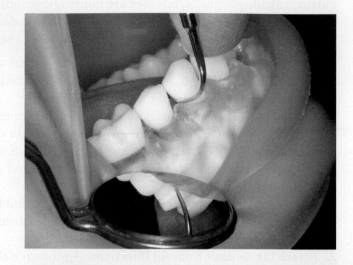

Correct Adaptation of Lateral Surface.
Correct adaptation of a lateral surface of the instrument tip parallel to the distal surface of an anterior tooth.

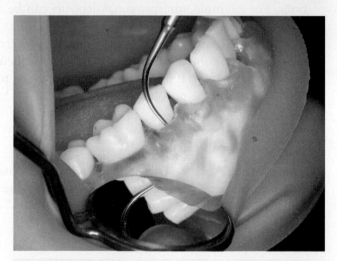

Correct Adaptation of Lateral Surface. The instrument tip can be positioned in a similar manner to that of a calibrated periodontal probe, with the point directed toward the junctional epithelium and the lateral surface against the tooth surface to be treated.

When using the tip in a point-up or point-down position the handle may be at a 50-degree angulation to the long axis of the tooth.

Correct Adaptation of the Back. When working with a magnetostrictive or sonic instrument, the back of the tip may be applied to the tooth surface with the point directed toward the junctional epithelium.

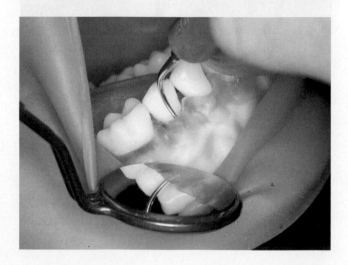

MOVING THE INSTRUMENT TIP

The powered instrument tip should be kept in constant motion when adapted to a tooth. There are two basic techniques for moving the vibrating instrument tip.

1. Calculus removal is accomplished using a series of gentle tapping motions against the deposit from different directions.
2. Subgingival deplaquing is accomplished using a series of gentle sweeping motions over the root surface. For deplaquing, short, overlapping strokes should cover every millimeter of the root surface.

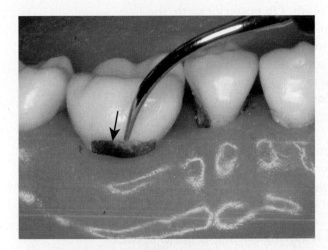

Tapping Motions for Calculus Removal. For calculus removal, a lateral surface or the back of the tip is adapted to the tooth surface to be instrumented.

The instrument tip is moved against the deposit in a series of light tapping motions. Only gentle tapping pressure is needed. Firm pressure greatly reduces the effectiveness of the instrument.

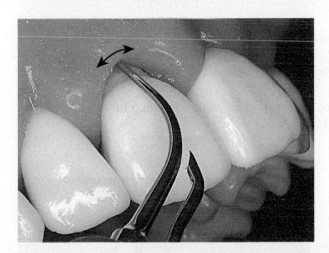

Sweeping Motions for Deplaquing. For subgingival deplaquing, a lateral surface or the back of the tip is adapted to the tooth surface and moved in a series of sweeping motions.

Imagine that you are using the side of a crayon (rather than the point) to color the entire root surface.

Box 24-1. Moving the Instrument Tip in Sweeping Motions

When using an electronically powered instrument tip, imagine that the tip is a crayon. Your goal is to gently color the entire root surface using the **side of a crayon tip**—rather than the point.

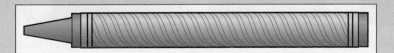

Section 7
Slim-Diameter Instrument Tips

THE STRAIGHT SLIM TIPS

1. **Use of Straight Slim-Diameter Tip on Anterior Teeth.** The straight slim-diameter instrument tip can be used on all surfaces of the anterior teeth. Because the roots of these teeth are not highly curved, the straight slim-diameter tip is effective for calculus removal even in deep periodontal pockets.

2. **Use of Straight Slim-Diameter Tip on Posterior Teeth.** On posterior teeth, the straight slim-diameter instrument tip is recommended for use on root surfaces located 4 mm or less below the cemento-enamel junction (CEJ). Because the straight tip does not adapt well to root curvatures and concavities, the slim tip is reserved for use in normal sulci and shallow periodontal pockets on posterior teeth.

3. **Orientation of the Instrumentation Tip to the Tooth Surface.** There are two basic techniques for adapting a straight slim-diameter instrument tip to a tooth:
   a. **Oblique Technique (Curet Position).**
      1) For the oblique technique, the working-end is positioned with the lateral surface in an oblique—almost horizontal—orientation to the long axis of the tooth. The tip is positioned in a similar manner to the working-end of a curet. The face of the working-end should be at a 0-degree angulation to the tooth surface.
      2) The oblique technique can be used when removing calculus deposits above or slightly below the gingival margin.
   b. **Vertical Technique (Probe Position).**
      1) For the vertical technique, the instrument tip is positioned in a manner similar to that of a calibrated periodontal probe, with the point directed toward the junctional epithelium. The instrument tip is in a vertical orientation to the long axis of the tooth.
      2) The vertical technique is used for calculus removal and deplaquing when instrumenting shallow or deep periodontal pockets.

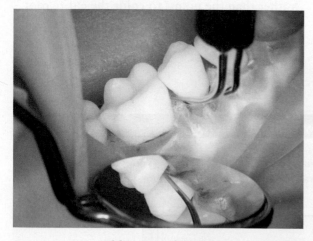

Oblique Technique

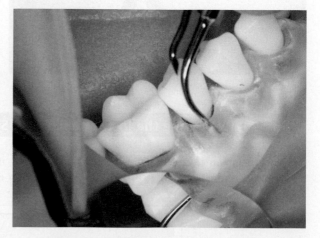

Vertical Technique

THE CURVED SLIM TIPS

A curved tip should be used for root surfaces located more than 4 mm below the CEJ.

1. When using magnetostrictive and sonic devices, it is best to adapt the back of the tip to the root surface. On posterior teeth, the back surface conforms best to the curved root surfaces.
2. When using a piezoelectric device, the lateral surfaces of the working-end should be used. Because of the linear tip motion pattern, only the lateral surfaces of the working-end are recommended for use with most piezoelectric devices.

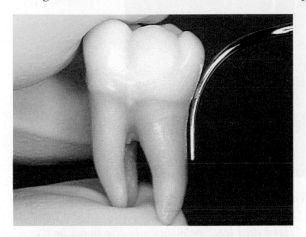

Curved Slim-Diameter Tips. Curved instrument tips were designed to facilitate adaptation to the curved root surfaces of posterior teeth. The back of the working-end adapts best to the curved root surfaces.

ORIENTATION OF CURVED SLIM TIPS

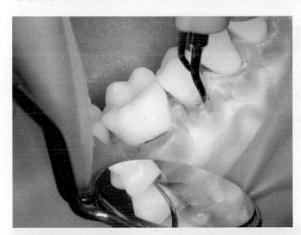

Oblique Technique. The curved slim-diameter tips can be adapted to the mesial and distal surfaces using the oblique technique. This orientation of the instrument tip is excellent for removing deposits apical to the contact area and deposits in the area of the CEJ.

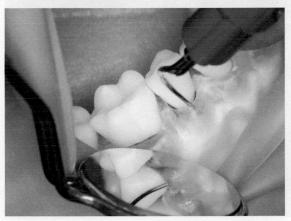

Vertical Technique. When using magnetostrictive or sonic instrument tips, the back of the working-end can be used for debridement. The back of the working-end conforms well to curved root surfaces in deep periodontal pockets.

TIP IDENTIFICATION

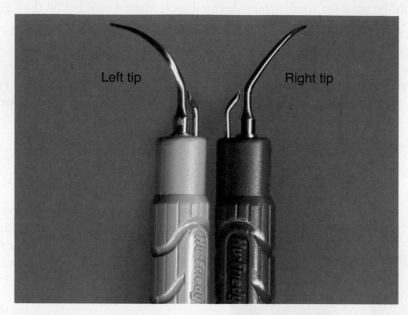

Left tip   Right tip

Identifying the Right and Left Curved Slim-Diameter Tips. To identify a curved tip, rotate the insert so the point is facing away from you and the back is facing toward you. The direction of the bend in the tip will identify the tip as right or left. *The terms "right and left" refer only to the bend in the design, not to a location for use in the mouth.*

Box 24-2. Instrumentation of Posterior Root Surfaces

For root surfaces located more than 4 mm apical to (below) the CEJ on posterior teeth:

1. Curved slim-diameter tips provide the best calculus removal and deplaquing.

2. The back of the working-end provides the best adaptation to subgingival root surfaces.

FURCATION SLIM TIPS

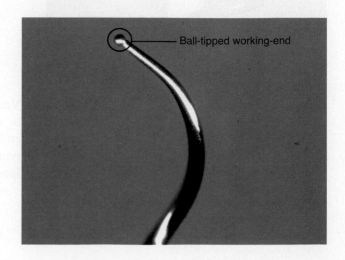

Ball-tipped working-end

Slim-Diameter Furcation Tip With Ball-End. Slim furcation tips have a ball end and are available in straight, right, and left designs.

FURCATION ENTRANCE

Slim-diameter instrument tips are more effective than hand instruments in treating class II and III furcations.[13, 16, 17] Standard Gracey curets are too wide to enter the furcation area of over 50 percent of all maxillary and mandibular molars.

1. The average facial furcation entrance of maxillary and mandibular first molars is from 0.63 to 1.04 mm in width.
2. The width of a new Gracey curet ranges from 0.76 to 1 mm. The diameter of a modified slim-diameter instrument tip is 0.55 mm or less in diameter.

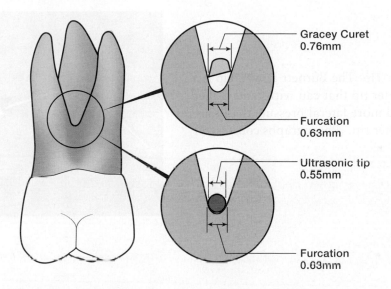

Gracey Curet
0.76mm

Furcation
0.63mm

Ultrasonic tip
0.55mm

Furcation
0.63mm

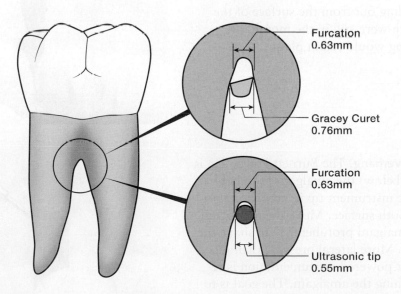

Furcation
0.63mm

Gracey Curet
0.76mm

Furcation
0.63mm

Ultrasonic tip
0.55mm

SMOOTHING AMALGAM OVERHANGS

Overhang removal is a recontouring procedure used to correct defective margins of restorations to provide a smooth surface that will deter bacterial accumulation. If a minor amalgam overhang is acting as a plaque trap and preventing effective plaque control, the excess amalgam can be removed using a specialized powered instrument tip for this purpose. The Burnett Power Tip (from Parkell USA and designed by Dr. Larry Burnett of Portland, Oregon) is a unique slim-diameter tip that can withstand higher power settings and more lateral pressure than a conventional slim-diameter tip. This tip is recommended for removing tenacious calculus deposits, smoothing amalgam overhangs, and removing orthodontic cement. The Burnett Power Tip is ideal for smoothing overhanging amalgam restorations. A conventional slim-diameter tip is not recommended for smoothing amalgam overhangs.

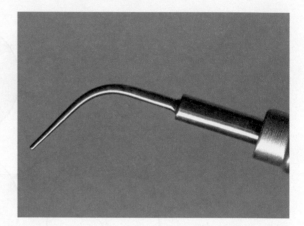

The Burnett Power Tip. The Burnett Power Tip is a unique slim-diameter tip that can withstand higher power settings and more lateral pressure than the typical slim-diameter tip. (Photographs courtesy of Parkell, USA.)

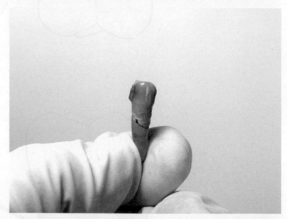

Amalgam Overhang. This tooth has an excess of amalgam protruding out from the surface of the tooth. If this tooth were still in the mouth, the amalgam overhang would retain plaque.

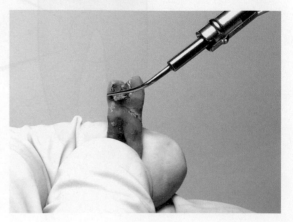

Smoothing the Overhang. The Burnett Power Tip is placed apical to (below) the amalgam protuberance. Position the instrument tip in an oblique orientation to the tooth surface. Move the tip up and down over the amalgam protuberance to shave the amalgam surface. More lateral pressure than is normally used for powered instrumentation is required for smoothing the amalgam. The goal is to have the amalgam restoration level with the root surface.

Section 8
Technique Practice: Slim Tips

STRAIGHT SLIM TIP—OBLIQUE TECHNIQUE

The straight slim-diameter instrument tip can be used on all surfaces of the anterior teeth. Because the roots of these teeth are not highly curved, the straight slim-diameter tip is effective for calculus removal even in deep periodontal pockets. The oblique technique is effective for removing calculus deposits located above or slightly below the gingival margin.

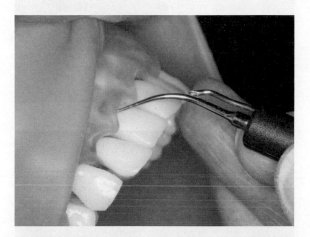

1. **Oblique Technique.** Position the straight-slim tip in an oblique orientation to the long axis of a maxillary central incisor. Insert the working-end slightly beneath the gingival margin leading with the convex back of the working-end toward the gingival margin.

   An oblique technique can be used for calculus removal above and slightly below the gingival margin.

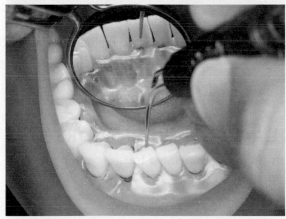

2. **INCORRECT Adaptation—Oblique Technique on Lingual Surfaces of Mandibular Anteriors.** Adapt the straight slim tip to the lingual surface of a mandibular anterior tooth using a traditional intraoral finger rest. Note that traditional intraoral finger rest makes it difficult to adapt the lateral surface of the instrument tip to the lingual surface of a mandibular anterior tooth.

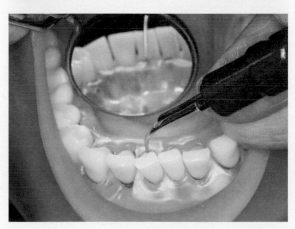

3. **Correct Adaptation—Mandibular Anteriors.** Rotate the instrument handpiece to the side of the mouth and establish a finger rest several teeth away. Establishing a finger rest on the posterior teeth makes it easier to correctly adapt the lateral surface of the instrument tip to the lingual surface of a mandibular anterior tooth.

STRAIGHT SLIM TIP—VERTICAL TECHNIQUE ON ANTERIORS

Because the roots of anterior teeth are not highly curved, the straight slim-diameter tip is effective for calculus removal even in deep periodontal pockets.

1. **Vertical Technique—With Lateral Surface.** Position a straight slim tip in a similar manner to a periodontal probe with the lateral surface against the tooth surface being debrided.

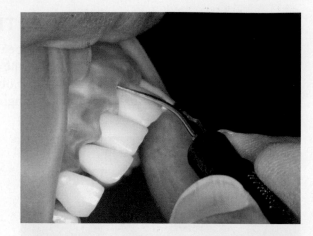

2. **Vertical Technique—With Back of Tip.** Adapt the back of the instrument tip to the facial surface of an anterior tooth.

   When working with a magnetostrictive ultrasonic or sonic instrument tip, the back of the working-end can be used to remove calculus deposits. Use of the back is not recommended with piezoelectric instrument tips.

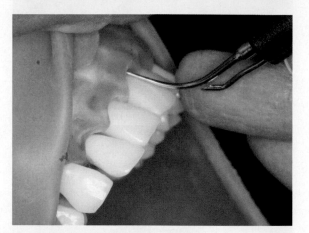

STRAIGHT SLIM TIP—VERTICAL TECHNIQUE ON POSTERIORS

On posterior teeth, the straight slim-diameter instrument tip is recommended for use on root surfaces located 4 mm or less below the cemento-enamel junction (CEJ).

1. **Posterior Tooth—with Lateral Surface.** Adapt the lateral surface of the straight slim tip to the facial surface of a molar. Use light lateral pressure as you make a combination of strokes across the tooth surface. Start at the CEJ and work toward the base of the pocket, covering every square millimeter of the root surface.

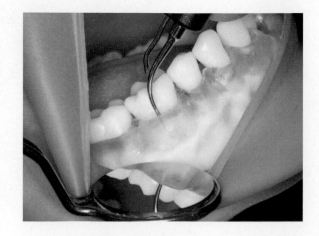

EFFICIENT SEQUENCE FOR CURVED TIPS ON POSTERIOR SEXTANTS

Curved tips come in right and left styles and both tips are needed to instrument the entire dentition. Instrumentation is accomplished most efficiently by completing all surfaces with the right instrument tip before switching to the left instrument tip. For example, the clinician can use the right tip in the oblique position to remove deposits above and slightly below the gingival margin. Next, the right tip can be used in the vertical position for subgingival debridement.

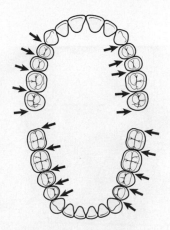

A—Oblique Technique with Right Tip

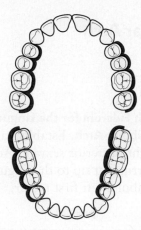

B—Vertical Technique with Right Tip

Right Tip. A, The proximal surfaces indicated by the red arrows can be debrided with the right slim-diameter tip using an oblique technique. In this position, the tip can remove calculus deposits located above and slightly below the gingival margin. **B,** The red line indicates the tooth surfaces that can be instrumented with the right slim-diameter tip using the vertical technique.

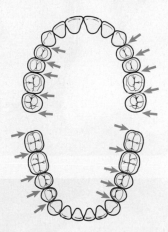

A—Oblique Technique with Left Tip

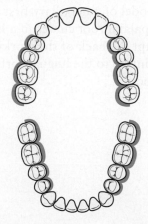

B—Vertical Technique with Left Tip

Left Tip. A, The proximal surfaces indicated by the teal arrows can be debrided with the left slim-diameter tip using an oblique technique. In this position, the tip can remove calculus deposits located above and slightly below the gingival margin. **B,** The teal line indicates the tooth surfaces that can be instrumented with the left-slim diameter tip using the vertical technique.

CURVED SLIM TIPS—CROSS ARCH FULCRUM FOR LINGUAL ASPECTS

The best adaptation to the lingual aspect of the mandibular and maxillary posterior teeth is achieved by adapting the back of the working-end to the tooth surface being treated. It can be difficult to adapt the back of the working-end to the lingual surfaces using a standard fulcrum. A cross arch fulcrum on the opposite side of the arch from the treatment area allows adaptation of the back of the instrument tip to the lingual aspects of the mandibular and maxillary arches.

Mandibular Arch

1. **Cross Arch Fulcrum for the Lingual Aspects of the Mandibular Arch.** Establish a finger rest on the right posterior sextant. Adapt the back of the instrument tip to the lingual aspect of the mandibular left first molar.

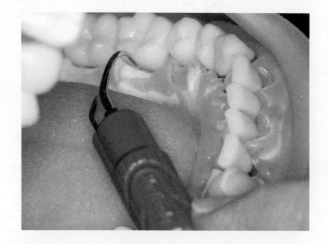

Maxillary Arch

2. **Palatal Roots of Maxillary Molars.** Obtain an acrylic model of a maxillary first molar. Note how the palatal root curves in a lingual direction. Adapt the back of the working-end of a curved slim tip to the lingual surface of the palatal root.

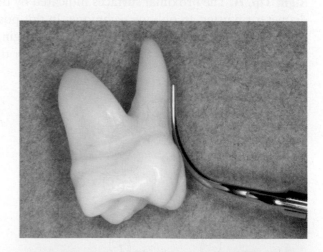

3. **Cross Arch Fulcrum for the Lingual Aspects of the Maxillary Arch.** Establish a finger rest on the maxillary right posteriors. Adapt the back of the instrument tip to the lingual aspect of the maxillary first molar.

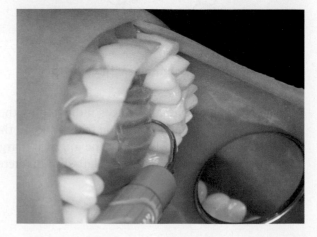

CURVED SLIM TIPS—OBLIQUE TECHNIQUE

The curved slim tips can be used with the oblique technique to remove calculus deposits above and slightly beneath the gingival margin from the mesial and distal surfaces of posterior teeth.

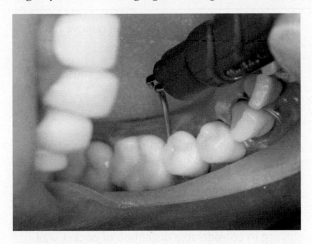

1. **Oblique Technique—Lingual Aspect.** Adapt the lateral surface of the right-slim tip to the proximal surfaces of the mandibular right posterior teeth, lingual aspect.

   Use tapping, horizontal strokes with light pressure to remove interproximal deposits.

CURVED SLIM TIPS—ACCESSING A FURCATION

The best instruments for debriding furcation areas are the curved slim-diameter tips and the curved furcation tips. The easiest way to locate the furcation area is to *deactivate* the ultrasonic instrument tip (remove foot from foot pedal). Use of a deactivated instrument tip provides the clinician with improved tactile sensitivity.

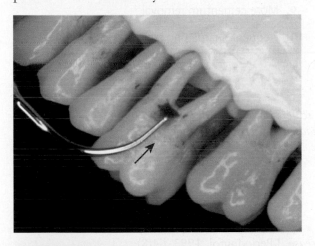

1. **Locate the Furcation Area.** Insert an inactivated instrument tip beneath the gingival margin near the distofacial line angle. Move the instrument tip in an oblique direction until you detect the entrance to the furcation.

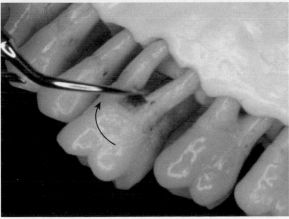

2. **Enter the Roof of the Furcation Area.** Once you have located the entrance to the furcation, turn the instrument working-end while rotating the wrist. This twisting motion allows the instrument tip to access the roof of the furcation.

   Activate the instrument tip. Roll the ball of the working-end back and forth across the entire roof of the furcation.

TABLE 24-9. Summary Sheet: Comparison of Powered and Hand Instrumentation

Electronically Powered Instrumentation	Hand Instrumentation
1. Several mechanisms of action; can disrupt bacteria from a distance	1. One mechanism of action; can remove only what it touches
2. Flushing action removes debris and bacteria from pocket	2. Some debris remains in pocket to cause irritation to tissue
3. Small tip size (0.3–0.55 mm)	3. Larger in size (0.76–1.0 mm)
4. Light lateral pressure and relaxed grasp used for calculus removal	4. Moderate to firm lateral pressure needed for calculus removal
5. Less time needed for calculus removal	5. More time needed for calculus removal
6. Easily inserted in pocket with minimal distention (stretching) of pocket wall away from the tooth	6. Must be positioned apical to deposit, resulting in considerable distention of pocket wall
7. Instrument tip can remove calculus deposit from above	7. Curet must be positioned beneath the deposit for removal
8. Less tissue trauma, faster healing rate	8. More tissue trauma, slower healing rate
9. Less cementum removal	9. More cementum removal
10. No sharpening required	10. Frequent sharpening required

SUGGESTED READING

Drisko, C.L., et al., *Position paper: sonic and ultrasonic scalers in periodontics. Research, Science and Therapy Committee of the American Academy of Periodontology.* J Periodontol, 2000. 71(11): 1792–1801.

REFERENCES

1. Copulos, T.A., et al., *Comparative analysis between a modified ultrasonic tip and hand instruments on clinical parameters of periodontal disease.* J Periodontol, 1993. 64(8): 694–700.

2. Drisko, C.L., *Scaling and root planing without overinstrumentation: hand versus power-driven scalers.* Curr Opin Periodontol, 1993: 78–88.

3. Kepic, T.J., T.J. O'Leary, and A.H. Kafrawy, *Total calculus removal: an attainable objective?* J Periodontol, 1990. 61(1): 16–20.

4. Drisko, C.L., et al., *Position paper: sonic and ultrasonic scalers in periodontics. Research, Science and Therapy Committee of the American Academy of Periodontology.* J Periodontol, 2000. 71(11): 1792–1801.

5. Breininger, D.R., T.J. O'Leary, and R.V. Blumenshine, *Comparative effectiveness of ultrasonic and hand scaling for the removal of subgingival plaque and calculus.* J Periodontol, 1987. 58(1): 9–18.

6. Leon, L.E. and R.I. Vogel, *A comparison of the effectiveness of hand scaling and ultrasonic debridement in furcations as evaluated by differential dark-field microscopy.* J Periodontol, 1987. 58(2): 86–94.

7. Oosterwaal, P.J., et al., *The effect of subgingival debridement with hand and ultrasonic instruments on the subgingival microflora.* J Clin Periodontol, 1987. 14(9): 528–533.

8. Thornton, S. and J. Garnick, *Comparison of ultrasonic to hand instruments in the removal of subgingival plaque.* J Periodontol, 1982. 53(1): 35–37.

9. Checchi, L. and G.A. Pelliccioni, *Hand versus ultrasonic instrumentation in the removal of endotoxins from root surfaces in vitro.* J Periodontol, 1988. 59(6): 398–402.

10. Badersten, A., R. Nilveus, and J. Egelberg, *Effect of nonsurgical periodontal therapy. I. Moderately advanced periodontitis.* J Clin Periodontol, 1981. 8(1): 57–72.

11. Fine, D.H., et al., *Studies in plaque pathogenicity. II. A technique for the specific detection of endotoxin in plaque samples using the limulus lysate assay.* J Periodontal Res, 1978. 13(2): 127–133.

12. Fine, D.H., et al., *Studies in plaque pathogenicity. I. Plaque collection and limulus lysate screening of adherent and loosely adherent plaque.* J Periodontal Res, 1978. 13(1): 17–23.

13. Bower, R.C., *Furcation morphology relative to periodontal treatment. Furcation entrance architecture.* J Periodontol, 1979. 50(1): 23–27.

14. Bower, R.C., *Furcation morphology relative to periodontal treatment. Furcation root surface anatomy.* J Periodontol, 1979. 50(7): 366–374.

15. Bader, H., *Scaling and root planing: evolution or revolution?* Dent Today, 1991. 10(9): 54, 56–57.

16. Hou, G.L., et al., *The topography of the furcation entrance in Chinese molars. Furcation entrance dimensions.* J Clin Periodontol, 1994. 21(7): 451–456.

17. Holbrook, W.P., et al., *Bacteriological investigation of the aerosol from ultrasonic scalers.* Br Dent J, 1978. 144(8): 245–247.

18. Dragoo, M.R., *A clinical evaluation of hand and ultrasonic instruments on subgingival debridement. 1. With unmodified and modified ultrasonic inserts.* Int J Periodontics Restorative Dent, 1992. 12(4): 310–323.

19. Jacobson, L., J. Blomlof, and S. Lindskog, *Root surface texture after different scaling modalities.* Scand J Dent Res, 1994. 102(3): 156–160.

20. Ritz, L., A.F. Hefti, and K.H. Rateitschak, *An in vitro investigation on the loss of root substance in scaling with various instruments.* J Clin Periodontol, 1991. 18(9): 643–647.

21. Buchanan, S.A. and P.B. Robertson, *Calculus removal by scaling/root planing with and without surgical access.* J Periodontol, 1987. 58(3): 159–163.

22. Caffesse, R.G., P.L. Sweeney, and B.A. Smith, *Scaling and root planing with and without periodontal flap surgery.* J Clin Periodontol, 1986. 13(3): 205–210.

23. Rateitschak-Pluss, E.M., et al., *Non-surgical periodontal treatment: where are the limits? An SEM study.* J Clin Periodontol, 1992. 19(4): 240–244.

24. Stambaugh, R.V., et al., *The limits of subgingival scaling.* Int J Periodontics Restorative Dent, 1981. 1(5): 30–41.

25. Waerhaug, J., *Healing of the dento-epithelial junction following subgingival plaque control. II: As observed on extracted teeth.* J Periodontol, 1978. 49(3): 119–134.26.   Shiloah, J. and L.A. Hovious, *The role of subgingival irrigations in the treatment of periodontitis.* J Periodontol, 1993. 64(9): 835–843.

27. Walmsley, A.D., W.R. Laird, and P.J. Lumley, *Ultrasound in dentistry. Part 2—Periodontology and endodontics.* J Dent, 1992. 20(1): 11–17.

28. Young, N.A., *Periodontal debridement: re-examining non-surgical instrumentation. Part I: A new perspective on the objectives of instrumentation.* Semin Dent Hyg, 1994. 4(4): 1–7.

29. Chapple, I.L., et al., *Effect of instrument power setting during ultrasonic scaling upon treatment outcome.* J Periodontol, 1995. 66(9): 756–760.

30. Nosal, G., et al., *The penetration of lavage solution into the periodontal pocket during ultrasonic instrumentation.* J Periodontol, 1991. 62(9): 554–557.

31. Walmsley, A.D., W.R. Laird, and A.R. Williams, *Dental plaque removal by cavitational activity during ultrasonic scaling.* J Clin Periodontol, 1988. 15(9): 539–543.

32. Walmsley, A.D., et al., *Effects of cavitational activity on the root surface of teeth during ultrasonic scaling.* J Clin Periodontol, 1990. 17(5): 306–312.

33. Walmsley, A.D., W.R. Laird, and A.R. Williams, *A model system to demonstrate the role of cavitational activity in ultrasonic scaling.* J Dent Res, 1984. 63(9): 1162-1165.

34. Thilo, B.E. and P.C. Baehni, *Effect of ultrasonic instrumentation on dental plaque microflora in vitro.* J Periodontal Res, 1987. 22(6): 518–521.

35. Baehni, P., et al., *Effects of ultrasonic and sonic scalers on dental plaque microflora in vitro and in vivo.* J Clin Periodontol, 1992. 19(7): 455–459.

36. Harrel, S.K., *Clinical use of an aerosol-reduction device with an ultrasonic scaler.* Compend Contin Educ Dent, 1996. 17(12): 1185–1193; quiz 1194.

37. Harrel, S.K., J.B. Barnes, and F. Rivera-Hidalgo, *Reduction of aerosols produced by ultrasonic scalers.* J Periodontol, 1996. 67(1): 28–32.

38. Fine, D.H., et al., *Efficacy of preprocedural rinsing with an antiseptic in reducing viable bacteria in dental aerosols.* J Periodontol, 1992. 63(10): 821–824.

39. Fine, D.H., et al., *Reduction of viable bacteria in dental aerosols by preprocedural rinsing with an antiseptic mouthrinse.* Am J Dent, 1993. 6(5): 219–221.

40. Veksler, A.E., G.A. Kayrouz, and M.G. Newman, *Reduction of salivary bacteria by pre-procedural rinses with chlorhexidine 0.12%.* J Periodontol, 1991. 62(11): 649–651.

41. *Recommended clinical guidelines for infection control in dental education institutions.* J Dent Educ, 1991. 55(9): 617–621.

42. Adams, D., et al., *The cardiac pacemaker and ultrasonic scalers.* Dent Health (London), 1983. 22(1): 6–8.

43. Bohay, R.N., et al., *A survey of magnetic fields in the dental operatory.* J Can Dent Assoc, 1994. 60(9): 835–840.

44. Rams, T.E. and J. Slots, *Antibiotics in periodontal therapy: an update.* Compendium, 1992. 13(12): 1130, 1132, 1134 passim.

45. Drisko, C.H., *Root instrumentation. Power-driven versus manual scalers, which one?* Dent Clin North Am, 1998. 42(2): 229–244.

46. Atlas, R.M., J.F. Williams, and M.K. Huntington, *Legionella contamination of dental-unit waters.* Appl Environ Microbiol, 1995. 61(4): 1208–1213.

47. Williams, J.F., et al., *Microbial contamination of dental unit waterlines: prevalence, intensity and microbiological characteristics.* J Am Dent Assoc, 1993. 124(10): 59–65.

48. Christensen, R.P., et al., *Efficiency of 42 brands of face masks and 2 face shields in preventing inhalation of airborne debris.* Gen Dent, 1991. 39(6): 414–421.

Section 9
Skill Application

PRACTICAL FOCUS
Periodontal Assessment Case: Mr. Burlington

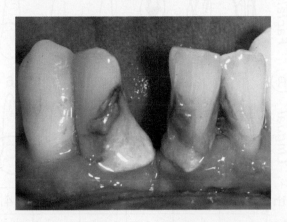

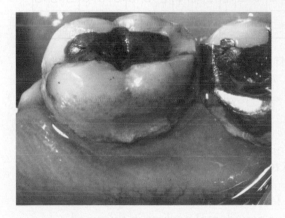 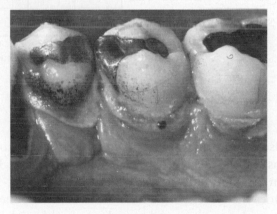

Mr. Burlington: Assessment Data
1. Generalized heavy bleeding upon probing
2. Deposits
   a. Medium- to large-sized supragingival calculus on all surfaces
   b. Subgingival calculus deposits—medium-sized deposits on all surfaces

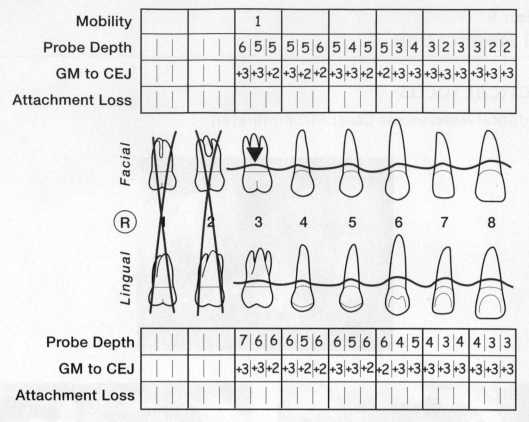

				6	5	5	5	5	6	5	4	5	5	3	4	3	2	3	3	2	2

	Mobility						1																	
Probe Depth		| |		| |	6	5	5	5	5	6	5	4	5	5	3	4	3	2	3	3	2	2
GM to CEJ		| |		| |	+3	+3	+2	+3	+2	+2	+3	+3	+2	+2	+3	+3	+3	+3	+3	+3	+3	+3
Attachment Loss		| |		| |	| |		| |		| |		| |		| |		| |

Facial   Ⓡ   1   2   3   4   5   6   7   8   *Lingual*

Probe Depth		| |		| |	7	6	6	6	5	6	6	5	6	6	4	5	4	3	4	4	3	3
GM to CEJ		| |		| |	+3	+3	+2	+3	+2	+2	+3	+3	+2	+2	+3	+3	+3	+3	+3	+3	+3	+3
Attachment Loss		| |		| |	| |		| |		| |		| |		| |		| |

Mr. Burlington: Periodontal Chart for Maxillary Right Quadrant.

Mr. Burlington: Case Questions

1. Use the information recorded on Mr. Burlington's chart to calculate the attachment loss on the facial and lingual aspects for teeth 3 to 8. Enter the loss of attachment on Mr. Burlington's chart.

2. Does the assessment data indicate normal bone levels or bone loss in this quadrant? Does the assessment data indicate healthy sulci or periodontal pockets in this quadrant? Explain which data you used to make these determinations.

3. Do you expect to instrument any root concavities or furcation areas while debriding the teeth in this quadrant? If so, indicate which teeth will probably have root concavities and/or furcation areas to be instrumented.

4. Based on the assessment information, develop a Calculus Removal Plan. Photocopy the Calculus Removal Plan form in Module 18 or create a similar form for yourself on tablet paper.
   a. Determine how many appointments you will need for calculus removal.
   b. List the treatment area(s) to be completed at each appointment.
   c. List appropriate hand and powered instruments for use at each appointment. Indicate the sequence in which the instruments will be used and the size and location of the deposits that each instrument will remove.

Student: _____   Date: _____

Evaluator: _____

DIRECTIONS FOR STUDENT: Use **Column S.** Evaluate your skill level as: **S** (satisfactory) or **U** (unsatisfactory).

DIRECTIONS FOR EVALUATOR: Use **Column E.** Indicate: **S** (satisfactory) or **U** (unsatisfactory). Each **S** equals I point, each **U** equals 0 points.

CRITERIA:	S	E
Equipment Preparation:		
Connects device to electrical and water sources; disinfects, applies barriers; flushes water line for 2 minutes		
Holds handpiece in upright position until entirely filled with water and seats a universal or straight insert; repeats procedure when changing inserts **(omit this criterion if using piezoelectric or sonic device)**		
Clinician and Patient Preparation:		
Uses protective attire for self and patient; provides patient with pre-procedural rinse		
Explains procedure to the patient including purpose, noise, water spray/evacuation; encourages patient to ask questions and provides appropriate answers; obtains informed consent		
Instrumentation Technique with All Tips:		
Uses evacuation effectively, positioning patient's head and saliva ejector to collect pooled water		
Adjusts power and water settings as appropriate for instrument tip		
Uses a gentle grasp and establishes an appropriate extra- or intraoral fulcrum		
Correctly adapts working-end to the tooth surface being treated		
Keeps the tip in motion using light overlapping, multidirectional, brushlike strokes		
Cups patient's lips and cheeks to collect water; deactivates tip occasionally to allow complete evacuation		
Universal or Straight Slim-Diameter Tip:		
Demonstrates oblique technique on maxillary anteriors, facial aspect		
Demonstrates vertical technique on mandibular anteriors, lingual aspect		
Right and Left Curved Slim-Diameter Tips:		
Identifies right and left tips		
Selects correct tip for oblique technique on the lingual aspect of mandibular left posteriors		
Demonstrates tapping strokes and cross-arch fulcrum for the mandibular left posteriors, lingual aspect		
Selects correct tip for vertical technique on facial aspect of mandibular left posteriors		
Demonstrates sweeping strokes and cross arch fulcrum for the mandibular left posteriors, lingual aspect		
Prepares device for next use; packages appropriate items for autoclaving		
OPTIONAL GRADE PERCENTAGE CALCULATION Total **S**'s in each E column.		

Sum of **S**'s _____ divided by Total Points Possible (**17 or 18**) equals the Percentage Grade _____

SKILL EVALUATION MODULE 24 ULTRASONIC AND SONIC INSTRUMENTATION

Student: _____

EVALUATOR COMMENTS

_____

_____

_____

_____

_____

_____

_____

_____

_____

_____

_____

_____

_____

_____

_____

_____

_____

_____

_____

_____

Box for sketches pertaining to written comments.

Debridement of Dental Implants

Module Overview

This module describes dental implant systems and discusses the specialized periodontal instruments used for the instrumentation of dental implant abutment posts and supporting structures.

Module Outline

Key Terms

Dental implant
Implant fixture
Abutment post

Learning Objectives

1. Describe the dental implant system.

2. Describe the characteristics of an instrument for debridement of a dental implant.

3. List four types of working-end designs for plastic implant instruments.

4. Remove deposits from dental implant structures using appropriate instruments.

Section 1
Dental Implantology

INTRODUCTION TO DENTAL IMPLANTS

A dental implant is a nonbiologic (artificial) device surgically inserted into or onto the jawbone to (1) replace a missing tooth or (2) provide support for a prosthetic denture. Understanding basic implant anatomy is a prerequisite for understanding instrumentation techniques for the maintenance of dental implants.

1. The implant fixture is the portion of the implant that is surgically placed into the bone. The fixture acts as the "root" of the implant and needs a period of 3 to 6 months to be fully surrounded and supported by bone.
2. The abutment post is a titanium post that protrudes through the tissue into the mouth and supports a crown or denture for replacement of a missing tooth or teeth.
3. Titanium is used for the abutment post because this metal is extremely biocompatible (not rejected by the body), allows tissue healing around the implant, and is a poor conductor of heat and electricity. The major disadvantage of titanium is that it scratches easily.

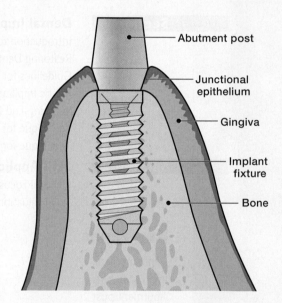

Dental Implant. The components of a dental implant system.

- Abutment post
- Junctional epithelium
- Gingiva
- Implant fixture
- Bone

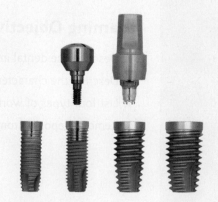

Titanium Implant Screws. Various diameter titanium implant screws. (© 2007 Implant Innovations, Inc. Used by permission, all rights reserved.)

RESTORING DENTAL IMPLANTS

The abutment post must be covered by a crown or connected to a prosthetic denture so that the implant system can function like a natural tooth or teeth. Modern dental implants may be difficult to recognize because they often have the same appearance as the crowns and fixed bridges that are used to restore natural teeth. For this reason, the patient's chart should be clearly labeled so that all dental team members are alerted to the fact that this patient has dental implants.

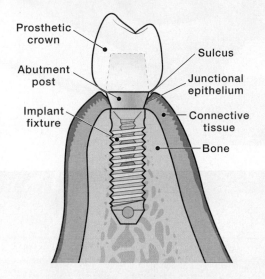

Prosthetic Crown Supported by Dental Implant. When an implant is used to replace a single missing tooth, the implant abutment is covered with a prosthetic crown.

In the mouth, this implant system would be difficult to distinguish from a natural tooth that had been crowned. For this reason, the location of dental implants should be clearly indicated in the patient chart.

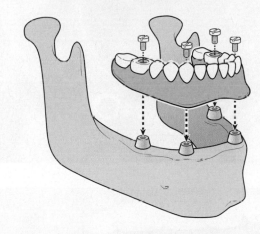

Dentist-Retrievable Prosthesis. For an edentulous patient, one restorative option is a prosthesis that is similar to a full denture except that it is attached by screws to the top of the abutment posts. Today, this restorative option is seldom used because the patient cannot remove the prosthesis from the mouth, making plaque removal difficult and time-consuming.

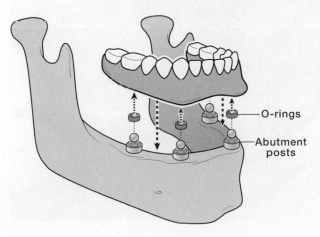

Removable Prosthesis. A more common restorative option for an edentulous patient is a removable prosthesis that is similar to a traditional full denture. In this instance, the denture is attached to the abutment posts by O-rings, magnets, or clips. The patient can remove the prosthesis for cleaning and overnight.

Patient with Dental Implants. An edentulous patient with four dental implants that support a removable mandibular prosthesis.

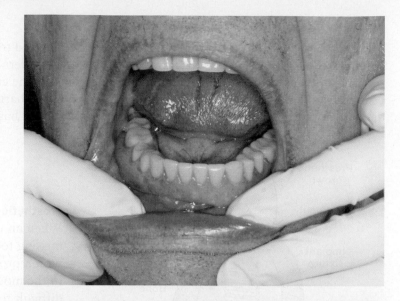

Underside of Prosthesis. The underside of the removable prosthesis showing the O-rings used to secure the prosthesis to the abutment posts.

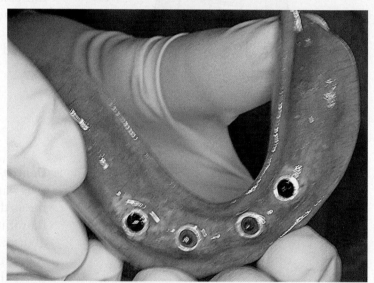

Dental Implants. This patient has four abutment posts on his mandibular arch that support the removable prosthesis.

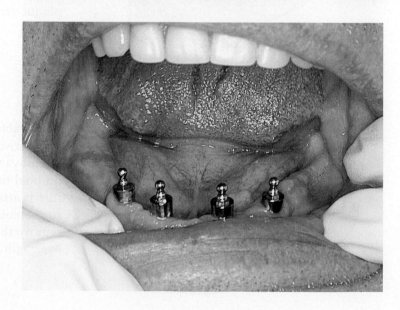

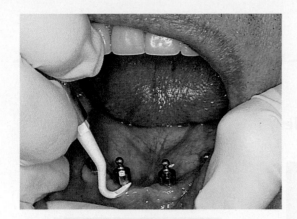

Sickle- and Curet-Shaped Working-Ends.
Sickle- and curet-shaped working-ends adapt well to abutment posts and single implant crowns.

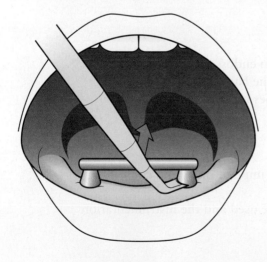

Crescent-Shaped Working-End. The crescent-shaped working-end is used to clean the surface of the abutment post using vertical strokes.

TECHNIQUE FOR DEBRIDEMENT OF FIXED PROSTHESIS

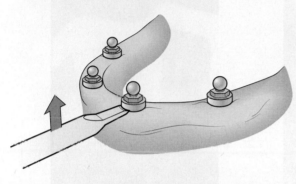

Contra-Angled Crescent-Shaped Working-End.
Contra-angled instruments with crescent-shaped working-ends are used to clean the abutment posts that are linked together with a bar. The bar helps to support a mandibular prosthesis.

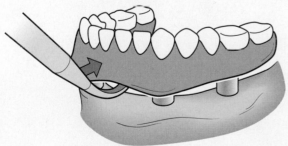

Contra-Angled Hoe-Shaped Working-End.
Contra-angled instruments with hoe-like working-ends are used to clean the underside of a fixed prosthesis.

Section 2
Skill Application

PRACTICAL FOCUS
Periodontal Assessment Case: Mrs. Marple

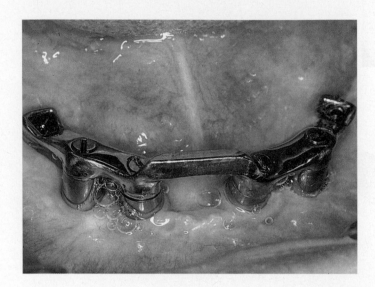
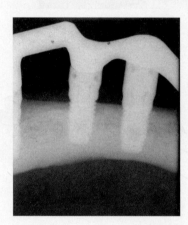

Mrs. Marple: Assessment Data
1. Full maxillary denture.
2. On the mandibular arch, the patient has four titanium endosseous implants.
3. The abutment posts are linked together with a bar. The bar helps to support a mandibular prosthetic denture because the patient does not have enough bone to support a mandibular denture.

Mrs. Marple: Case Questions
1. Select appropriate instruments for debriding the four implant posts and connecting bar.
2. Indicate the sequence in which the instruments will be used and the instrumentation technique used with each instrument.

SKILL EVALUATION MODULE 25	DEBRIDEMENT OF DENTAL IMPLANTS

Student: _____　　　Instrument 1 = _____

Evaluator: _____　　　Instrument 2 = _____

Date: _____　　　Instrument 3 = _____

MODULE DIRECTIONS: Demonstrate the use of plastic instruments on a typodont with dental implants. If a typodont with dental implants is not available, a simple alternative can be constructed using nails and wooden blocks. Hammer a long nail partway into a small wooden block. A portion of the nail extending above the wooden block can be used to represent the abutment post of a dental implant.

DIRECTIONS FOR STUDENT: Use **Column S.** Evaluate your skill level as: **S** (satisfactory) or **U** (unsatisfactory).

DIRECTIONS FOR EVALUATOR: Use **Column E.** Indicate: **S** (satisfactory) or **U** (unsatisfactory). Each **S** equals 1 point, each **U** equals 0 points.

	1		2		3	
CRITERIA:	S	E	S	E	S	E
Explains use of the instrument						
Demonstrates instrumentation strokes using light pressure						
Demonstrates instrumentation strokes using the correct stroke direction						
OPTIONAL GRADE PERCENTAGE CALCULATION Total **S**'s in each E column.						

Sum of **S**'s _____ divided by Total Points Possible (**9**) equals the Percentage Grade _____

EVALUATOR COMMENTS

_____

_____

_____

_____

_____

_____

_____

_____

_____

_____

_____

_____

_____

_____

Cosmetic Polishing Procedures

Module Overview

This module discusses historical perspectives of polishing and the evidence-based change from polishing as a routine to a nonessential procedure. Indications and contraindications for coronal polishing are presented as well as the adverse effects of polishing. Two coronal polishing methods are described: the rubber cup method and the air-powder method.

Module Outline

Key Terms

Coronal polishing

Therapeutic procedure

Aerosols

Splatter

Bacteremia

Extrinsic stain

Chlorhexidine stain

Tobacco stain

Intrinsic stain

Selective polishing

Rubber cup polishing

Right-angle

Contra-angle

Reusable angle

Disposable angle

Abrasive agent

Grit

Air-powder polishing

Learning Objectives

1. Discuss the American Dental Hygienists' Association Position Paper on polishing.

2. Define the term *therapeutic procedure,* and explain why stain removal is a cosmetic rather than a therapeutic procedure.

3. List three adverse effects of coronal polishing.

4. Define the terms *extrinsic* and *intrinsic stain,* and give examples of each.

5. List the indications and contraindications for coronal polishing.

6. Demonstrate the correct technique for securing a rubber cup to a prophylaxis angle with a threaded head.

7. List and describe five factors that can be controlled to minimize loss of tooth structure during coronal polishing.

8. List special considerations and contraindications to be observed when using the air-powder method of stain removal.

9. Describe the correct nozzle angulation for use of an air-powder device on (1) facial and lingual surfaces of the anterior teeth, (2) facial and lingual surfaces of posterior teeth, and (3) occlusal surfaces.

10. Demonstrate the correct technique for coronal polishing to remove stain using a rubber polishing cup and dental floss.

11. Demonstrate the correct technique for flossing a patient's teeth.

12. Explain the rationale for not routinely polishing the teeth as part of an oral prophylaxis.

SUGGESTED READINGS

1. American Dental Hygienists' Association Position on Polishing Procedures online at http://www.ADHA.org.

2. Gutkowski, S., *Whether they need it...or not! Are you compelled to polish every tooth? Dental researchers advise a re-evaluation of methods, materials, and modalities.* RDH, November 2001: 50–56.

Section 1
Introduction to Stain Removal

HISTORICAL PERSPECTIVES ON CORONAL POLISHING

Coronal polishing is a cosmetic procedure designed to remove extrinsic stains from the enamel surfaces of the teeth. Stain removal is a nonessential procedure undertaken for esthetic reasons—to improve the appearance of the anterior teeth. A therapeutic procedure is a dental procedure used to maintain health or treat a disease to restore health. There is no therapeutic benefit to coronal polishing because dental stains do not directly contribute to periodontal disease, dental caries, or any other disease. Historically, all teeth were polished at the completion of the oral prophylaxis. Today, researchers agree that coronal polishing is not necessary on a routine basis. In fact, over time, polishing can remove tooth structure causing morphological changes in the teeth. The principles of evidence-based care indicate that routine polishing of all teeth is a "tradition" that should be discontinued. It is poor healthcare to lead a patient to believe that coronal polishing is a therapeutic procedure, when coronal polishing is, at best, a cosmetic procedure with no health benefits and, at worst, a procedure that damages the tooth surfaces.

TABLE 26-1. Historical Perspectives on Coronal Polishing	
Date	**Treatment Approach**
The past	Coronal polishing was a routine part of the oral prophylaxis.
	We believed the following:
	1. Tooth Surface. It was important to have smooth, stain-free tooth surfaces to impede the buildup of new plaque.
	2. Fluoride. Stains and plaque must be removed before a fluoride treatment to allow adequate uptake of fluoride in the enamel.
	3. Sealants. It was necessary to polish tooth surfaces before sealant placement to ensure proper acid etching and sealant penetration.
Today	Coronal polishing is a nonessential cosmetic procedure with little therapeutic benefit. Instead of polishing the teeth, time is better spent in teaching techniques for personal plaque control.
	Research has shown the following:
	1. Tooth Surface. Thorough brushing and flossing at home can produce the same effect as polishing.
	a. Rather than smoothing tooth surfaces, polishing actually scratches and grooves tooth surfaces.
	b. Cementum and dentin are softer than enamel; therefore, these surfaces scratch more easily than enamel surfaces.
	c. Fluoride in the outer layers of enamel is removed by polishing, making the tooth more vulnerable to decay.
	2. Fluoride. Polishing does not improve the uptake of fluoride.
	3. Sealants. The use of an explorer and forceful rinsing are as effective as polishing before sealant placement.

ADVERSE EFFECTS OF CORONAL POLISHING

The practice of routinely polishing the teeth came into question when research findings showed that over time routine polishing is detrimental to the tooth surface. The adverse effects of coronal polishing include:

1. Aerosol Production and Splatter. Contaminated aerosols and splatter present a hazard to the clinician, the patient, and other dental personnel and patients in the dental office.
   a. Dental aerosols are invisible airborne particles dispersed into the surrounding environment by dental equipment such as dental handpieces and electronically powered instruments. Microorganisms in the dental aerosols have been shown to survive for up to 24 hours.
   b. Splatter consists of airborne particles that land on people and objects. Unlike aerosols, splatter from polishing often is visible after it lands on objects such as eyewear, uniforms, skin, hair, or other surfaces. Polishing splatter is composed of polishing paste, microorganisms, and saliva.
   c. Power-driven equipment should not be used for a patient with a known communicable condition that could be spread by aerosols.
   d. Power-driven equipment should not be used for a patient with high susceptibility to infection such as individuals with respiratory or pulmonary disease or immunocompromised or debilitated individuals.
   e. Patients and dental team members need eyewear to protect their eyes from splatter. Constituents of commercial prophylaxis pastes may include various chemicals that can cause a severe inflammatory response in the eye.
2. Creation of Bacteremia. Bacteremia is the presence of bacteria in the bloodstream.
   a. Bacteria from the oval cavity are introduced into the bloodstream during hand or powered instrumentation and polishing. The health history must be prepared initially, reviewed, and updated at all appointments to identify patients who are at risk for bacteremia.
   b. Patients who are susceptible to bacteremia need premedication with antibiotics before coronal polishing. Examples of individuals who are susceptible to bacteremia include those with damaged or abnormal heart valves, prosthetic heart valve, prosthetic joint replacement, rheumatic heart disease, congenital heart disease, cardiac bypass surgery within the last 6 months, and dialysis patients.
3. Iatrogenic Damage to Tooth Surfaces
   a. Stain removal with an abrasive agent removes the surface layer of enamel where the fluoride content is greatest and most protective.
   b. The cemento-enamel junction has a thin cementum or dentin surface that can be easily abraded or removed with an abrasive agent.
   c. Polishing generates heat. Care must be taken to use a wet polishing agent with minimal pressure and low speed to prevent overheating of a tooth. Primary teeth have large pulp chambers that make these teeth particularly vulnerable to the heat generated during polishing.
   d. Coronal polishing can cause injury to the gingiva. Incorrect polishing technique can injure the gingival margin. In addition, during polishing, abrasive paste is forced into the gingival sulcus and even into the tissue itself. Some people have a negative tissue response to abrasive particles or chemicals in the paste that can result in delayed tissue healing.

TYPES OF STAINS

In determining the need for coronal polishing, the clinician must distinguish between stains that can be removed by polishing and those that cannot.

1. Stains that can be removed by polishing are extrinsic.
   a. Extrinsic stains occur on the external (outer) surfaces of the teeth.
   b. The most common extrinsic stains are chlorhexidine stain and tobacco stain.
      1) **Chlorhexidine stain** is caused by the use of antimicrobial mouth rinses that contain chlorhexidine. Chlorhexidine causes a yellowish-brown stain on the cervical and proximal tooth surfaces, restorations, and the surface of the tongue.
      2) **Tobacco stain** is a tenacious dark brown or black stain that results from cigarette or cigar smoking or the use of chewing tobacco.
2. Stains that cannot be removed by polishing.
   a. Intrinsic stains occur *within the enamel* of the tooth and cannot be removed by polishing. Intrinsic stains may be endogenous (occurring during tooth development) or exogenous (acquired after tooth eruption).
   b. Examples of endogenous intrinsic stains are tetracycline stain and dental fluorosis.
   c. Examples of exogenous intrinsic stains are stains from silver amalgams, nonvital teeth, and endodontic (root canal) treatment.

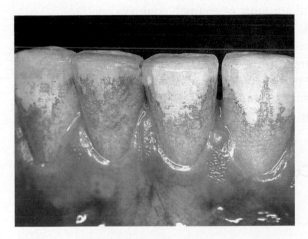

Chlorhexidine Stain

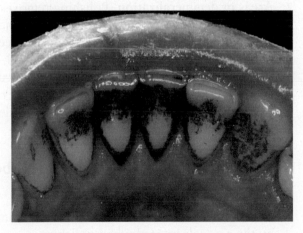

Tobacco Stain

INDICATIONS FOR CORONAL POLISHING

Coronal polishing is indicated to improve the esthetic appearance of tooth surfaces that are visible when the patient smiles or engages in conversation. Selective polishing means that only those stained tooth surfaces with an objectionable appearance are polished. Selective polishing stresses daily patient self-care for the removal of plaque biofilms.

1. Debridement with hand or powered instruments is completed first. As much stain as possible is removed during periodontal debridement. Sonic and ultrasonic instruments are excellent for stain removal.
2. The patient uses a toothbrush, dental floss, or other interdental aids to remove plaque. The clinician plays a supportive role by providing instruction and guidance to the patient.
3. Each patient is evaluated individually to determine whether cosmetic polishing is necessary.

CONTRAINDICATIONS FOR CORONAL POLISHING

Dental Contraindications for Rubber Cup and Air-Powder Polishing

1. **Lack of stain.** Tooth surfaces that either have no extrinsic stain or have stains that are not visible when the patient smiles or engages in conversation should not be polished.
2. **Sensitive teeth.** Application of fluoride is one treatment for dental sensitivity. Polishing removes the fluoride-rich outer layers of enamel that should be preserved.
3. **Exposed cementum or dentin.** Areas of exposed cementum or dentin should not be polished because polishing removes significant amounts of these structures. Polishing should be confined to stained enamel surfaces.
4. **Restored tooth surfaces.** Restorative materials are not as hard as enamel and therefore are scratched easily by the abrasive agent. Air-powder polishing should be avoided around most types of restorative materials because of the possibility of scratching, eroding, pitting, or margin leakage.
5. **Newly erupted teeth.** Because the mineralization of newly erupted teeth is incomplete, polishing should be avoided.
6. **Implant abutments.** Titanium abutments should not be polished. The implant superstructure—prosthetic crown or denture—can be polished if needed for stain removal; however, stain-free superstructures should not be polished.
7. **Areas of demineralization.** Polishing removes small amounts of enamel; conservation of demineralized enamel surfaces is indicated.
8. **Gingiva that is enlarged, soft, spongy, or bleeds easily.** Cosmetic polishing is not recommended for any patient with inflamed, enlarged, soft, spongy, or bleeding tissue. The abrasive particles can enter the sulcus or periodontal pocket resulting in increased inflammation, and the action of the rotating cup can further traumatize the tissue. Cosmetic polishing should be scheduled for a separate appointment after tissue healing has occurred.

Systemic Contraindications for Rubber Cup and Air-Powder Polishing

1. **Communicable disease.** Patients with a communicable disease that could be spread by the aerosols created when polishing.
2. **Susceptibility to infection.** Patients with a high susceptibility to infection that can be transmitted by contaminated aerosols (those with respiratory or pulmonary disease; debilitated, immunosuppressed, or immunocompromised individuals).

Special Considerations with Air-Powder Polishing

In addition to all the contraindications listed above, the air-powder polishing technique is contraindicated for a patient with:

1. A restricted sodium diet—because of the high sodium content of the powder.
2. A respiratory disease or other condition that limits swallowing such as multiple sclerosis, amyotrophic lateral sclerosis, muscular dystrophy, or paralysis.
3. Renal disease or metabolic disorders and in individuals on diuretics or long term-steroid therapy—because the high sodium content of the powder could cause an electrolyte imbalance in these individuals. Electrolytes are minerals such as potassium, calcium, sodium, and magnesium that are needed to keep the body's balance of fluids at the proper level.

Section 2
Rubber Cup Method of Stain Removal

The most common technique for stain removal is rubber cup polishing. This technique uses an abrasive polishing agent and a slowly revolving polishing cup to abrade stain from the tooth surfaces. Another term for this method of polishing is *power-driven polishing*.

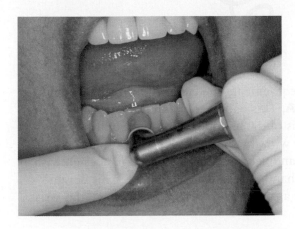

Rubber Cup Polishing. A rubber cup filled with a polishing agent is used to remove extrinsic stain from the teeth.

COMPONENTS OF THE POLISHING SYSTEM

This polishing system comprises (1) a dental handpiece, (2) a prophylaxis angle, and (3) various angle attachments.

1. **Dental handpiece (handle).** A slow-speed dental handpiece is used for polishing. The handpiece is air driven and attaches to the dental unit slow-speed handpiece line.
2. **Prophylaxis angle (shank).** The prophylaxis angle, commonly called a *prophy angle*, is used to hold a prophy cup or other attachment used for polishing the teeth.
   a. Design. Prophylaxis angles may be either right-angled or contra-angled in design.
      1) A right-angle has a straight shank.
      2) A contra-angle has a bent shank. A contra-angle allows the clinician to maintain a neutral wrist position and facilitates access to the proximal surfaces of teeth.
   b. Types. Prophylaxis angles are available in reusable and disposable designs. Reusable prophy angles must be properly cleaned and sterilized between each use to prevent cross-contamination. For this reason, many clinicians prefer to use disposable prophy angles that are discarded after a single use.

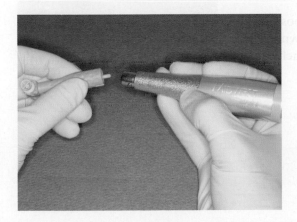

Dental Handpiece and Prophylaxis Angle. The prophylaxis angle connects to a dental handpiece. The angle holds attachments that are used to remove stain from the teeth.

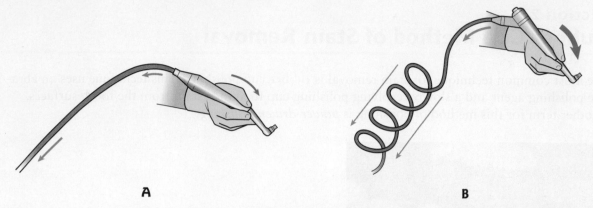

A

B

Handpiece Hose Attachment. When purchasing dental equipment, one factor the clinician should consider is the design of a handpiece hose attachment. **A,** This handpiece has a good ergonomic design with the hose attachment aligned with the long axis of the handpiece and a straight hose with no coils. This design aligns the weight of the handpiece with the long axis of the arm, placing less stress on the clinician's arm, wrist, and hand. **B,** This handpiece has a poor ergonomic design with the hose attachment at an angle to the long axis of the handpiece and a coiled hose. This design causes the weight of the handpiece and the hose to pull against the clinician's arm, hand, and wrist.

Reusable Right-Angle. Shown here is a reusable right-angle that must be autoclaved after each use.

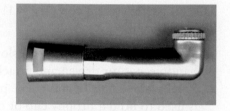

Disposable Right-Angle. This right-angle is disposable and should be discarded after a single use.

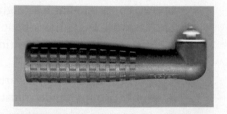

Contra-Angle. A contra-angle facilitates neutral wrist position and access to proximal surfaces. The contra-angle shown in the photograph is reusable and must be autoclaved after each use.

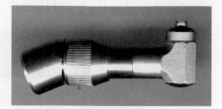

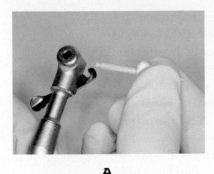
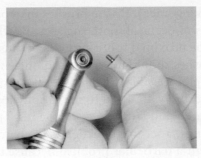
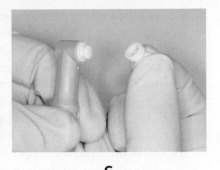

A   B   C

Prophylaxis Angle Head Designs. The head of a prophylaxis angle can have a (**A**) latch design, (**B**) threaded head, or (**C**) button-ended head.

3. **Prophy cup attachments (working-ends).**
   a. **Natural or synthetic rubber.** Prophy cups are made from natural or synthetic rubber. Non-latex cups are used for latex-sensitive patients.
   b. **Internal cup design.** Internal cup design affects the cleaning ability of the cup and the amount of paste that can be held on the tooth surface. Prophy cups are available in a wide variety of designs. For example, Young Dental manufactures over 20 variations of prophy cups. Cups come in standard ribbed, curved ribbed, and webbed interior designs.
   c. **Length and diameter.** Prophy cups come in standard lengths, shorter lengths (for children and adults with small mouths), and smaller-diameter versions (for access to rotated or overlapping anterior teeth or orthodontic appliances). The length of the cup affects visibility (shorter cups allow the clinician to see around the cup better while polishing) and the ability to reach posterior tooth surfaces (shorter cups are easier to use in the confined space of the posterior regions of the mouth).
   d. **Flexibility.** Cups are available in soft and firm styles. Natural rubber cups are more flexible and allow the cup to flare and conform better to the contours of the teeth.

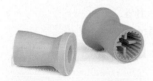

Standard Webbed Cup. Cups with divided webbed interiors provide efficient stain removal. Webbed cups are less flexible and hold less abrasive paste than ribbed cups. (Courtesy of Young Dental.)

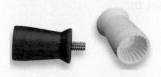

Standard Ribbed Cup. A ribbed interior cup design allows the cup to flex and follow the tooth contours. (Courtesy of Young Dental.)

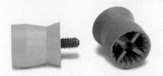

Petite Webbed Cup. A petite cup is shorter than a standard web cub. This design facilitates access in hard to reach areas. (Courtesy of Young Dental.)

4. **Bristle brush attachments (working-ends).** Bristle brushes may be used to remove stains from the pits and fissures of occlusal tooth surfaces. Bristle brushes should not be used on facial, lingual, or proximal tooth surfaces because the bristles could lacerate the gingival tissue. Brushes should never be used on cementum or dentin.

5. **Securing attachments to the angle.** Special care must be taken to ensure that the rubber cup or bristle brush is securely attached to the prophylaxis angle.

   a. If the cup falls off, the patient could swallow or inhale it. If a cup or brush is aspirated (inhaled) into the lungs, a serious infection is likely to develop.

   b. Screw-on attachments present a particular problem because they will come off while polishing if the handpiece is run in reverse. This problem can be avoided by running the handpiece to slowly thread the cup into the head of the prophy angle. If the handpiece is running in the forward direction, the cup or brush will secure itself to the angle. If the handpiece is running in the reverse direction, the angle will not accept the cup.

MINIMIZING LOSS OF TOOTH STRUCTURE

There are five factors that can be controlled to minimize the loss of tooth structure during the polishing procedure: (1) abrasiveness of the prophylaxis paste, (2) adaptation of the rubber cup, (3) pressure, (4) speed, and (5) application time.

1. **Abrasive Agent.** Abrasive agents are substances in prophylaxis pastes that remove extrinsic stains by scratching and abrading the tooth surface.

   a. Brands of prophylaxis paste vary considerably in levels of abrasiveness. The larger the size of the abrasive particles in a paste, the deeper the scratches produced. Smaller abrasive particles produce a finer scratch. Particle size is also referred to as grit.

   b. Manufacturers label pastes with descriptive terms such as "extra fine, fine, medium, coarse, and extra coarse." Unfortunately, there is no standard definition of these terms, so clinicians must rely on the recommendations of the manufacturer when selecting a particular paste for a task.

   c. The clinician should use a prophylaxis paste with the smallest particle size that will remove the stain.

      1) Select an extra-fine or fine-grit paste for most polishing tasks.

      2) Medium grit is the largest abrasive particle size that should be used. If a medium-grit paste does not remove the stain, the clinician should reevaluate the stain to confirm that it is not intrinsic stain.

2. **Rubber Cup Adaptation**

   a. The rubber cup should be adapted parallel to the tooth surface being polished.

   b. Adapting the rubber cup at an acute angle to the tooth surface increases the scratching of the tooth surface.

3. **Pressure.** The rubber cup should be applied using *just enough pressure to make the cup flare slightly.*

4. **Speed of Application**

   a. The rubber cup should rotate at the slowest speed possible, using only enough speed to keep the rubber cup from stopping.

   b. The speed is too fast if the handpiece makes a high-pitched "whining" sound.

5. **Application Time.** The rubber cup should be applied to a tooth surface only 1 or 2 seconds before moving the cup to another area of the tooth.

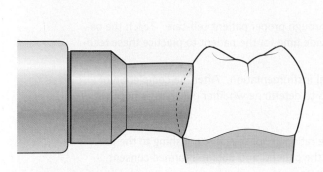

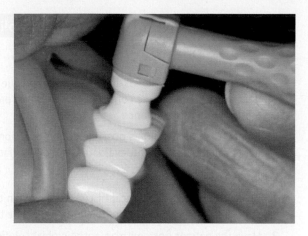

Correct Adaptation and Flaring of the Rubber Cup. The rubber cup should be adapted parallel to the tooth surface being treated and sufficient pressure applied to flare the rim of the cup.

A MODIFIED APPROACH TO POLISHING

Most adult patients are accustomed to having their teeth polished at the end of each check-up appointment. In fact, many adult patients mistakenly believe that the polishing procedure rather than the periodontal instrumentation is the therapeutic part of an oral prophylaxis.

1. Education plays an important role in the patient's understanding of cosmetic polishing. The rationale for selective polishing should be explained to patients. This explanation can be brief, covering several key points:
   a. The patient must remove plaque on a daily basis because plaque re-forms within 24 hours after being removed.
   b. Stain is not responsible for any problems in the mouth but can be removed to improve the appearance of the teeth.
   c. Polishing is a cosmetic procedure with no health benefits; in fact if done routinely, it can damage the tooth surfaces.
2. When patients understand the rationale for selective polishing, most are willing to do without or minimize polishing. In fact, many patients dislike the sensation of having their teeth polished or the taste of the gritty polishing paste. Some patients experience tooth sensitivity for several days after having their teeth polished.
3. Many patients enjoy the fresh feeling in their mouths after polishing. For these patients, the clinician might use a modified approach to the polishing procedure.
   a. A fine-grit prophylaxis paste is used to remove stain that is visible when the patient smiles or engages in conversation.
   b. After stain removal, the clinician rinses the mouth and attaches a new prophy cup. A new prophy cup is used whenever changing from a more abrasive to a less abrasive polishing agent.
   c. Using regular toothpaste, the clinician quickly and lightly polishes the remaining teeth in the mouth. Toothpaste is much less abrasive than prophylaxis paste but still provides the patient with that "just polished" feeling.
   d. After any polishing procedure, all tooth surfaces should be rinsed thoroughly and flossed.

Box 26-1. Procedure for Rubber Cup Polishing

Before Polishing

1. Discuss the importance of daily removal of plaque through proper patient self-care. Teach the patient appropriate plaque control techniques and provide time for the patient to practice these techniques with your guidance.

2. Remove as much stain as possible during periodontal instrumentation. After the completion of periodontal debridement, evaluate the tooth surfaces to determine whether polishing is necessary.

Patient Preparation

1. Review the patient's medical history, and explain the rationale for selective polishing to the patient. Explain the rubber cup polishing procedure to the patient, and obtain informed consent.

2. Have the patient rinse with an antimicrobial solution.

3. Provide the patient with protective eyewear.

Clinician Preparation. Use all appropriate protective equipment including a high-BFE (bacterial filtration efficiency) mask, protective eyewear, face shield, gloves, and a long-sleeved gown.

Rubber Cup Polishing Procedure

1. Position the patient in a supine position.

2. Cup the patient's lip or cheek, and use an evacuator tip or saliva ejector throughout the polishing procedure.

3. Select extra-fine or fine-grit paste for most polishing tasks. Use a latex-free cup with a latex-sensitive patient. Fill the rubber cup with paste, and establish a secure fulcrum. Rest the handpiece in the V-shaped area of your hand between the index finger and thumb.

4. Hold the rubber cup so that the rim is almost in contact with, but not touching, the tooth surface. Activate the foot pedal and regulate the speed so the cup rotates at a slow, steady speed.

5. Adapt the cup to the cervical-third of the crown, applying just enough pressure to make the rim of the cup flare slightly. The cemento-enamel junction is susceptible to abrasive damage, so take care when moving the cup into the sulcus.

6. Using a wiping motion, draw the cup across the tooth surface while moving from the cervical-third of the crown toward the incisal edge. Most surfaces can be polished in 2 to 3 seconds using steady speed and light intermittent pressure.

7. Apply the cup to the proximal surfaces by flaring the cup rim as far interproximally as possible. The cup is adapted to the proximal surfaces by repositioning the entire handpiece.

8. Refill the cup frequently with paste. An empty cup will not polish the tooth surface and generates excessive heat. Before refilling the cup, first remove saliva from the cup by slowly spinning it against a dry gauze square.

9. Polish several teeth, then rinse the tooth surfaces thoroughly.

10. After polishing, floss the entire mouth to remove abrasive particles from between the teeth. Thoroughly rinse the entire mouth to loosen and remove particles from around the gingival margin; use an evacuation tip to remove the particles and water from the mouth.

Section 3
Air-Powder Method of Stain Removal

A second technique for stain removal is air-powder polishing. This technique uses a mixture of warm water, sodium bicarbonate powder, and air for extrinsic stain removal. The sodium bicarbonate powder is the abrasive agent used to remove stain from the tooth surfaces. Air-powder polishing is indicated for patients with heavy amounts of stain, especially chlorhexidine stain. Other terms for air-powder polishing include airbrasive polishing and air polishing.

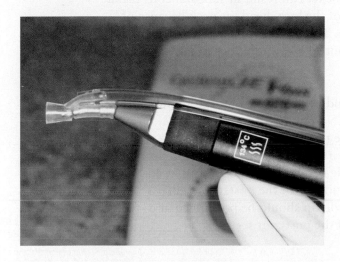

Polisher Handpiece. The handpiece nozzle of-fan air-powder polishing device. The handpiece delivers a mixture of warm water, sodium bicarbonate powder, and air to the tooth surface

AIR-POWDER POLISHING DEVICES

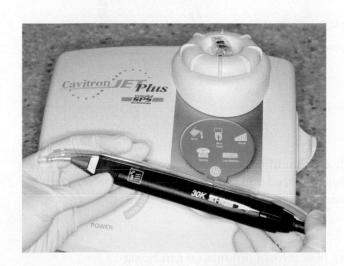

Stand Alone Air-Powder Polishing Device. This air-powder polishing device has an electric generator that provides power to the handpiece.

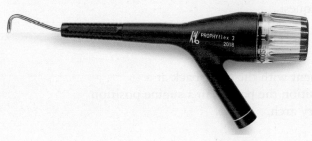

Air-Powder Polishing Device. This device connects to the dental unit handpiece tubing. (Courtesy of KaVo America Corporation)

TECHNIQUE FOR AIR-POWDER POLISHING

Precise angulation of the nozzle tip should be maintained throughout the air-powder polishing procedure.

1. **Dangers of Incorrect Nozzle Angulation**
   a. **The nozzle tip should never be directed at the soft tissues of the cheeks, lips, gingival margin, or tongue. Directing the nozzle tip at the soft tissues can result in severe tissue sloughing.**
   b. Never angle the powder spray directly into the sulcus or pocket. Directing the powder-spray directly into the sulcus or pocket can result in subcutaneous facial emphysema, a sudden unilateral swelling of the face, head, or neck because of the presence of air in the connective tissue. Treatment of subcutaneous facial emphysema consists of analgesics for pain control and antibiotics to prevent a secondary infection.

2. **Correct Technique for Positioning the Nozzle**
   a. Distance from Tooth. The nozzle tip should be held 3 to 4 mm from the tooth surface.
   b. Adaptation for Anterior Teeth. The nozzle tip should be positioned at a 60-degree angle to the facial and lingual surfaces of the anterior teeth.
   c. Adaptation for Posterior Teeth. The nozzle tip should be positioned at an 80-degree angle to the facial and lingual surfaces of the posterior teeth.
   d. Adaptation to Occlusal Surfaces. The nozzle tip should be positioned at a 90-degree angle to the occlusal surfaces of the posterior teeth.

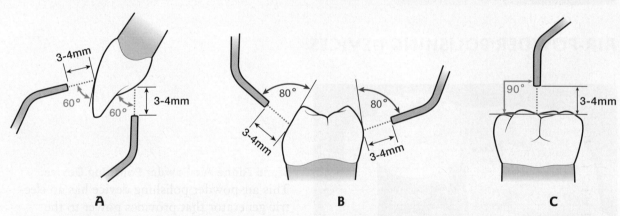

Correct Angulation of the Nozzle Tip. The nozzle tip should be positioned 3 to 4 mm away from the tooth surface. **A,** Correct 60-degree angulation for the facial and lingual surfaces of anterior teeth. **B,** Correct 80-degree angulation for the facial and lingual surfaces of posterior teeth. **C,** Correct angulation of nozzle tip for the occlusal surfaces.

3. Aerosol Control. The research literature shows that aerosol production can be significantly reduced through the following techniques:
   a. Correct positioning of the nozzle tip.
   b. Use of high-velocity evacuation. The evacuator should be held as close to the handpiece nozzle as possible.
   c. Correct patient positioning. Position the patient with the chair back at a 45-degree angle for most tooth surfaces. Position the patient in a supine position to polish the lingual surfaces on the maxillary arch.

d. **Correct patient head position.** The patient's head should be turned all the way to the side. For example, when a right-handed clinician polishes the lingual surfaces on the right side of the mouth, the patient's head should be turned as far to the right as possible.

e. **Tissue cupping.** The clinician should cup the lip or cheeks to contain the powder slurry for evacuation.

Box 26-2. Procedure for Air-Powder Polishing

Preparation

1. Follow the manufacturer's recommendations for power settings, powder-to-water ratio, and maintenance of the air-powder polishing device.

2. Review the patient's medical history, explain the procedure to the patient, and obtain informed consent.

3. Have the patient rinse with an antimicrobial solution.

4. Provide the patient with protective eyewear.

5. Use all appropriate protective equipment including a high-BFE (bacterial filtration efficiency) mask, protective eyewear, face shield, gloves, and a long-sleeved gown.

Air-Powder Polishing Procedure

1. Position the patient's chair back at a 45-degree angle, and ask the patient to turn to the side. If treating the maxillary lingual surfaces, position patient in a supine position.

2. Evaluate the tooth surfaces, and determine an efficient plan for polishing only those tooth surfaces with objectionable esthetics.

3. Cover the patient's lips with a non-petroleum lubricant. Place a gauze square on the patient's lip near the area to be treated.

4. Cup the patient's lip or cheek and use an evacuator tip or saliva ejector throughout the polishing procedure.

5. Position the nozzle tip 3 to 4 mm from the tooth surface, and establish the recommended angulation of the nozzle tip to the tooth surface being treated. Center the nozzle tip on the middle and incisal thirds of the tooth crown.

6. Activate the foot pedal. Use a constant circular sweeping motion, going from interproximal surface to interproximal surface on the tooth. Polish each tooth for only 1 or 2 seconds.

7. Polish several teeth, then rinse all tooth surfaces thoroughly.

8. After polishing, floss the entire mouth to remove abrasive particles from between the teeth. Thoroughly rinse the entire mouth to loosen and remove particles from around the gingival margin; use an evacuation tip to remove the particles and water from the mouth.

After Treatment

1. Wear a mask, eyewear, and face shield while cleaning the equipment. Follow the manufacturer's recommendations for disinfection of the unit and handpiece hose.

2. Remove the nozzle from the handpiece. Clean inside the nozzle tip; most manufacturers provide a special tool for this purpose. Use the air syringe to blow any residual powder from the nozzle tip.

3. Sterilize the nozzle and handpiece according to the manufacturer's recommendations.

Section 4
Technique Practice: Polishing

TECHNIQUE PRACTICE: PART 1

Directions:

1. Begin this technique practice by using the rubber cup on the *mandibular first molar, facial aspect.*

2. Photocopy Box 26-1 Procedure for Rubber Cup Polishing on page 608. Follow the steps listed in this box to practice the polishing technique. After gaining some experience in using the rubber cup on the first molar, refer to Part 2 of this technique practice on page 614 to practice polishing all the sextants of the dentition. Even though you may rarely polish a patient's entire dentition, you need to be proficient in the polishing technique for all areas of the mouth.

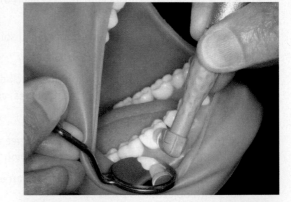

1. **Facial Aspect of First Molar.** Begin your practice by polishing the facial aspect of the first molar. Right-handed clinicians should practice on the mandibular right first molar, left-handed clinicians on the mandibular left first molar.

   Rest the handpiece in the V-shaped area of your hand between the index finger and thumb.

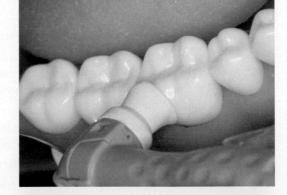

2. **Activate the Handpiece.** Establish an intraoral fulcrum. Hold the rubber cup so that the rim is almost in contact with the distofacial line angle of the molar. Regulate the speed so that the cup rotates at a slow, steady speed. Adapt the cup to the tooth, applying just enough pressure to make the cup rim flare slightly. Apply light, intermittent pressure.

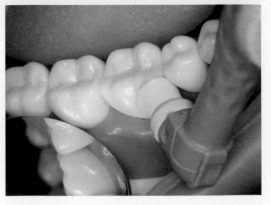

3. **Adapt the Cup.** Reposition the entire handpiece to adapt the cup to the facial and mesial surfaces. Keep the cup moving; resting it in one area for any length of time will generate heat.

   Flare the rim of the cup onto the mesial surface and beneath the contact area.

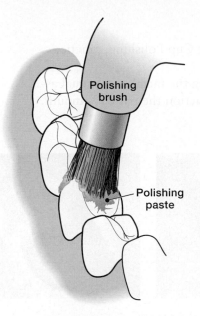

Polishing brush

Polishing paste

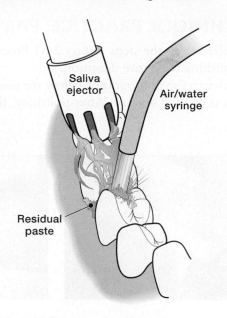

Saliva ejector

Air/water syringe

Residual paste

Occlusal Surfaces

Irrigate and Evacuate

4. **Occlusal Surfaces.** Use either a rubber cup or a bristle brush to polish the occlusal surface of the molar. Angle the cup or brush to adapt to the occlusal planes and into the grooves and fissures.

5. **Irrigate and Evacuate.** Use the air/water syringe to rinse the residual paste from around the molar. Suction to remove the paste and water from the patient's mouth.

Dental floss can be used in two ways during the polishing procedure.

1. First, dental floss—or dental tape—and prophylaxis paste can be used to remove stain from the proximal surfaces.
   a. Place some of the paste between the teeth coronal to the contact area.
   b. Insert the floss past the contact area. Wrap the floss around a proximal surface, and use the floss in a back-and-forth motion against the tooth to remove the stain. Repeat the process for the other proximal surface bordering the embrasure space.

2. Second, floss should always be used to remove abrasive particles from between the teeth at the completion of the polishing procedure.

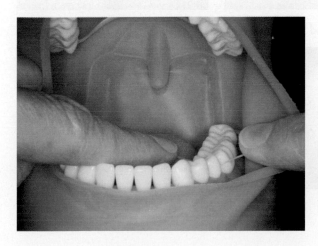

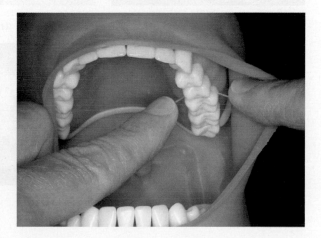

TECHNIQUE PRACTICE: PART 2

1. Referring to the steps in Box 26-1 Procedure for Rubber Cup Polishing, practice polishing the entire dentition.
2. Refer to the photographs below for guidance in accessing the facial and lingual aspects of each sextant. After polishing, floss, rinse, and suction the patient's mouth.

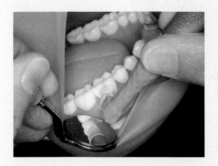
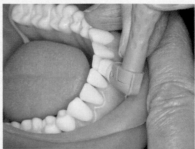
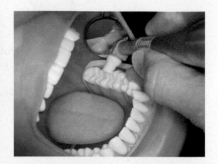

Mandibular Facial and Lingual Aspects

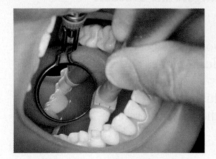
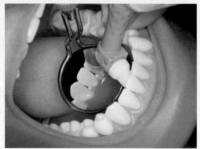
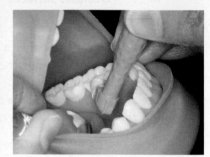

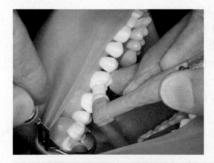
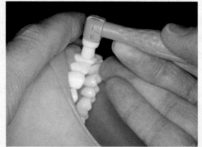
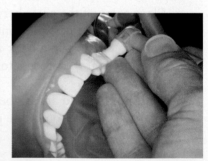

Maxillary Facial and Lingual Aspects

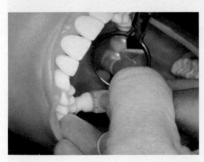
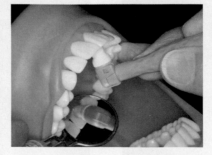
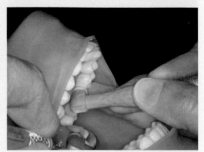

Skill Application

SKILL EVALUATION MODULE 26 RUBBER CUP POLISHING

Student: _____

Evaluator: _____

Date: _____

Area 1 = _____
Area 2 = _____
Area 3 = _____
Area 4 = _____

DIRECTIONS FOR STUDENT: Use **Column S.** Evaluate your skill level as **S** (satisfactory) or **U** (unsatisfactory).

DIRECTIONS FOR EVALUATOR: Use **Column E.** Indicate: **S** (satisfactory) or **U** (unsatisfactory). Each **S** equals 1 point, each **U** equals 0 points.

CRITERIA:	Area 1 S	Area 1 E	Area 2 S	Area 2 E	Area 3 S	Area 3 E	Area 4 S	Area 4 E
Clinician and Patient Preparation:								
Uses protective attire for self and patient; provides patient with pre-procedural rinse								
Explains the rationale for selective polishing and the polishing procedure to the patient; encourages patient to ask questions and provides appropriate answers; obtains informed consent								
Polishing Technique:								
Uses evacuation effectively, positioning patient's head and saliva ejector to facilitate evacuation								
Attaches cup to prophy angle and checks that cup is securely attached to angle								
Rests handpiece in the V-shaped area of hand and establishes a secure fulcrum								
Holds cup with rim near, but not touching, tooth surface; activates cup and regulates speed so that cup rotates at a slow, steady speed								
Adapts the cup to tooth, applying enough pressure to make rim flare slightly								
Uses a wiping motion to draw the cup across the tooth surface, moving from cervical-third of crown toward the incisal/occlusal surface. Uses light intermittent pressure.								
Applies cup to the proximal surfaces, flaring the cup rim as far interproximally as possible								
Refills the cup frequently with paste; before refilling cup, spins it against a gauze square to remove saliva								
Polishes several teeth, then rinses the tooth surfaces thoroughly								
Flosses to remove abrasive particles from between teeth; rinses and evacuates mouth								

OPTIONAL GRADE PERCENTAGE CALCULATION
Total **S**'s in each E column.

Sum of **S**'s _____ divided by Total Points Possible (**46**) equals the Percentage Grade _____

SKILL EVALUATION MODULE 26 | RUBBER CUP POLISHING

Student: _____

EVALUATOR COMMENTS

_____
_____
_____
_____
_____
_____
_____
_____
_____
_____
_____
_____
_____
_____
_____
_____
_____

Box for sketches pertaining to written comments.

Glossary

Abscess of the periodontium—a localized collection of pus in the periodontal tissues.

Abutment post—a titanium post that protrudes through the tissue into the mouth and supports a crown or denture for replacement of a missing tooth or teeth.

Acoustic turbulence—the swirling effect produced within the confined space of a periodontal pocket by the continuous stream of fluid flowing over an electronically powered instrument tip. This intense swirling effect disrupts the plaque biofilm.

Active tip area—the portion of an electronically powered instrument tip that is capable of doing work. The active tip area ranges from approximately 2 to 4 mm of the length of the instrument tip.

Adaptation—the positioning of the first 1 or 2 mm of the lateral surface in contact with the tooth. Correct adaptation of the working-end to the tooth surface requires positioning the working-end so that only the leading-third of the working-end is in contact with the tooth surface.

Advanced fulcrum—a variation of an intraoral or extraoral finger rest used to gain access to root surfaces within deep periodontal pockets. Examples include the modified intraoral, cross-arch, opposite arch, finger on finger, and finger assist fulcrums.

Aerosols—invisible airborne particles dispersed into the surrounding environment by dental equipment such as dental handpieces and electronically powered instruments. Microorganisms in the dental aerosols have been shown to survive for up to 24 hours. See also *splatter*.

Air-powder polishing—a technique for extrinsic stain removal that uses a mixture of warm water, sodium bicarbonate powder, and air. The sodium bicarbonate powder is the abrasive agent used to remove stains from the tooth surfaces.

Alveolar bone—the bone that surrounds the roots of the teeth. It forms the bony sockets that support and protect the roots of the teeth.

Alveolar mucosa—the apical boundary, or lower edge, of the gingiva. It can be distinguished easily from the gingiva by its dark red color and smooth, shiny surface.

Amplitude—see *frequency*.

Angle—formed by two straight lines that meet at an endpoint. The size of an angle is measured in degrees using a protractor. The 90-degree angle and the 45-degree angle are common reference points in instrumentation.

Angulation—the relation between the face of a calculus removal instrument and the tooth surface to which it is applied. For insertion beneath the gingival margin, the face-to-tooth surface angulation should be an angle between 0 and 40 degrees. For calculus removal, the face-to-tooth surface angulation should be an angle between 45 and 90 degrees.

Anterior surfaces toward the clinician—the surfaces of the anterior teeth that are closest to the clinician.

Anterior surfaces away from the clinician—the surfaces of the anterior teeth that are farthest from the clinician.

Apical—toward the tooth apex.

Area-specific curet—a periodontal instrument used to remove light calculus deposits from the crowns and roots of the teeth. Area-specific curets have long, complex functional shanks for root surface debridement within periodontal pockets. Each area-specific curet is designed for use only on certain teeth and tooth surfaces. These curets have only one working cutting edge that is used for calculus removal.

Aspect—a tooth, sextant, quadrant, or dental arch may be divided into two aspects: (1) a facial aspect and (2) a lingual aspect.

Aspects toward the clinician—the aspects of the posterior sextants that are closest to the clinician.

Aspects away from the clinician—the aspects of the posterior sextants that are farthest from the clinician.

Assessment stroke—an instrumentation stroke used to evaluate the tooth or the health of the periodontal tissues.

Attached gingiva—the part of the gingiva that is tightly connected to the cementum on the cervical-third of the root and to the periosteum (connective tissue cover) of the alveolar bone.

Automatically tuned—an ultrasonic device that does not allow the clinician to adjust the vibration frequency of the instrument tip. See also *tuning* and *manually tuned*.

Back—the portion of the instrument working-end that is opposite the face. Sickle scalers have a pointed back, and curets have a rounded back.

Bacteremia—the presence of bacteria in the bloodstream. Bacteria from the oval cavity are introduced into the bloodstream during hand or powered instrumentation and polishing.

Balanced instrument—a periodontal instrument that has working-ends that are aligned with the long axis of the handle.

Basic extraoral fulcrum—an extraoral fulcrum in which the clinician's dominant hand rests against the patient's chin or cheek.

Bifurcation—see *furcation*.

Biofilm—a well-organized community of bacteria that adheres to surfaces and is embedded in an extracellular slime layer. Biofilms form rapidly on any wet surface and usually consist of many species of bacteria, as well as other organisms and debris.

Burnished calculus—a calculus deposit that has had the outermost layer removed. Burnished calculus is difficult to remove because the cutting edge tends to slip over the smooth surface of the deposit.

Calculus—mineralized bacterial plaque, covered on its external surface with a living layer of plaque biofilm. Because the surface of a calculus deposit is irregular and is always covered with disease-causing bacteria, dental calculus plays a significant role in causing periodontal disease.

Calculus removal work stroke—an instrumentation stroke used to remove calculus deposits.

Calibrated periodontal probe—a type of periodontal probe that is marked in millimeter increments and is used to evaluate the health of the periodontal tissues.

Carious lesion—a decayed area on the tooth crown or root.

Cavitation—the formation of tiny bubbles in the water exiting from an electronically powered instrument tip. When these tiny bubbles collapse, they produce shock waves that destroy bacteria by tearing the bacterial cell walls. See also *acoustic turbulence.*

Chlorhexidine stain—a yellowish-brown stain on the cervical and proximal tooth surfaces, restorations, and the surface of the tongue caused by the use of antimicrobial mouth rinses that contain chlorhexidine.

Circuit scaling—see *gross scaling.*

Clinical attachment level (CAL)—the estimated position of the structures that support the tooth as measured with a periodontal probe. The clinical attachment level provides an estimate of a tooth's stability and the loss of bone support.

Clinical attachment loss (CAL)—the extent of periodontal support that has been destroyed around a tooth.

Closed angle—angulation of the working-end at an angle between 0 and 40 degrees for insertion beneath the gingival margin into the sulcus or pocket.

Col—a valley-like depression in the portion of the interdental gingiva that lies directly apical to (beneath) the contact area of two adjacent teeth.

Color-coded reference marking—a colored band on the WHO probe located 3.5 to 5.5 mm from the probe tip. This reference marking is used when performing the PSR screening examination. See also *Periodontal Screening and Recording System* and *WHO probe.*

Complex shank—a shank that is bent in two planes (front to back and side to side) to facilitate instrumentation of posterior teeth. Also termed a straight shank. See also *simple shank.*

Concavity—see *root concavity.*

Contra-angle—a prophylaxis angle that has a bend in the shank.

Coronal—toward the tooth crown.

Cross-arch fulcrum—an advanced intraoral fulcrum in which the finger rest is established on opposite side of arch from the treatment area.

Cross section—formed by cutting through an object, usually at right angles to its longest dimension. A sickle scaler is triangular in cross section; a curet is semicircular in cross section.

Curet—a periodontal instrument used to remove calculus deposits from the crown and roots of the teeth. Its working-end has a rounded back, rounded toe and is semicircular in cross section. See also *universal curet* and *area-specific curet.*

Cutting edge—a sharp edge formed where the face and lateral surfaces of a working-end meet. Cutting edges may be **straight** or **curved**. See also *sharp cutting edge* and *dull cutting edge.*

Decay—*See dental caries.*

Dental calculus—mineralized bacterial plaque, covered on its external surface with a living layer of plaque biofilm. Because the surface of a calculus deposit is irregular and is always covered with disease-causing bacteria, dental calculus plays a significant role in causing periodontal disease.

Dental caries—a decayed area on the tooth crown or root.

Dental endoscope—an illuminated optic instrument that is inserted into the periodontal pocket to provide the clinician with direct vision of subgingival root conditions.

Dental implant—a nonbiologic (artificial) device surgically inserted into or onto the jawbone to (1) replace a missing tooth or (2) provide support for a prosthetic denture.

Dental mirror—the working-end of a dental mirror has a reflecting mirrored surface used to view tooth surfaces that cannot be seen directly.

Dentinal hypersensitivity—a short, sharp painful reaction that occurs when some areas of exposed dentin are subjected to a mechanical stimulus (touch of toothbrush bristles), thermal stimulus (ice cream), or chemical stimulus (acidic grapefruit).

Dentinal tubule—a long tunnel running through the dentin extending from the pulp chamber to dentinoenamel junction (in the crown) or the dentinocemental junction (in the root). This tube is filled with a cellular extension of the odontoblast called the odontoblastic process.

Deplaquing—the disruption or removal of the subgingival plaque biofilm and its products from root surfaces and the pocket space.

Design name—identifies the school or individual originally responsible for the design or development of a periodontal instrument or group of instruments.

Design number—a number designation that, when combined with the design name, provides an exact identification of the working-end of a periodontal instrument.

Digital motion activation—moving the instrument by flexing the thumb, index, and middle fingers. See also *motion activation* and *wrist motion activation*.

Drive finger—the finger used to turn the instrument handle while holding the instrument in a modified pen grasp. Either the index finger <u>or</u> the thumb acts as the drive finger to turn the instrument. The finger used to roll the handle determines the direction in which the working-end will turn.

Dull cutting edge—the rounded surface that results when metal is worn away from the cutting edge of an instrument.

Edema—abnormal swelling resulting from fluid accumulating in the tissues.

Electronically powered instrumentation—instrumentation using the rapid energy vibrations of a powered instrument tip to fracture calculus from the tooth surface and clean the environment of the periodontal pocket. See also *sonic devices, piezoelectric ultrasonic devices,* and *magnetostrictive ultrasonic devices.*

Endoscope—an illuminated optic instrument used to view the interior of a body cavity or organ. See also *dental endoscope.*

Ergonomics—the science of adjusting the design of tools, equipment, tasks, and environments for safe, comfortable, and effective human use.

Evidence-based care—clinical care that is based on the best available scientific evidence.

Explorer—a fine wirelike periodontal instrument used to locate calculus deposits, tooth surface irregularities, defective margins, and carious lesions.

Explorer tip—the 1 to 2 mm of the side of the explorer working-end that is used for calculus detection.

Exposed dentin—dentin that has been exposed to the oral cavity owing to an absence of the enamel or cementum that normally covers it. Dentin may be exposed on a tiny or extensive area of the tooth.

Extended lower shank—a shank that is 3 mm longer than a standard lower shank.

Extraoral fulcrum—a stabilizing point outside the patient's mouth (e.g., against the patient's chin or cheek). See also *basic extraoral fulcrum.*

Extrinsic stains—stains that occur on the external (outer) surfaces of the teeth.

Face—the portion of the instrument working-end that is opposite the back; on sickle scales and curets, the face is bounded by the cutting edges.

Face at 90-degree angle to lower shank—a design characteristic of the cross sections of sickle scalers and universal curets. This design feature means that the working-end has two level cutting edges, both of which can be used for calculus removal.

Fibers of the gingiva—a network of fibers that brace the free gingiva against the tooth and unite the free gingiva with the tooth root and alveolar bone.

File—an instrument used to crush large calculus deposits. Its working-end has several cutting edges.

Finger assist fulcrum—an advanced fulcrum in which a finger of the nondominant hand is used to concentrate lateral pressure against the tooth surface and help control the instrument stroke.

Fingerlike formation—a long narrow deposit of calculus running parallel or oblique to the long axis of the tooth.

Finger-on-finger fulcrum—an advanced intraoral fulcrum in which the finger of the nondominant hand serves as the resting point for the dominant hand.

Finger rest—the place where the fulcrum finger rests and pushes against during instrumentation.

Flexible shank—an instrument shank that is thinner in diameter. Flexible shanks enhance the amount of tactile information transmitted to the clinician's fingers.

Fluid lavage—the action produced within the confined space of a periodontal pocket by the constant stream of fluid that exits near the point of an electronically powered instrument tip. This fluid lavage produces a flushing action that washes debris, bacteria, and unattached plaque from the periodontal pocket.

Free gingiva—the unattached portion of the gingiva that surrounds the tooth in the region of the cemento-enamel junction (CEJ). The free gingiva is also known as the unattached gingiva or the marginal gingiva.

Frequency—how many times an electronically powered instrument tip vibrates per second.

Fulcrum—a stabilizing point for the clinician's hand during instrumentation. In periodontal instrumentation, the ring finger serves as the fulcrum finger, acting as a "support beam" for the weight of the hand during instrumentation. See also *intraoral fulcrum, extraoral fulcrum,* and *advanced fulcrum.*

Full-mouth debridement—calculus removal that is completed in a single appointment or in two appointments within a 24-hour period.

Full-mouth disinfection—full-mouth debridement combined with the use of professionally applied topical antimicrobial therapy.

Functional shank—the portion of the instrument shank that allows the working-end to be adapted to the tooth surface. The functional shank begins below the working-end and extends to the last bend in the shank nearest the handle.

Furcation—the place on a multirooted tooth where the root trunk divides into separate roots. The furcation is termed a **bifurcation** on a two-rooted tooth and a **trifurcation** on a three-rooted tooth.

Furcation area—the space apical to the root trunk between two or more roots. In health, the furcation area cannot be probed because it is filled with alveolar bone and periodontal ligament fibers.

Furcation involvement—a loss of alveolar bone and periodontal ligament fibers in the space between the roots of a multirooted tooth.

Furcation probe—a type of periodontal probe used to evaluate the bone support in the furcation areas of bifurcated and trifurcated teeth.

Gingiva—the tissue that covers the cervical portions of the teeth and the alveolar processes of the jaws. See also *free gingiva* and *attached gingiva.*

Gingival fibers—a network of fibers that brace the free gingiva against the tooth and unite the free gingiva with the tooth root and alveolar bone.

Gingival margin—the thin rounded edge of the free gingiva that meets the tooth.

Gingival pocket—a deepened sulcus that results from swelling of the gingival tissues.

Gingival recession—movement of the gingival margin from its normal position, usually with underlying loss of bone, resulting in the exposure of a portion of the root surface. In recession, the gingival margin is apical to the cemento-enamel junction, and the papillae may be rounded or blunted.

Gingival sulcus—the space between the free gingiva and the tooth surface.

Gingivitis—a bacterial infection that is confined to the gingiva. It results in damage to the gingival tissues that is reversible. See also *periodontitis.*

Gross scaling—a method of planning multiple calculus removal appointments that advocated removing only the large-sized calculus deposits from the entire mouth at the first appointment. Gross scaling is no longer recommended because of the undesirable consequences that can result from incomplete calculus removal.

Handle—the part of a periodontal instrument used for holding the instrument.

Handle roll—the act of turning the instrument handle slightly between the thumb and index finger to readapt the working-end to the next segment of the tooth.

Horizontal—parallel to ground level; level with the ground.

Horizontal strokes—instrumentation strokes that are perpendicular to the long axis of the tooth; used (a) at the line angles of posterior teeth, (b) in furcation areas, and (c) within pockets that are too narrow to permit vertical or oblique strokes.

Implant—see *dental implant.*

Implant fixture—the portion of the implant that is surgically placed into the bone. The fixture acts as the "root" of the implant and needs a period of 3 to 6 months to be fully surrounded and supported by bone.

Indirect illumination—the use of the mirror surface to reflect light onto a tooth surface in a dark area of the mouth.

Indirect vision—the use of a dental mirror to view a tooth surface or intraoral structure that cannot be seen directly.

Insertion—the action of moving the working-end beneath the gingival margin into the sulcus or pocket. Curets are the primary calculus removal instruments for subgingival instrumentation. The working-end is inserted at an angle between 0 and 40 degrees.

Instrumentation zones—a series of imaginary narrow tracts on the root surface used to assist the clinician in systematically removing calculus deposits from subgingival root surfaces. Each instrumentation zone is only as wide as the toe-third of the instrument's cutting edge.

Interdental gingiva—the portion of the gingiva that fills the area between two adjacent teeth apical to (beneath) the contact area.

Intraoral fulcrum—a stabilizing point inside the patient's mouth against a tooth surface.

Intrinsic stains—stains that occur within the enamel of the tooth and cannot be removed by polishing. Intrinsic stains may be endogenous (occurring during tooth development) or exogenous (acquired after tooth eruption).

Junctional epithelium—a specialized type of epithelium that attaches the gingiva to the tooth surface. The junctional epithelium forms the base of a gingival sulcus or periodontal pocket.

Knurling—texturing, as on the handle of a periodontal instrument.

Lateral pressure—the act of applying equal pressure with the index finger and thumb inward against the instrument handle to press the working-end against a calculus deposit or tooth surface before and throughout an instrumentation stroke.

Lateral surfaces—the surfaces on either side of the instrument face.

Leading-third—the portion of the working-end that is kept in contact with the tooth surface during instrumentation.

Ledge—a long ridge of calculus running parallel to the gingival margin.

Level of attachment—see *clinical attachment level.*

Limited use-life—an item that must eventually be discarded after a certain amount of use, such as a sickle scaler or curet. The working-end of a sickle scaler or a curet becomes worn and must eventually be replaced.

Line angle—an imaginary line formed where two tooth surfaces meet.

Long axis—an imaginary straight line that passes through the center of a tooth and divides the tooth symmetrically.

Long junctional epithelium—the primary pattern of healing that occurs after periodontal debridement. There is no new formation of periodontal ligament or bone.

Loss of attachment (LOA)—damage to the structures that support the tooth. Loss of attachment occurs in periodontitis and is characterized by (1) relocation of the junctional epithelium to the tooth root, (2) destruction of the fibers of the gingiva, (3) destruction of the periodontal ligament fibers, and (4) loss of alveolar bone support from around the tooth.

Lower cutting edge—the cutting edge of an area-specific curet that is used for periodontal debridement. See also *working cutting edge.*

Lower shank—another term for the terminal shank; the portion of the functional shank nearest to the working-end. It provides an important visual clue when selecting the correct working-end of an instrument.

Lubricant—a substance such as water or oil that is applied to the surface of a sharpening stone to reduce friction between the stone and the instrument during sharpening.

Magnetostrictive ultrasonic device—an electronically powered device that uses the rapid energy vibrations of a powered instrument tip to fracture calculus from the tooth surface and clean the environment of the periodontal pocket. A magnetostrictive ultrasonic device consists of a portable unit that contains an electronic generator, a handpiece, and interchangeable instrument inserts. The instrument tip of a magnetostrictive instrument vibrates 18,000 to 42,000 cycles per second.

Magnification loupes—magnification of the treatment area through surgical telescopes that can be a technological aid during periodontal instrumentation.

Manually tuned—an ultrasonic device that has a tuning control knob or button that can be used to set the vibration frequency of the tip at a level above or below the resonant frequency. See also *tuning* and *automatically tuned.*

Metal burs—minute pieces of metal that project from the cutting edge of an incorrectly sharpened instrument working-end.

Midline—an imaginary line that divides an anterior tooth into two equal halves.

Millimeter—a unit of length equal to one thousandth of a meter or 0.0394 inch. The abbreviation for millimeters is mm.

Miniature working-end—a curet that has a *shorter, thinner working-end* and a *longer lower shank* in comparison to the design of a standard Gracey curet.

Mirror—the working-end of a dental mirror has a reflecting mirrored surface used to view tooth surfaces that cannot be seen directly.

Mobility—the loosening of a tooth in its socket. Mobility may result from loss of bone support to the tooth. Most periodontal charts include boxes for documenting tooth mobility. **Horizontal tooth mobility** is the ability to move the tooth in a facial-lingual direction in its socket. **Vertical tooth mobility** is the ability to depress the tooth in its socket.

Modified intraoral fulcrum—an advanced intraoral fulcrum that uses an altered point of contact between the middle and ring fingers in the grasp.

Modified pen grasp—the recommended grasp for holding a periodontal instrument. This grasp allows precise control of the working-end, permits a wide range of movement, and facilitates good tactile conduction.

Motion activation—the act of moving the instrument to produce an instrumentation stroke on the tooth surface. See also *wrist motion activation* and *digital motion activation*.

Moving instrument technique—a method of instrument sharpening accomplished by moving the working-end over a stabilized sharpening stone.

Moving stone technique—a method of instrument sharpening accomplished by moving a sharpening stone over the working-end of a stabilized instrument.

Mucogingival junction—the clinically visible boundary where the pink attached gingiva meets the red, shiny alveolar mucosa.

Multidirectional strokes—instrumentation strokes that are made using a combination of vertical, oblique, and horizontal strokes; used for assessment or debridement of a subgingival tooth surface.

Musculoskeletal disorder (WMD)—an injury, affecting the musculoskeletal, peripheral nervous, and neurovascular systems, which is caused or aggravated by prolonged repetitive forceful or awkward movements, poor posture, ill-fitting chairs and equipment, or a fast-paced workload.

Nabers probe—see *furcation probe*.

Neutral position—the ideal positioning of the body while performing work activities that is associated with decreased risk of musculoskeletal injury. It is generally believed that the more a joint deviates from the neutral position, the greater the risk of injury.

Neutral wrist position—the ideal positioning of the wrist while performing work activities that is associated with decreased risk of musculoskeletal injury.

Nonworking cutting edge—a cutting edge on the working-end of an area-specific curet that is not used for calculus removal.

Oblique—line that has a slanting or sloping direction or position; inclined.

Oblique strokes—instrumentation strokes that are diagonal to the long axis of the tooth; used most commonly on facial and lingual surfaces.

Oblique technique—using the working-end of an electronically powered instrument with the lateral surface in an oblique almost horizontal orientation to the long axis of the tooth. The tip is positioned in a similar manner to the working-end of a curet.

Odontoblastic process—a thin tail of cytoplasm from a cell in the tooth pulp that enters a dentinal tubule and extends from the pulp to the dentoenamel or dentocementum junction.

Opposite arch fulcrum—an advanced intraoral fulcrum in which the finger rest is established on the opposite arch from the treatment area.

Overhang removal—recontouring procedures that correct defective margins of restorations to provide a smooth surface that deters bacterial accumulation. If a minor amalgam overhang is acting as a plaque trap and preventing effective plaque control, the excess amalgam can be removed using a specialized powered instrument tip for this purpose.

Overhanging restoration—an area of a restoration in which an excess of restorative material projects beyond the tooth surface.

Paired working-ends—a double-ended instrument with working-ends that are exact mirror images of each other. See also *unpaired working-ends*.

Parallel lines—lines that run in the same direction and will never meet or intersect one another.

Pellicle—a thin coating of salivary proteins that attach to the tooth surface within minutes after a professional cleaning. The pellicle provides a sticky surface for attachment of plaque and dental calculus to the tooth surface.

Periodontal attachment system—a group of structures that work together to attach the teeth to the skull. The periodontal attachment system is comprised of the junctional epithelium, fibers of the gingiva, periodontal ligament fibers, and alveolar bone.

Periodontal assessment—a fact-gathering process designed to provide a complete picture of a patient's periodontal health status.

Periodontal debridement—the removal or disruption of bacterial plaque, its products, and plaque retentive calculus deposits from coronal surfaces, root surfaces, and within the pocket. Periodontal debridement includes instrumentation of every square millimeter of root surface for removal of plaque and calculus, but does not include the deliberate, aggressive removal of cementum.

Periodontal disease—a bacterial infection of the periodontium. Periodontal disease that is limited to an inflammation of the gingival tissues is called **gingivitis**. Periodontal disease that involves the gingiva, periodontal ligament, bone, and cementum is called **periodontitis**.

Periodontal file—an instrument used to crush large calculus deposits. Its working-end has several cutting edges.

Periodontal ligament fibers—the fibers that surround the root of the tooth. These fibers attach to the bone of the socket on one side and to the cementum of the root on the other side.

Periodontal pocket—a deepened gingival sulcus where the junctional epithelium is attached to the root surface somewhere apical to (below) the cemento-enamel junction. In periodontal pockets, there is destruction of alveolar bone and the periodontal ligament fiber bundles.

Periodontal probe—see *probe*.

Periodontal Screening and Recording (PSR)—an efficient easy-to-use screening system for the detection of periodontal disease.

Periodontitis—a bacterial infection of all parts of the periodontium including the gingiva, periodontal ligament, bone, and cementum. It results in irreversible destruction (permanent damage) to the tissues of the periodontium. See also *gingivitis*.

Periodontium—the functional system of tissues that surrounds the teeth and attaches them to the jawbone. These tissues include the gingiva, periodontal ligament, cementum, and alveolar bone.

Perpendicular lines—two lines that intersect (meet) to form a 90-degree angle.

Piezoelectric ultrasonic device—an electronically powered device that uses the rapid energy vibrations of a powered instrument tip to fracture calculus from the tooth surface and clean the environment of the periodontal pocket. A piezoelectric ultrasonic device is comprised of a portable electronic generator, a handpiece, and instrument inserts. The instrument tip of a piezoelectric instrument vibrates 24,000 to 34,000 cycles per second.

Pivoting—a swinging motion of the hand and arm carried out by balancing on the fulcrum finger. The hand pivot is used to assist in maintaining adaptation of the working-end.

Placement stroke—an instrumentation stroke used to position the working-end of an instrument apical to a calculus deposit or at the base of a sulcus or pocket.

Posterior aspects toward the clinician—the aspects of the posterior sextants that are closest to the clinician.

Plaque biofilm—a well-organized community of bacteria that adheres tenaciously to tooth surfaces, restorations, and prosthetic appliances. Research investigations have shown that the primary cause of most periodontal diseases is the bacterial plaque biofilm.

Plaque retentive factors—conditions that foster the establishment and growth of plaque biofilms, such as calculus deposits and overhanging restorations.

Plastic instruments—instruments made of plastic that are used for the assessment and debridement of implant teeth.

Pointed junction—see *sharp cutting edge.*

Polishing—a cosmetic procedure to remove extrinsic stains from the enamel surfaces of the teeth. Stain removal is a nonessential procedure undertaken for esthetic reasons to improve the appearance of the anterior teeth. See also *selective polishing.*

Position of the instrument face—the position that the face of an instrument is placed in for the purpose of instrument sharpening.

Posterior aspects away from the clinician—the aspects of the posterior sextants that are farthest from the clinician.

Precision-thin instrument tip—see *slim-diameter instrument tip.*

Pre-procedural rinse—an antimicrobial or antiseptic mouthrinse used before a treatment procedure to reduce the number of bacteria introduced into the patient's bloodstream and to control aerosols going into the surrounding environment.

Probe—a slender assessment instrument used to evaluate the health of the periodontal tissues. See also *calibrated probe* and *furcation probe.*

Probing—the act of walking the tip of a probe along the junctional epithelium within the sulcus or pocket for the purpose of assessing the health status of the periodontal tissues.

Probing depth—a measurement of the depth of a sulcus or periodontal pocket. It is determined by measuring the distance from the gingival margin to the base of the sulcus or pocket with a calibrated periodontal probe.

Quadrant—one fourth of the combined dental arches. There are two maxillary quadrants and two mandibular quadrants.

Recontouring—the process of removing metal from the back and toe to restore the curved surfaces of a curet's working-end.

Repetitive task—a task that involves the same fundamental movement for more than 50 percent of the work cycle.

Resonant frequency—the level at which a magnetostrictive instrument insert vibrates naturally. See also *frequency*.

Retraction—use of a mirror head or finger to hold the patient's cheek, lip, or tongue so that the clinician can view tooth surfaces or other structures that are otherwise hidden from view by these soft tissue structures.

Right angle—another term for a 90-degree angle. The sides of a right angle are bounded by two lines that are perpendicular to each other and measure exactly 90 degrees.

Right-angle—a prophylaxis angle with a straight shank.

Rigid shank—an instrument shank that is larger in diameter and will withstand the pressure needed to remove heavy calculus deposits.

Ring—a ridge of calculus running parallel to the gingival margin that encircles the tooth.

Root concavity—a linear developmental depression in the root surface. Root concavities commonly occur on the proximal surfaces of anterior and posterior teeth and the facial and lingual surfaces of molar teeth. In health, root concavities are covered with alveolar bone and help to secure the tooth in the bone.

Root debridement stroke—an instrumentation stroke used to remove residual calculus deposits, bacterial plaque, and byproducts from root surfaces.

Root planing—a treatment procedure designed to remove cementum or surface dentin that is rough, impregnated with calculus, or contaminated with toxins or microorganisms.

Rounded surface—see *dull cutting edge*.

Rubber cup polishing—a polishing technique that uses an abrasive polishing agent and a slowly revolving polishing cup to abrade stain from the tooth surfaces.

Scaling—instrumentation of the crown and root surfaces of the teeth to remove plaque, calculus, and stains.

Selective polishing—the practice of polishing only those stained tooth surfaces that have an objectionable appearance. Selective polishing stresses daily patient self-care for the removal of plaque biofilms. See also *polishing*.

Self-angulated curet—a curet in which the face is tilted in relation to the lower shank, such as an area-specific curet. The tilted face causes one cutting edge to be lower than the other cutting edge on a working-end. This feature positions the working cutting edge in correct angulation to the root surface.

Sextant—one sixth of the combined dental arches. There are two anterior sextants and four posterior sextants.

Shank—a rod-shaped length of metal located between the handle and the working-end of a dental instrument. See also *complex, simple, rigid,* and *flexible*.

Sharp cutting edge—a fine line formed by the pointed junction of the instrument face and lateral surface. See also *dull cutting edge, visual evaluation, tactile evaluation,* and *sharpening test stick*.

Sharpening—the procedure to restore a sharp cutting edge on a calculus removal instrument. See also *sharp cutting edge, moving instrument technique,* and *moving stone technique*.

Sharpening stone—natural or synthetic stone made of abrasive particles that is used to restore a sharp cutting edge on a calculus removal instrument. See also *stone angulation*.

Sharpening test stick—a plastic or acrylic rod used to evaluate the sharpness of a cutting edge.

Sickle scaler—a periodontal instrument used to remove calculus deposits from the crowns of the teeth. Its working-end has a pointed back and pointed tip and is triangular in cross section. Sickle scalers are available in **anterior** and **posterior** designs.

Simple shank—a shank that is bent in one plane (front to back). See also *complex shank*.

Slim-diameter instrument tip—sonic or ultrasonic instrument tip that is smaller in size than the working-end of a Gracey curet.

Sonic device—an electronically powered device that uses the rapid energy vibrations of a powered instrument tip to fracture calculus from the tooth surface. Sonic devices consist of a handpiece that attaches to the dental unit's high-speed handpiece tubing and interchangeable instrument tips. The instrument tip of a sonic device vibrates between 3000 and 8000 cycles per second (3 to 8 kHz).

Spicule—an isolated, minute particle or speck of calculus.

Splatter—airborne particles that land on people and objects. Unlike aerosols, splatter often is visible once it lands on objects such as eyewear, uniforms, skin, hair, and other surfaces.

Stabilization—the act of preparing for an instrumentation stroke by locking the joints of the ring finger and pressing the fingertip against a tooth surface to provide control for the instrumentation stroke.

Stone angulation—an angulation of the stone between 70 and 80 degrees to the instrument face during instrument sharpening.

Stroke—how far an electronically powered instrument tip moves during one cycle. Another term for stroke is amplitude. Ultrasonic electronically powered devices have a *power knob* that is used to change the length of the stroke. Higher power delivers a longer, more forceful stroke; lower power delivers a shorter, less forceful stroke.

Subgingival instrumentation—the use of an instrument apical to (below) the gingival margin. See also *supragingival instrumentation*.

Supine position—the position of the patient during dental treatment, with the patient lying on his or her back in a horizontal position and the chair back nearly parallel to the floor.

Supragingival instrumentation—use of an instrument coronal to (above) the gingival margin.

Support beam—descriptive term for the ring finger in the modified pen grasp. The ring finger supports the weight of the hand during instrumentation.

Surfaces toward the clinician—the surfaces of the teeth that are closest to the clinician.

Surfaces away from the clinician—the surfaces of the teeth that are farthest from the clinician.

Tactile evaluation—a method of evaluating cutting edge sharpness by testing the cutting edge against a plastic or acrylic rod known as a sharpening test stick. A dull cutting edge slides over the surface of the stick. A sharp cutting edge scratches the surface of the test stick. See also *sharpening test stick* and *visual evaluation*.

Tactile sensitivity—the clinician's ability to feel vibrations transmitted from the instrument working-end with his or her fingers as they rest on the shank and handle.

Terminal shank—another term for the lower shank; the portion of the functional shank nearest to the working-end. It provides an important visual clue when selecting the correct working-end of an instrument.

Therapeutic procedure—a dental procedure used to maintain health or treat a disease to restore health.

Thin-diameter instrument tip—see *slim-diameter instrument tip*.

Tip of working-end—a pointed working-end, such as that found on a sickle scaler.

Tip-third of working-end—the portion of the working-end of a sickle that is kept in contact with the tooth surface during instrumentation. See also *toe-third of working-end* and *leading-third of working-end*.

Thin veneer—a thin, smooth coating of calculus on a portion of the root surface.

Tobacco stain—a tenacious dark-brown or black stain on the teeth that results from cigarette or cigar smoking or the use of chewing tobacco.

Toe of working-end—a rounded working-end, such as that found on a curet.

Toe-third of working-end—the portion of the working-end of a curet that is kept in contact with the tooth surface during instrumentation. See also *tip-third of working-end* and *leading third of working-end*.

Transillumination—the use of the mirror surface to reflect light through the anterior teeth.

Trifurcation—see *furcation*.

Tuning—adjusting the length of the stroke made by an electronically powered instrument. See also *automatically tuned* and *manually tuned*.

Two-point contact—the method of correct adaptation of a periodontal file to the tooth with the working-end on the calculus deposit and the lower shank resting against the tooth. Two-point contact provides the additional stability and leverage needed when using a file.

Universal curet—a periodontal instrument used to remove calculus deposits from the crown and roots of the teeth. The working-end of a universal curet has a rounded back, rounded toe, and two working cutting edges, and it is semicircular in cross section. Universal curets are one of the most frequently used and versatile of all the debridement instruments.

Unpaired working-ends—a double-ended instrument with working-ends that are dissimilar, such as an explorer-probe combination. See also *paired working-ends*.

Vertical—a line that is perpendicular to level ground; upright.

Vertical strokes—instrumentation strokes that are parallel to the long axis of the tooth; used on the mesial and distal surfaces of posterior teeth.

Vertical technique—using the working-end of an electronically powered instrument in a manner similar to that of a calibrated periodontal probe, with the point directed toward the junctional epithelium. The instrument tip is in a vertical orientation to the long axis of the tooth. The vertical technique is used for calculus removal and deplaquing when instrumenting shallow or deep periodontal pockets.

Visual—able to be seen by the eyes, especially as opposed to being registered by one of the other senses.

Visual evaluation—examination of a cutting edge to evaluate sharpness accomplished by holding the working-end under a light source, such as the dental light or a high-intensity lamp. A dull cutting edge reflects light because it is rounded and thick. The reflected light appears as a bright line running along the edge of the face. A sharp cutting edge is a line with no thickness and does not reflect the light. See also *tactile evaluation.*

Walking stroke—the movement of a calibrated probe around the perimeter of the base of a sulcus or pocket.

Water-cooled instrument tip—sonic or ultrasonic instrument tip that is cooled by a constant stream of water that exits near the point of the instrument tip.

WHO probe—the probe used with the Periodontal Screening and Recording (PSR) System for periodontal assessment. The WHO probe has a colored band (called the reference marking) located 3.5 to 5.5 mm from the probe tip. This color-coded reference marking is used when performing the PSR screening examination.

Working cutting edge—a cutting edge that is used for periodontal debridement. Universal curets have two working cutting edges per working-end; area-specific curets have one working cutting edge per working-end.

Working-end—the part of a dental instrument that does the work of the instrument. The working end begins where the instrument shank ends.

Wrist motion activation—the act of rotating the hand and wrist as a unit to provide the power for an instrumentation stroke. See also *motion activation* and *digital activation.*

Index

Page numbers in *italic* designate figures; page numbers followed by "t" designate tables; page numbers followed by "b" designate boxes; *(see also)* designates related topics or more detailed lists of subtopics.